T0329786

NETWORK
MEDICINE

We wish to dedicate this book to the students
and teachers who have influenced our scientific paths
and led us to embark on this new journey

Contents

Preface

Mankind has sought rational explanations for the causes of illness since first recognizing symptoms of disease. Early cultures attempted to account for disease as a consequence of an imbalance among internal humors or of divine punishment for unacceptable behavior. With the advent of the formal disciplines of pathology and histology, coupled with more rigorous assessment of phenotype, the era of clinicopathological correlation began, linking, for the first time, objective abnormalities in tissue or organ function with disease syndromes. By the middle of the previous century, the disciplines of physiology and biochemistry matured, phenotypes became more quantitative, and the earliest molecular causes of disease were identified. All of these efforts, however, followed a conventional reductionist approach to the discovery of the etiology of disease: It was assumed that one or a very limited number of molecular abnormalities would be responsible for every disease, no matter the complexity of the phenotype. In this era of modern genomics, big data, and quantitative phenotypic complexity, we are now poised to think about the causes of disease in a truly integrative fashion. No gene product exerts its effect on phenotype in isolation. Understanding the molecular context—the integrated linkage diagram or network among all gene products in a cell—is essential for understanding the true bases for phenotype and pathophenotype. This goal is the primary purpose of the newly defined field of network medicine.

Representing the marriage of systems biology and network science, network medicine proposes a disciplinary structure and investigative strategy that can be used to dissect the causes of all human diseases. Network medicine embraces the complexity of multifactorial influences on disease, which can be driven by nonlinear effects and molecular and statistical interactions. The development of comprehensive and affordable -omics platforms provides the data types for network medicine, and graph theory and statistical physics provide the theoretical framework to analyze networks. While network medicine offers a fundamentally different approach toward understanding disease etiology, it will eventually lead to key differences in how diseases are treated—with multiple molecular targets that may require manipulation in a coordinated, dynamic fashion.

In this text, we and our contributing authors present the elements of network medicine, which include the application of modern -omics technologies, network analysis, and dynamic systems analysis to complex molecular networks within which genetic variants exist that alter the system's behavior in an integrative context. The multidisciplinary nature of network medicine research, which includes network science, systems biology, molecular biology, biostatistics, and bioinformatics, creates important opportunities and challenges. Even among experienced network science researchers, no single investigator can have complete mastery of network methods, clinical phenotyping, molecular characterization, and bioinformatic approaches. Thus, network medicine requires a team-based approach to medical research.

Our goals in this book are to provide an introduction to the major fields and network approaches to complex diseases (Chapters 1 to 6), to provide more detailed reviews of progress in the analysis of specific -omics data types using network-based approaches (Chapters 7 to 13), and to consider how network medicine will influence disease treatment (Chapters 14 to 16). Readers interested only in specific topics may choose to read relevant chapters selectively, but mastering the basic network concepts reviewed in Chapters 1 and 2 would greatly assist in understanding the subsequent chapters. We believe that network medicine, which will ultimately redefine all of human disease and provide rational approaches to therapeutic development, represents the true future of modern molecular medicine.

We hope that this book will be useful for medical researchers and quantitative scientists—both students at the beginning of their careers and experienced investigators who are well established. We are particularly hopeful that those at the beginning of their investigative careers will turn to network medicine as a way forward in understanding complex diseases and that this book will help them in this journey. We also hope that clinicians will find useful information here as well; although network medicine does not yet influence treatment of most of the conditions discussed, it increasingly influences our understanding of disease pathobiology. As progress continues, we expect that network medicine strategies will lead to new treatment approaches and provide useful insights into treatment responses and adverse events.

As in any multi-authored book, the success of the endeavor relates to the commitment and creativity of the collaborating authors; we are extremely thankful for the diligent and careful work of each of our contributors. They represent an important resource as we enter the network medicine era. Many of the chapters in this book evolved from the "Introduction to Network Medicine" course developed by Harvard Catalyst (The Harvard Clinical and Translational Science Center). We would also like to thank our colleagues at Harvard University Press, Michael Fisher and Janice Audet, who provided outstanding support for this project, and Stephanie Tribuna and Justin Tribuna for expert editorial assistance. Finally, we wish to thank our families for their patience and unwavering support during this project.

Scientific Basis of Network Medicine

Edwin K. Silverman and Joseph Loscalzo

Introduction

This chapter reviews the key concepts in molecular biology for readers without much background in biology and includes an introduction to network science for readers without prior experience in systems biology. Without an understanding of the terminology and basic principles in these fields, the remaining chapters of this book will be difficult to follow. We will provide only an overview of basic principles, but we will cite references to other sources for in-depth discussion of these topics.

Basic Principles of Molecular Biology

Overview of Molecular Biology

Living organisms are composed of multiple types of molecules that are organized in cells to perform specific biological functions. Each multicellular organism comprises different cell types that are carefully placed within organs and tissues during development. The fundamental instructions for each organism are encoded within the sequence of their deoxyribonucleic acid (DNA), composed of four different types of nucleotides—adenine, guanine, thymine, and cytosine—in eukaryotic organisms. DNA is a double helical structure, which, in humans, includes a linear sequence of about 3 billion nucleotide bases. The DNA molecules are organized into chromosomes (normal humans have 22 pairs of autosomal chromosomes and 2 sex chromosomes) inherited from the parents after molecular recombination of parental chromosomes during the process of meiosis. About 1% of the genome encodes the sequence for approximately 20,000 genes that specify proteins; messenger ribonucleic acid (mRNA) is transcribed from the DNA of these protein-coding genes. The mRNA is translated into proteins, composed of amino acids; proteins are the primary building blocks of cells. Thus, the central dogma of molecular biology is: DNA is transcribed to RNA, and RNA is translated to protein (Figure 1–1).

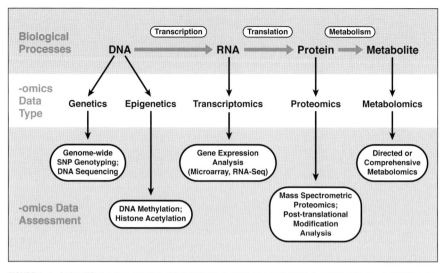

FIGURE 1–1. A simplified representation of key biological processes and related -omics data types. DNA is transcribed to RNA, and mRNA is translated to proteins, which can then undergo post-translational modifications. Proteins can function as enzymes to catalyze reactions between different types of metabolites; metabolites also serve as building blocks for other key molecules in the cell. The -omics data types that can be extracted from these biological processes, including genetics, epigenetics, transcriptomics, proteomics, and metabolomics, will be discussed in detail in subsequent chapters. SNP = single-nucleotide polymorphism.

Not surprisingly, the molecular and cellular processes in biological systems are more complicated than the central dogma may imply. Every cell of an organism inherits the same DNA sequence, and a network of interacting factors determines whether that cell will differentiate into, for example, a lung epithelial cell or a cardiac muscle cell, and whether the organ in which that cell resides will develop into a lung or a heart. Epigenetic changes to the DNA sequence, such as the addition to or removal from cytosines of methyl groups, can have profound effects on gene regulation. For transcription to occur, the DNA molecule, which is tightly wound within the nucleus of the cell, needs to be unwound and bound by a group of molecules that compose the transcriptional machinery. Post-translational modification of histone proteins (histone "marks") can either facilitate or impair access to the transcriptional machinery. These histone marks, DNA methylation, RNA methylation, and noncoding, regulatory RNAs (vide infra) comprise the elements of epigenetic regulation, viz., determinants of phenotype that do not depend on the intrinsic genetic sequence of DNA itself. After the DNA sequence of a gene has been transcribed into RNA, this primary RNA transcript is processed by splicing to remove the noncoding intronic regions located between the protein-coding exons. For many genes, alternative splicing can occur, with the selective exclusion of specific exons—resulting in distinct mRNA, and ultimately protein, sequences derived from that gene.

After translation of the mRNA into a primary amino acid sequence, secondary structures such as sheets and helixes are formed, and the protein folds into a tertiary structure that may become a subunit of a larger protein complex (quaternary structure). In addition, a variety of post-translational modifications of protiens may occur, such as the addition of carbohydrate side chains or ubiquitin molecules that can influence protein function and fate. Small molecules that can be building blocks for larger biochemical structures (e.g., amino acids), sources of energy (e.g., sugars), or breakdown products are referred to as metabolites. Biochemical reactions that produce or alter metabolites are often catalyzed by enzymes, which are proteins with specific molecular functions.

The DNA sequences of different people are quite similar; common sites of genetic variation, which most often involve single-base-pair differences in the DNA sequence (single-nucleotide polymorphisms, or SNPs), occur on average only about once every 300 bases. Thus, there are about 10 million locations in the genome that commonly vary between individuals. There are many more rare genetic variants, which often are unique to an individual. If a genetic variant alters part of the DNA sequence that encodes an amino acid within a protein, a different amino acid may be incorporated that may lead to altered biological functionality of that variant protein. Genetic variants can also influence regions of the genome that regulate nearby or distant genes. Krebs, Goldstein, et al. (2012), Lodish, Berk, et al. (2016), and Watson, Baker, et al. (2013) provide excellent overviews of the basic principles of molecular biology.

Key Molecular Players in Gene Regulation

Even in the brief and simplified description of molecular biology provided above, it is clear that multiple types of molecules must be coordinated in organized processes for living organisms to function. Some of the coordinators of gene regulation include the key molecular participants in biological networks. For example, transcription factors are proteins that bind to the DNA sequence and influence the transcription of other genes. The binding locations can be upstream, downstream, or within coding regions, and those regulatory elements fall into several major classes that influence gene expression. Enhancers increase gene expression, while silencers reduce gene expression. Insulators function as enhancer-blockers or barriers that limit the effects of enhancers or silencers (Raab and Kamakaka 2010).

Although only a small percentage of the DNA encodes exons within genes that include the protein-coding sequence, much of the remaining DNA sequence shows a low level of transcription. The functional impact of these noncoding genomic regions is largely unknown, but an important group of regulatory molecules are noncoding RNAs. Noncoding RNAs include microRNAs and long-noncoding RNAs (lncRNAs), which have important gene regulatory functions. In addition to gene regulatory networks, other key networks in molecular biology include signal transduction networks, protein–protein interaction networks, and metabolic networks (Junker 2008).

Overview of Major -omics Data Types

In order to identify a comprehensive set of interactions between genes and proteins, the development of large-scale datasets that capture the biological activities of cells is essential (Figure 1–1). We will briefly discuss: (1) transcriptomics—the gene expression signals in RNA; (2) proteomics—the protein components of a biological sample; (3) metabolomics—the metabolites produced in biochemical reactions; and (4) microbiomics—the microbiological (typically bacterial) components of an organ or other biological sample. All of these -omics approaches require substantial bioinformatics support and sophisticated statistical analyses.

Transcriptomics was made feasible by microarray assays that allowed detection of thousands of expressed transcripts in one experiment. A probe attached to an array platform is used to interrogate selected types of RNA. Typically, the various mRNA species are the focus of these assays, although microRNA and other RNA types can also provide valuable information. Increasingly, transcriptomic studies are being performed with sequencing of RNA (RNA-seq), which does not require capturing specific RNA transcripts in order to perform quantitation (Guigo 2013).

Proteomic studies can provide complementary information to transcriptomics, since the correlation between mRNA and protein levels within a cell or other biological sample is often surprisingly low. The development of robust, high-throughput proteomic analysis has been technically challenging, but recently developed mass spectrometric approaches, such as selected reaction monitoring (SRM), are promising tools for quantitative proteomics assessment (Brusniak, Chu, et al. 2012). In addition to measurements of protein levels, assessment of post-translational protein modifications can also be performed (Hein, Sharma, et al. 2013).

Metabolomic studies have been enabled by the recent development of reliable, high-throughput assay systems for large panels of metabolites (Artati, Prehn, et al. 2012). Metabolomics can reflect many of the cellular functional activities and provide information about dynamic changes, such as metabolite conversion events known as "flux," within a biological system. Other terms are used to describe analyses of specific metabolite classes, such as "lipidomics," which is the study of (small-molecule) lipids. Nontargeted, comprehensive metabolomics typically involves quantitative assessments of a very large number of metabolites, including unidentified analytes, while targeted metabolomics focuses on measuring a preselected set of metabolites.

Microbiomics involves the assessment of the presence and/or abundance of various microorganisms within a biological system of interest, such as the human intestine (Faust and Raes 2012). The identification of bacterial species using 16S ribosomal sequencing or whole-genome sequencing has revolutionized this field, since culturing and conventionally speciating the microorganism is no longer required. Determination of microbial abundance is complex, as it requires accurate taxonomic identification of the nucleotide sequence and appropriate statistical analysis to quantify the relative abundance of each taxonomic group.

Basic Principles of Network Science

Definitions of Key Network Terms

Excellent reviews of network science principles have been provided by others (Alon 2007; Schreiber 2008; Steuer and Lopez 2008; Newman 2010; Yu, Huang, et al. 2011; Barzel, Sharma, et al. 2013; Barabasi 2016). In this section, we will present some of the key terminology that will be used throughout this book. A more detailed and theoretical discussion of network science principles is provided in Chapter 2.

Networks are composed of nodes (also known as vertexes) that are connected by edges (also known as links) (Figure 1–2). Networks can be used to visualize and analyze a broad range of biological processes, with nodes in the network representing a biological entity (e.g., gene, protein, or disease) and edges representing the relationships and/or interactions between entities (e.g., physical interactions, transcriptional activation, correlations in gene expression levels, or metabolic conversions by enzymes). Key nodes that include multiple edges are often referred to as "hubs." Graph theory is used to describe and analyze networks.

Edges can be undirected (indicating a connection or interaction between two nodes) or directed (indicating a specific direction of the interaction between two nodes; typically represented with an arrow drawn from one node to another). Edges can also be unweighted (in which an edge is placed if a threshold of evidence for a connection or interaction is reached) or weighted (in which the strength of the interaction is indicated by the weight [e.g., depicted by variable thickness] assigned to the edge). We will focus on simple networks in which single edges connect different nodes, but edges connecting a node to itself (self-edges) or multiple edges connecting two nodes can be included in more complex networks.

A network can be completely specified by the whole list of edges between nodes; such "edge lists" can be used to improve computational efficiency (Schreiber 2008). However, a more typical network representation is that of an "adjacency matrix," in which both the rows and the columns of the matrix (each

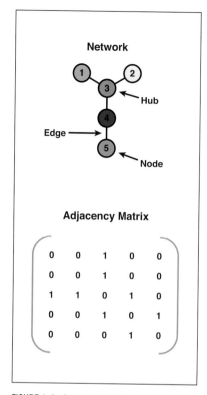

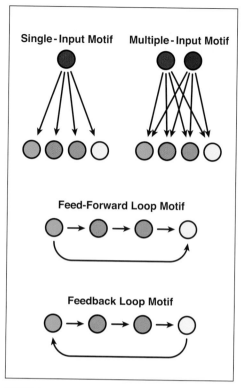

FIGURE 1–2. A network with five nodes is shown at the top, and the corresponding adjacency matrix for this network is shown on the bottom.

FIGURE 1–3. Some common network motifs are shown, including single-input, multiple-input, feed-forward loops, and feedback loops. (Adapted from Yu, H., J. Huang, et al. (2011). Network analysis to interpret complex phenotypes. In: M. Dehmer, F. Emmert-Streib, A. Graber, and A. Salvador, eds., Applied Statistics for Network Biology. Weinheim, Germany: Wiley-VCH, pp. 3–12.)

having a dimension equal to the number of nodes) correspond to the nodes of the network. The adjacency matrix includes values of 0 if an edge is not present between two nodes and a nonzero value (1 for a simple network) if an edge is present in an unweighted network. When there are no self-edges, the diagonal elements of the adjacency matrix are zero. The adjacency matrix of such a simple undirected network is symmetric (Figure 1–2). For a weighted network, the adjacency matrix includes values based on the magnitude of the connection weight. For a directed network, the adjacency matrix is asymmetric, conventionally assigning a value of 1 (in an unweighted network) in the matrix location for an edge running from one node to another (Newman 2010).

Network motifs are characteristic network patterns or subgraphs associated with specific biological functions. Some common network motifs, shown in Figure 1–3, include: (1) single-input motifs—one node regulates multiple other nodes; (2) multiple-input motifs—multiple nodes regulate multiple other nodes; (3) feed-forward loops—multiple upstream nodes regulate a downstream node together; and (4) feedback loops—a downstream node regulates an upstream node. More complex motifs can produce specific biological responses. For example, oscillations in regulatory systems can be produced either by the combination of a negative feedback loop from a gene regulated by a transcription factor in conjunction with positive autoregulation by that transcription factor or by multiple repressors that negatively regulate each other in a cycle (a "repressilator") (Alon 2007). Larger, highly connected components of the network, which may be composed of multiple motifs that perform a specific biological function, are referred to as "network modules."

Commonly Used Network Metrics

For a particular node in the network, the number of edges directly linked to that node is the "degree" of that node. The frequencies of the degree values in the network constitute the "degree distribution" for the network, which corresponds to the probability that a randomly selected node has a specific degree value (Figure 1–4).

The maximum number of edges within an entire simple network composed of n nodes is $\frac{1}{2}(n)(n-1)$; the density of the network is the fraction of these total possible edges that exist (Newman 2010). Many biological networks have low density values and are referred to as "sparse." Since the simple histogram approach for assessing the nature of the degree distribution can be inaccurate for some networks, other approaches, such as the use of the cumulative degree distribution, have been proposed (Steuer and Lopez 2008). For directed networks, the number of inward-pointed edges to a node specifies the "in-degree" while the number of outward-pointed edges from that node specifies the "out-degree." Determining that a particular motif or module is overrepresented within a network typically requires comparing it to randomly generated networks with similar degree distributions. A variety of metrics have been used to identify the most important or central node in a network; one of the most commonly used is "degree centrality," which refers to the node with the highest degree.

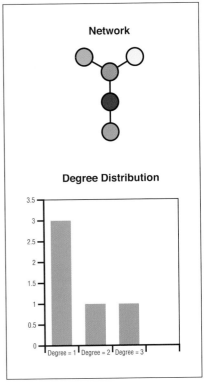

FIGURE 1–4. The degree distribution for the undirected network in Figure 1–1 is shown.

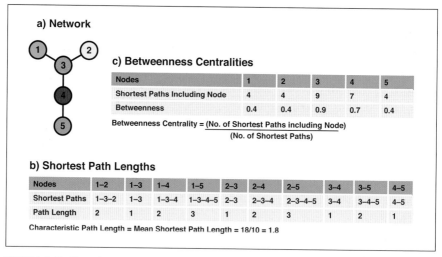

a) Network

c) Betweenness Centralities

Nodes	1	2	3	4	5
Shortest Paths Including Node	4	4	9	7	4
Betweenness	0.4	0.4	0.9	0.7	0.4

$$\text{Betweenness Centrality} = \frac{\text{(No. of Shortest Paths including Node)}}{\text{(No. of Shortest Paths)}}$$

b) Shortest Path Lengths

Nodes	1–2	1–3	1–4	1–5	2–3	2–4	2–5	3–4	3–5	4–5
Shortest Paths	1–3–2	1–3	1–3–4	1–3–4–5	2–3	2–3–4	2–3–4–5	3–4	3–4–5	4–5
Path Length	2	1	2	3	1	2	3	1	2	1

Characteristic Path Length = Mean Shortest Path Length = 18/10 = 1.8

FIGURE 1–5. For the undirected network in Figure 1–1, the shortest path lengths, characteristic path length, and betweenness centralities are shown.

A "path" within a network is a connection between two nodes that follows the edges; the length of the path is quantified as the number of edges that are included in the path. The minimum number of edges that must be traversed to travel between two nodes in a network is referred to as the "shortest path length" or "geodesic path." If there is a path between every node in the network, then that network is called "connected." The mean shortest path length among all of the nodes in a connected network is also known as the "characteristic path length." Many biological networks demonstrate the "small world effect," in which the path lengths between nodes are surprisingly small (Watts and Strogatz 1998). The "betweenness" or "betweenness centrality" of a particular node or edge assesses how often that network component is present within the group of shortest paths in the network; it is calculated as the number of shortest paths in the network that pass through that node or edge divided by the total number of shortest paths in the network. These network metrics are demonstrated in Figure 1–5.

The "clustering coefficient" is another metric frequently used to characterize network structure; it describes the probability that two nodes that are connected to another node are directly connected themselves within the network. The average clustering coefficient for the entire network describes the mean value of these probabilities, while a local clustering coefficient refers to that probability for a specific node.

Network Properties

Some of the key network properties are reviewed in this section on random versus scale-free networks.

The earliest network models, developed by Erdős and Rényi, were based on an equal probability of connections between nodes in the network (Steuer and Lopez 2008). Thus, the degree distribution of these random, undirected networks followed a Poisson distribution (Loscalzo 2012) (Figure 1–6). Many networks that have been studied in biological and other contexts have degree distributions that follow a power law; in such networks, most of the nodes have a low degree value, but a small number of nodes (the hubs mentioned above) have very high degree values—much higher than would be expected with a Poisson distribution of degree values. The probability of a specific degree value (referred to as k) in scale-free networks is directly proportional to $k^{-\gamma}$, where γ typically has values between 2 and 3 in biological networks (Barabasi 2016). When graphed using logarithmic axes (probability of k vs. k), the degree distribution of a scale-free network is linear with slope $-\gamma$

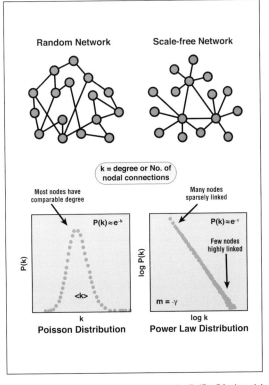

FIGURE 1–6. A random network based on the Erdős–Rényi model is shown on the left, and a scale-free network is shown on the right. The degree distribution of the random network follows a Poisson distribution, while the degree distribution of the scale-free network follows a power law. For the scale-free network, the slope of the line (m) is given by the negative value of the exponent γ. (Reprinted with permission from Loscalzo, J. (2012). Personalized cardiovascular medicine and drug development: time for a new paradigm. Circulation 125(4): 638–45.)

(Barzel, Sharma, et al. 2013). These networks are described as scale-free because the slope of this power law distribution is invariant with respect to size, a property that represents a key feature of evolving molecular networks. The characteristic path length of scale-free networks is substantially less than that of random networks. Scale-free networks are remarkably robust to loss of a random node in the network, while still maintaining their topological characteristics such as average path length. However, scale-free networks can be disabled by losing a small number of hub nodes—so they are susceptible to attack by processes such as infection or malignant transformation that affect these key network components.

Cyclic versus Acyclic Networks

In a directed network, a closed loop of directed edges can form a cycle. Directed acyclic networks (also known as directed acyclic graphs), which do not include any cycles, have an adjacency matrix with all of its nonzero elements above the diagonal. All of the eigenvalues of the adjacency matrix for directed acyclic graphs are zero. An undirected network without a closed loop is referred to as a "tree"; trees provide only one path between any pair of nodes.

Static versus Dynamic Networks

Many of the networks that will be discussed in this book are static networks that provide topological descriptions of relationships among network components. However, the dynamic relationships between components can also be captured in a network context. By analogy, the network of highways in the United States provides a topological network, while the flow of traffic along the highways denotes a dynamic network. Network dynamics can be analyzed using a variety of approaches ranging from fully deterministic, using ordinary differential equations for each rate process defined by a link, to methods that are less deterministic, yielding a range of possible solutions to system dynamics, such as flux balance analysis and structural kinetic models. Importantly, dynamic analyses of scale-free networks do not require knowledge of every rate and stoichiometric parameter, as these systems are overdetermined from a (bio)engineering perspective. Another dimension to dynamic network modeling could be provided by allowing for a nonstatic topology in which the network can be dynamically rewired based on environmental exposures or disease; however, additional research is required in this area (Yu, Huang, et al. 2011).

Deterministic versus Stochastic Networks

Although most networks models developed to date have been deterministic, ignoring the impact of random biological noise on network behavior, these stochastic events can have important effects on biological processes such as gene expression. For example, Burga, Casanueva and colleagues (2011) showed that stochastic effects in gene expression of an ancestral gene duplication in a model organism (the worm *Caenorhabditis elegans*) led to differential effects of inherited mutations. Biological noise can result from intrinsic influences, such as having a limited number of molecules involved in a particular process (e.g., receptors or enzymes), or extrinsic processes, such as environmental exposures. Various stochastic modeling approaches, such as the stochastic simulation algorithm, have been applied in gene regulatory networks; these methods have been reviewed by Tian (2011).

Types of Networks

Many different types of networks are used in network medicine. Several of the major types of networks will be described in this section.

Structural networks depict the topological relationships between biological entities that have a known relationship, such as a protein–protein interaction network. In structural networks, biological entities are represented as nodes and the presence of a biological relationship is indicated by an edge.

Correlation networks have been used for transcriptomic and metabolomic data in which the nodes correspond to the biological entity and the undirected edges correspond to the magnitude of the correlation based on multiple experiments (e.g., measurements in many people)—either as a weighted edge or the presence/absence of an edge based on a correlation threshold (Junker 2008). The -omics data to be used in a correlation network analysis are typically normalized to adjust for technical variability. Standard correlation coefficients, such as Pearson and Spearman, may be used in correlation networks. Partial correlation coefficients can be used to assess the extent of correlation between two nodes after adjusting for all of the other network relationships (Chu, Weiss, et al. 2009). More complex association measures, such as mutual information, may also be used in correlation networks (Steinhauser, Krall, et al. 2008).

Bayesian networks employ directed acyclic graphs, which are quite computationally intensive to analyze. In order to limit the network search space, Djebbari and Quackenbush (2008) used seed genes (selected from previous publications or from protein–protein interaction databases) to create Bayesian transcriptomic networks.

The networks that we have described thus far have only a single type of node. Networks that are composed of two different types of nodes are referred to as "bipartite." In a bipartite network (or graph), edges connect one type of node to another—never two nodes of the same type. Bipartite networks can be directed or undirected. Higher-order networks comprising more than two types of nodes are also possible to conceive theoretically and may be useful in biomedical applications, as well.

Molecular Medicine in a Network Context

Networks can be applied in many different contexts in molecular medicine. Some examples are provided below, and other chapters in this book will provide many additional applications of networks to molecular biology and medicine.

Protein–protein interaction networks have been the main type of network used to describe the cellular molecular interactome, which will be discussed in detail in Chapter 3. The protein interactions, which constitute the edges in these networks, can be determined by bioinformatics methods to predict protein relationships or by experiments to demonstrate biological relationships, such as yeast two-hybrid screens or tandem affinity purification assays (Carvunis, Roth, et al. 2013). Protein–protein interactions can occur in many contexts, including between subunits in a functional protein complex; between an enzyme and a protein substrate; and between a receptor and a ligand. Post-translational modifications of proteins, which will be discussed in Chapter 9, can also be included in protein–protein interaction networks.

In genetic regulatory networks (discussed in Chapter 8), the genes are typically denoted by nodes in a directed bipartite network, where a regulator (such as a transcription factor or another genetic regulator such as a noncoding RNA) binds to DNA at specific locations in the general vicinity of the coding sequence for another gene and regulates transcription of that gene. Regulation can either increase or decrease gene expression, depending on the type of regulatory element bound. Some of the DNA binding locations are immediately adjacent to (or within) the coding gene sequence, while other binding sites can be located many thousands of base pairs away from the coding sequence. Key regulatory motifs, such as feedback loops, can often be identified in genetic regulatory networks (Bulyk and Walhout 2013).

Metabolic networks depict the chemical reactions (both spontaneous and catalyzed by enzymes) that convert one biochemical entity into another. A metabolic network could be depicted as a bipartite network with substrates as one type of node and chemical reactions as another type of node (Steuer and Lopez 2008). Alternatively, the nodes could all be metabolites, which are connected by an edge only if they are both involved in a biochemical reaction. Metabolomics and related networks will be discussed in Chapter 11 and have been reviewed by other authors (Palsson 2006; Hefzi, Palsson, et al. 2013).

Microbiomics networks have been used to study the ecological relationships between different species or other taxonomic groups of microorganisms (Artati, Prehn, et al. 2012). Based on presence/absence or quantitative microbiomics abundance data, microbial networks can be built to capture ecological relationships between species. For example, pairwise relationships can be analyzed by assessing the similarity in co-occurrence of different microbial species across multiple biological samples, and a network of statistically significant pairwise relationships can then be constructed. Alternatively, more complex relationships between the abundance of multiple microbial species can be determined with regression or association rule mining approaches. Microbiomics networks will be discussed in Chapter 16.

Environmental factors are key determinants of many human diseases and likely influence all of the -omics measurements described above; however, they are often difficult to identify and measure. Recent efforts to analyze a comprehensive set of environmental exposures inside and outside the body (the "exposome") have been proposed (Wild 2012). Faisandier, Bonneterre, and colleagues (2011) used a comprehensive dataset including occupational health problems and environmental exposures to study the occupational component of the exposome. They built an undirected network in which the occupational health problems, constituted by a disease state with specific occupational exposures, were the network nodes. The edges were weighted based on the number of environmental hazards shared between occupational health problems. For non-Hodgkin's lymphoma, they found that the occupational exposome network had scale-free properties.

Conclusion

There is not a single biological network within a cell or an organism; rather, there are multiple interdependent networks that vary over time (Barzel, Sharma, et al. 2013). Gao, Buldyrev, and colleagues (2012) reviewed approaches that have attempted to study complex systems of interdependent networks. Percolation theory from physics has been applied to study two interdependent networks, and cascading failures can result from perturbations of systems with this design. This approach has been extended to systems of more than two networks ("networks of networks" as shown in Figure 1–7), with analysis of the dynamic effects of failures in key interdependent nodes. Failure of a key dependent node in one network can lead to additional failures in related networks. Further research will be required to apply this approach to the multiple, dynamic biological networks involved in many human diseases. Barabási (2007) presented a framework in which human diseases can be viewed as a set of interacting networks, including social networks, disease networks, and molecular networks (Figure 1–8). Identifying and understanding the relationships between these different types of

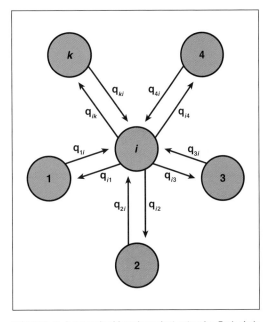

FIGURE 1–7. A network of interdependent networks. Each circle represents a separate network; each of the networks labeled 1 to k on the exterior of the diagram has bidirectional interdependencies with the central network denoted by i. (Reprinted with permission from Gao, J., S. V. Buldyrev, et al. (2012). Networks formed from interdependent networks. Nature Physics 2012; 8: 40–48.)

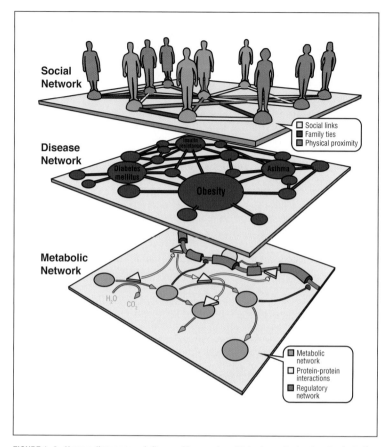

FIGURE 1–8. Human diseases are influenced by a series of interdependent networks, including social networks, which specify interactions between people; disease networks, which analyze relationships between disease entities; and molecular networks, which include protein–protein interactions, genetic regulatory networks, and metabolic networks. (Reprinted with permission from Barabási, A. L. (2007). Network medicine—from obesity to the "diseasome." N Engl J Med **357**(4): 404–7.)

networks will be essential to improving the diagnosis and treatment of human diseases.

References

Alon, U. (2007). An Introduction to Systems Biology: Design Principles of Biological Circuits, Boca Raton, FL: Chapman and Hall.

Artati, A., C. Prehn, et al. (2012). Assay tools for metabolomics. In: K. Shure, ed., Genetics Meets Metabolomics. New York: Springer Science and Business Media, pp. 13–38.

Barabási, A. L. (2007). Network medicine—from obesity to the "diseasome." N Engl J Med **357**(4): 404–7.

Barabási, A. L. (2016). Network Science. Cambridge: Cambridge University Press.

Barzel, B., A. Sharma, et al. (2013). Graph theory properties of cellular networks. In: M. Walhout, M. Vidal, and J. Dekker, eds., Handbook of Systems Biology. New York: Academic Press, pp. 177–93.

Brusniak, M. Y., C. S. Chu, et al. (2012). An assessment of current bioinformatic solutions for analyzing LC-MS data acquired by selected reaction monitoring technology. Proteomics **12**(8): 1176–84.

Bulyk, M. L., and M. Walhout (2013). Gene regulatory networks. In: M. Walhout, M. Vidal, and J. Dekker, eds., Handbook of Systems Biology. New York: Academic Press, pp. 65–88.

Burga, A., M. O. Casanueva, et al. (2011). Predicting mutation outcome from early stochastic variation in genetic interaction partners. Nature **480**(7376): 250–53.

Carvunis, A.-R., F. P. Roth, et al. (2013). Interactome networks. In: M. Walhout, M. Vidal, and J. Dekker, eds., Handbook of Systems Biology. New York: Academic Press, pp. 45–63.

Chu, J. H., S. T. Weiss, et al. (2009). A graphical model approach for inferring large-scale networks integrating gene expression and genetic polymorphism. BMC Syst Biol **3**: 55.

Djebbari, A., and J. Quackenbush (2008). Seeded Bayesian networks: constructing genetic networks from microarray data. BMC Syst Biol **2**: 57.

Faisandier, L., V. Bonneterre, et al. (2011). Occupational exposome: a network-based approach for characterizing occupational health problems. J Biomed Inform **44**(4): 545–52.

Faust, K., and J. Raes (2012). Microbial interactions: from networks to models. Nat Rev Microbiol **10**(8): 538–50.

Gao, J., S. V. Buldyrev, et al. (2012). Networks formed from interdependent networks. Nature Physics **8**: 40–48.

Guigo, R. (2013). The coding and the non-coding transcriptome. In: M. Walhout, M. Vidal, and J. Dekker, eds., Handbook of Systems Biology. New York: Academic Press, pp. 27–41.

Hefzi, H., B. O. Palsson, et al. (2013). Reconstruction of Genome-Scale Metabolic Networks. In: M. Walhout, M. Vidal, and J. Dekker, eds., Handbook of Systems Biology. New York: Academic Press, pp. 229–50.

Hein, M. Y., K. Sharma, et al. (2013). Proteomic analysis of cellular systems. In: M. Walhout, M. Vidal, and J. Dekker, eds., Handbook of Systems Biology. New York: Academic Press, pp. 3–25.

Junker, B. H. (2008). Networks in biology. In: B. H. Junker and F. Schreiber, eds., Analysis of Biological Networks. New York: Wiley-Interscience, pp. 3–14.

Krebs, J. E., E. S. Goldstein, et al. (2012). Lewin's Genes XI. Burlington, MA: Jones & Bartlett.

Lodish, H., A. Berk, et al. (2016). Molecular Cell Biology. New York: W. H. Freeman.

Loscalzo, J. (2012). Personalized cardiovascular medicine and drug development: time for a new paradigm. Circulation **125**(4): 638–45.

Newman, M. E. J. (2010). Networks: An Introduction. New York: Oxford University Press.

Palsson, B. O. (2006). Systems Biology: Properties of Reconstructed Networks. New York: Cambridge University Press.

Raab, J. R., and R. T. Kamakaka (2010). Insulators and promoters: closer than we think. Nat Rev Genet **11**(6): 439–46.

Schreiber, F. (2008). Graph theory analysis of biological networks. In: B. H. Junker and F. Schreiber, eds., Analysis of Biological Networks. New York: Wiley-Interscience, pp. 15–28.

Steinhauser, D., L. Krall, et al. (2008). Correlation networks. In: B. H. Junker and F. Schreiber, eds., Analysis of Biological Networks. New York: Wiley, pp. 305–33.

Steuer, R., and G. Z. Lopez (2008). Global network properties. In: B. H. Junker and F. Schreiber, eds., Analysis of Biological Networks. New York: Wiley-Interscience, pp. 31–63.

Tian, T. (2011). Stochastic modeling of gene regulatory networks. In: M. Dehmer, F. Emmert-Streib, A. Graber, and A. Salvador, eds., Applied Statistics for Network Biology. New York: Wiley-VCH, pp. 13–37.

Watson, J. D., T. A. Baker, et al. (2013). Molecular Biology of the Gene. San Francisco: Benjamin Cummings.

Watts, D. J., and S. H. Strogatz (1998). Collective dynamics of 'small-world' networks. Nature **393**(6684): 440–42.

Wild, C. P. (2012). The exposome: from concept to utility. Int J Epidemiol **41**(1): 24–32.

Yu, H., J. Huang, et al. (2011). Network analysis to interpret complex phenotypes. In: M. Dehmer, F. Emmert-Streib, A. Graber, and A. Salvador, eds., Applied Statistics for Network Biology. Weinheim, Germany: Wiley-VCH, pp. 3–12.

2

Introduction to Network Analysis

JÖRG MENCHE AND ALBERT-LÁSZLÓ BARABÁSI

Introduction

The mechanisms underlying human disease involve complex interactions across many levels of cellular organization, from protein–DNA interactions to signal transduction and metabolism. Despite the very different nature of the components and the diversity of the interactions between them, they have one important thing in common: they can all be described as networks. In the past decade, the emerging field of network science has established new paradigms and tools to analyze and understand systems of interacting components and their collective properties. In this chapter, we review the basic concepts and tools of network science and illustrate their application to the study of human disease.

Basic Network Properties

Networks are defined as a collection of components and their interactions. The components are called nodes or vertices and their interactions links or edges. Figure 2–1 shows examples of networks encountered in the study of human disease. Protein interaction networks (Rual, Venkatesan, et al. 2005; Stelzl, Worm, et al. 2005; Venkatesan, Rual, et al. 2009) are best described as undirected networks: two proteins are connected by an undirected link if they physically interact with each other. Most commonly, these links are unweighted, representing a yes/no relationship. In weighted networks the nodes and/or links carry an additional weight, representing, for example, the activity of an enzyme (node weight) or the flux of a reaction (link weight) in metabolic networks (Ideker, Thorsson, et al. 2001; Stelling, Klamt, et al. 2002; Forster, Famili, et al. 2003). Gene regulatory networks (Davidson and Levin 2005) are directed networks, as each interaction has a source and a target, for example, "the expression of gene A inhibits the expression of gene B." The regulatory mechanism is mediated by other molecules such as transcription factors or microRNAs. Networks that explicitly include two different types of nodes are

TABLE 2–1. Mathematical Symbols

C_i	Local clustering coefficient of node i
$<C>$	Mean clustering averaged over all nodes
d	Distance between two nodes (i.e., the length of the shortest path between them)
d_{max}	Diameter of a network (i.e., the largest d between all possible node pairs)
d_s	Shortest distance observed between a node and a given group of nodes
$<d>$	Mean distance averaged over all node pairs in the network
$<d_{AA}>$	Average of d_s for a group of nodes A
$<d_{AB}>$	Average of d_s between two groups of nodes A and B
γ	Exponent of the degree distribution in scale-free networks
k	Degree of a node (i.e., the number of links attached to it)
k_s	Number of links that a node has to a given set of seed genes
$<k>$	Average degree of all nodes in a network
$<k^2>$	Second moment of the degree distribution $P(k)$
l	Length of a path in a network
L	Number of links in a network
L_{max}	Maximal possible number of simple, undirected links in a network
m	Number of nodes in a subgraph
N	Number of nodes in a network
N_d	Number of genes associated with a certain disease
p	Probability that two nodes are connected in an Erdős–Rényi graph
p_c	Critical probability at which a giant component emerges
p_c^{bino}	Critical probability at which a giant component emerges in an Erdős–Rényi graph
$P(k)$	Distribution of the degrees of all nodes
r	Reset probability in a random walk on a network
$<S_{rand}^{degree}>$	Mean random expectation for the largest connected component size according to the degree-preserving randomizing method
σ	Standard deviation
s	Number of seed genes in the network
S	Size of the largest connected component
s_{AB}	Network-based separation of two groups of nodes A and B

called bipartite networks. Examples of such bipartite networks are networks in which diseases are connected to their associated genes (Goh, Cusick, et al. 2007) or symptoms (Zhou, Menche, et al. 2015).

Figure 2–2 illustrates the basic concepts and quantities frequently encountered in the characterization of unweighted, undirected networks (Barabási, 2016). Throughout this chapter, we illustrate the introduced concepts using the interactome (Menche, Sharma, et al. 2014) described in Figure 2–3.

Network size. The total number of nodes N is called the size of the network; L denotes the total number of links. In networks without multiple links between two nodes, the maximal possible number of links between N nodes is

$$L_{max} = \binom{N}{2} = \frac{N(N-1)}{2},\qquad (2\text{–}1)$$

in which case the network is fully connected. Most real networks are sparse, that is, only a small fraction of all possible links is present. The current version of the human interactome, for example, has $N = 13{,}460$ nodes and $L = 141{,}296$ links, which is less than 0.2% of all possible links.

Degree. The number of links a node has (i.e., the number of its direct neighbors) is called its degree k. The mean or average degree $<k>$ in a network is given by

$$\langle k\rangle = \frac{2L}{N}.\qquad (2\text{–}2)$$

The mean degree of the human interactome is $<k> \approx 21$.

Network paths. A network path refers to a sequence of links that connect two nodes A and B; its length l is simply given by the number of steps. The minimal number of links necessary to connect A and B is called the shortest path length and gives their network-based distance d. Note

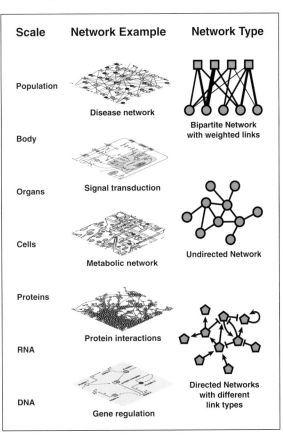

FIGURE 2–1. Networks relevant in human disease are shown. Network-based approaches to human disease involve different levels of organization. At every level we find systems that are best described in terms of networks, from gene regulatory networks at the molecular scale, to co-morbidity networks at the population scale. Depending on the complexity of the system and the desired level of detail in its representation, we can distinguish different network types. The most elementary network types are undirected and unweighted networks. More complex types may include a link directionality or link weights or use different types of nodes, describing the system as bipartite networks.

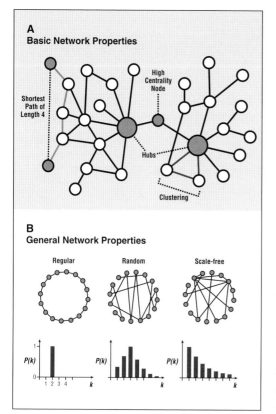

A
Basic Network Properties

High Centrality Node

Shortest Path of Length 4

Hubs

Clustering

B
General Network Properties

Regular   Random   Scale-free

$P(k)$ $P(k)$ $P(k)$

1 2 3 4 k k k

FIGURE 2–2. General network properties. A, Illustration of the fundamental concepts that characterize nodes and their relationship within a network. B, Three important classes of networks and their degree-distribution. In a regular network, all nodes have the same number of links. In a random network, each pair of nodes is connected with a given probability, hence their degree distribution, $P(k)$, follows the binomial distribution (3). In a scale-free network, $P(k) \sim k^{-\gamma}$; its main feature is the presence of a limited number of highly connected nodes, or *hubs*.

that there is typically a large number of shortest paths connecting most pairs of nodes within a network. Figure 2–3C shows the distribution $P(d)$ of all pairwise distances in the interactome.

Network diameter. The diameter d_{max} of a network is the longest of all shortest paths between any two nodes. Most real networks have a surprisingly small diameter, a property called the "small world" phenomenon, referring to the popular notion that everyone is connected to everyone else by only a small number of intermediate acquaintances. The diameter of the interactome, for example, is $d_{max} = 13$ and the mean distance of all protein pairs is $<d> = 3.4$, implying that on average any two proteins are connected via less than four intermediate links (see Figure 2–3B, C).

Degree distribution. The distribution $P(k)$ of the degrees of all nodes in a network can be used to distinguish classes of networks. Historically, the first networks to be studied were regular, like a square lattice, encountered, for example, in crystals. The degree distribution of regular networks typically has a single peak, implying that all nodes have the same number of neighbors (see Figure 2–2B).

Random networks. Many of the fundamental concepts used in modern network science are derived from *random networks* (Erdős 1959; Erdős and Rényi 1960). Consider a network of size N in which each of the possible L_{max} node pairs is connected by a link with a

A Global View of the Interactome

B Global Properties

Number of nodes N	13,460
Number of links L	141,296
Mean degree $\langle E \rangle$	21
Mean clustering $\langle G \rangle$	0.17
Mean shorest path $\langle e \rangle$	3.6
Diameter d_{max}	13

C Shortest-Path Distribution

D Degree Distribution

E Disease Neighborhoods within the Interactome

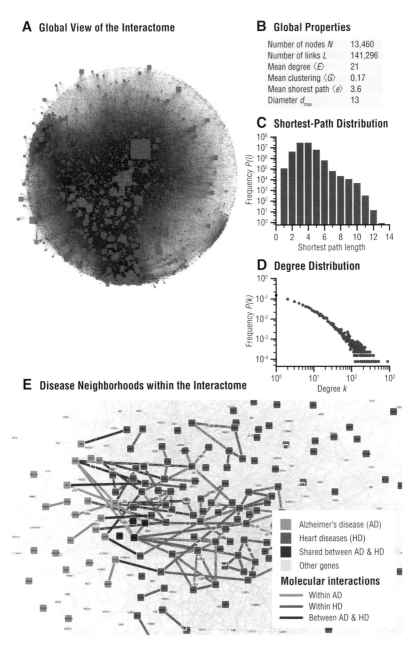

Alzheimer's disease (AD)
Heart diseases (HD)
Shared between AD & HD
Other genes

Molecular interactions
—— Within AD
—— Within HD
—— Between AD & HD

FIGURE 2–3. Overview of the interactome. The interactome represents a comprehensive map of all biologically relevant molecular interactions, for example, binary, regulatory, or signaling interactions. It includes data from high-throughput experiments, such as yeast two-hybrid, as well as literature-curated interactions. A, Global map of the interactome, illustrating its heterogeneity. Node sizes are proportional to their degree, that is, the number of links each node has to other nodes. B, Basic characteristics of the interactome. C, Distribution of the shortest paths within the interactome. The average shortest path is $\langle d \rangle = 3.6$. D, The degree distribution of the interactome is approximately scale-free. E, A local neighborhood of the interactome, illustrating the different types of connections and highlighting the proteins associated with two different diseases.

fixed probability p. In a random network, the probability for a node to have exactly k links follows the binomial distribution:

$$P(k) = \binom{N-1}{k} p^k (1-p)^{N-1-k}. \tag{2-3}$$

An important property of the degree distribution shown in Eq. (2–3) is that degrees much larger or much smaller than the average are absent, that is, most nodes in the network have a comparable number of links around $<k>$.

Scale-free networks. A key finding of network science is that for most real networks the degree distribution does not follow Eq. (2–3). Instead, as discovered in 1999 (Albert, Jeong, et al. 1999; Barabási and Albert 1999), many real-world networks are scale-free, exhibiting a power-law degree distribution:

$$P(k) \sim k^{-\gamma}. \tag{2-4}$$

A scale-free distribution decays more slowly for large k than does the binomial distribution (2–3). While the vast majority of nodes have only a few connections, there are some nodes in the network with a very large number of links, called hubs. For example, while more than 2000 proteins in the interactome have only a single link, 8 have more than 400 interactions, like *GRB2* ($k=872$), *YWHAZ* ($k=502$), and *TP53* ($k=450$) (see Figure 2–3D). The presence of hubs impacts many network properties. For example, they serve as shortcuts, connecting different parts of a network, making them not just "small," but "ultrasmall" (Cohen and Havlin 2003).

Centrality. A frequently used measure of node importance is its centrality (Freeman 1977; Wasserman and Faust 1994). For example, betweenness centrality measures the number of shortest paths that run through a node. Different centrality measures of a node generally correlate with each other, and hubs tend to have high centrality, as they are likely to lie on many shortest paths. Betweenness may reveal unexpected structural features within a network: low-degree nodes with high betweenness can, for example, hint at an underlying modular network structure (Girvan and Newman 2002).

Clustering coefficient. Clustering describes the tendency for two neighbors of a node to also be connected to each other. In a network, such a relationship is represented by a triangle (see

Figure 2–2A). The local clustering coefficient of node i (C_i) measures for node i of degree k_i the number of possible triangles present in its neighborhood:

$$C_i = \frac{2L_i}{k_i(k_i - 1)},$$

(2–5)

where L_i denotes the number of all connections between the neighbors of node i. C_i varies between $0 \leq C_i \leq 1$, where $C_i = 0$ indicates that there are no connections between the neighbors of node i, and $C_i = 1$ represents a fully connected subgraph around it. The local clustering coefficient, therefore, measures the local density of a network. The degree of clustering of a network is measured by averaging over all local clustering coefficients C_i:

$$\langle C \rangle = \frac{1}{N} \sum_{i=1}^{N} C_i.$$

(2–6)

In a random network, each link is present with the same probability p, regardless of whether or not the two nodes share a neighbor. Hence, the average clustering coefficient is $<C> = p$. This typically yields values orders of magnitudes below the ones observed in real networks. The interactome depicted in Figure 2–3, for example, exhibits strong clustering with $<C> = 0.17$, whereas the expected value for a random network of the same density is only $<C> = 0.0016$.

Analyzing the Properties of Node Groups

The quantities introduced above capture the global characteristics of networks based on the properties of single nodes or node pairs. Yet, many biological functions and their perturbations in disease states arise from the coordinated action of groups of molecules. Next, we introduce network measures to explore the properties of such node groups.

Motifs. Small recurrent subgraphs in a network are called motifs (Figure 2–4). They are defined as a subgraph that occurs more often in a network than expected by chance under an appropriately chosen null model (Milo, Shen-Orr, et al. 2002). Motifs have attracted considerable attention in gene regulatory networks, where they can be interpreted as molecular building blocks associated with certain functions. For example, a particularly simple motif found in the *Escherichia coli* regulatory network is a single node with an inhibitory self-loop, representing a transcription factor repressing its own expression. This motif has been shown to be beneficial for the dynamics of gene expression, leading to faster response to signals and enhanced stability against noise. Other motifs observed in regulatory networks include feed-forward loops, feedback loops, and oscillators.

The detection of motifs typically relies on network randomization (see section entitled "Randomizing the Network Topology" below) and is computationally challenging, limiting the size of motifs that can be systematically studied to, at most, 10 nodes. At the same time, the functional interpretation of larger motifs is difficult since their interface with the rest of the network increases, thereby impeding their analysis in isolation from the rest of the network.

Communities. Larger topological structures within networks are commonly explored in terms of communities (or modules) (Girvan and Newman 2002; Ravasz, Somera, et al. 2002; Fortunato 2010). A community is loosely defined as a subgraph with high local link density, so that nodes within the community have a higher number of links to each other than to nodes outside the community. A large number of definitions of communities appear in the literature, as well as algorithms to detect them (see Fortunato [2010] for a comprehensive review). Depending on the concrete application, one may, for example, choose between algorithms that allow for overlapping communities or distinct communities, determined by whether a node can belong to several communities at the same time (Palla, Derenyi, et al. 2005; Ahn, Bagrow, et al. 2010). Some algorithms can also reveal hierarchical community structures (Girvan and Newman 2002; Ahn, Bagrow, et al. 2010).

In biological networks, topological communities are often associated with certain biological processes. Using an algorithm from (Ahn, Bagrow, et al. 2010), more than 1112 communities with five or more nodes can be identified in the interactome, with more than half of them being significantly enriched with at least one biological process according to the gene ontology (GO) (Ashburner, Ball, et al. 2000) (see Figure 2–4B, C). Figure 2–4D shows an example of a community of 22 proteins that are connected via 120 links. The community contains all 5 proteins associated with ethanol metabolism, corresponding to highly significant enrichment ($p < 2 \times 10^{-6}$).

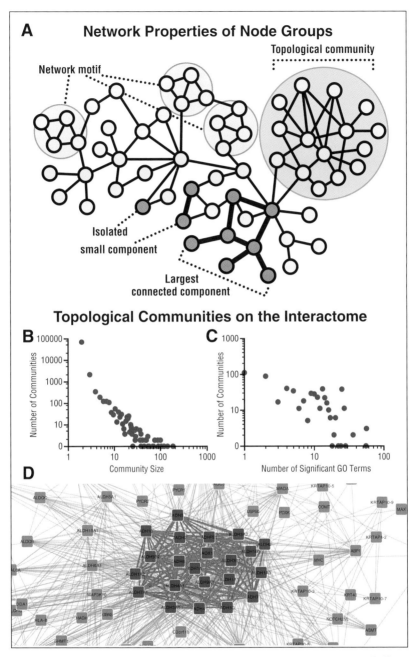

FIGURE 2–4. Properties of node groups. A, Illustration of collective node characteristics: (1) Motifs are small subgraphs that occur more often than expected by chance. (2) Topological communities are local areas of high link density. (3) Connectivity patterns with a given set of nodes, for example, proteins associated with the same disease. They can either be isolated, that is, not interacting with any other nodes of the set, or form connected components of different sizes. B–D, Topological communities on the interactome. The community-finding algorithm of (Ahn, Bagrow, et al. 2010) identified 92,510 communities, of which 1,112 consist of five or more nodes. C, 574 (51%) of these communities are significantly enriched with at least one gene ontology (GO) term (biological processes); the maximum number is 56 per community. D, Illustration of the community of the 22 densely interconnected genes associated with ethanol metabolism (GO:0006067).

Localization of biological function in networks. While in some cases there is a correspondence between topological communities and functional modules in biological networks, there are also important counterexamples: disease modules formed by proteins associated with a particular disease are generally not very densely interconnected within the interactome. This is due in part to the incompleteness of the current interactome and our incomplete list of disease genes (see also, section entitled "Network-Based Disease Gene Discovery" below). It is also possible, however, that disease modules and functional modules have different topological properties. Regardless of their link density, however, there is evidence that disease modules are highly localized in specific network neighborhoods. Two quantities allow us to measure the degree of network localization of a given set of nodes (Menche, Sharma, 2015):

1. *Size of the largest connected component S,* that is, the number of nodes that form a connected subgraph (see Figure 2–4). Many properties of this quantity can be understood analytically, indicating that its value is relatively sensitive to data incompleteness (see also section entitled "Network-Based Disease Gene Discovery" below). In extreme cases, a single missing link in the interactome or a single protein whose disease association is not known may destroy the connected component and leave many proteins isolated.

2. *Mean shortest distance.* As a complementary quantity that is less sensitive to network incompleteness, consider the distribution of shortest distances d_s: For each disease-associated node we determine the distances d to all other disease-associated nodes. Taking into account only the *shortest* distance d_s among them results in a distribution $P(d_s)$. The mean value $<d_s>$ can be interpreted as the diameter of the disease module. Note that in contrast to the diameter of the network as introduced above, here *diameter* refers to an average distance, instead of a maximal distance.

In order to interpret the values of S_i and d_s, a comparison with an appropriate random expectation is necessary (see Statistical Tools for Network Analysis). In a comprehensive study of 299 complex diseases, it was shown that proteins associated with 226 diseases exhibit significant localization in the interactome according to both measures (Menche, Sharma, et al. 2015). Furthermore, the more significant the localization of a disease module, the more similar are the molecular functions of the proteins involved in it.

Separation between diseases. The concept of network localization can be further generalized to examine the relation between different sets of nodes, like proteins associated with two different diseases. The network serves as a map, in which diseases are represented by different neighborhoods. The proximity and degree of overlap of two network neighborhoods has been found to be highly predictive of the pathobiological similarity of the corresponding diseases (Menche, Sharma, et al. 2015).

To quantify the distance of two sets of nodes A and B, we first compute the distribution $P(d_{AB})$ of all shortest distances d_{AB} between nodes A and B and the respective mean distance $<d_{AB}>$ (Figure 2–5). The network-based separation s_{AB} can be obtained by comparing the mean shortest distances $<d_{AA}>$ and $<d_{BB}>$ *within* the respective node sets A and B, to the mean shortest distance $<d_{AB}>$ *between* them (Figure 2–5):

$$s_{AB} = \langle d_{AB} \rangle - \frac{\langle d_{AA} \rangle + \langle d_{BB} \rangle}{2} \qquad (2\text{–}7)$$

A negative s_{AB} indicates topological overlap of the two node sets, whereas a positive s_{AB} indicates topological separation of the two node sets. Rheumatoid arthritis and multiple sclerosis, for example, are two closely related diseases with overlapping disease modules ($s_{AB} = -0.2$), whereas proteins associated with peroxisomal disorders are well separated from the multiple sclerosis proteins ($s_{AB} = 1.3$) (see Figure 2–5B). The network-based separation of disease-associated proteins has been studied for 44,551 pairs among 299 diseases, showing that only 7% of all pairs show network overlap. The degree of this overlap, however, is highly predictive for the pathobiological similarity of diseases: disease pairs with overlapping modules are associated with functionally similar genes that show elevated co-expression, are diseases that have similar symptoms, and are diseases with a high comorbidity. At the same time, nonoverlapping diseases lack any detectable clinical or molecular relationships.

Perturbations and Network Incompleteness

The structural characteristics of a network have important implications for the properties of the dynamic processes they support, like the speed and reliability of signals propagating through them. In general, two nodes in the network can communicate only if there is a path connecting them. An important property of networks is, therefore, their robustness, or resilience, against the breakdown of nodes or links that may break such paths.

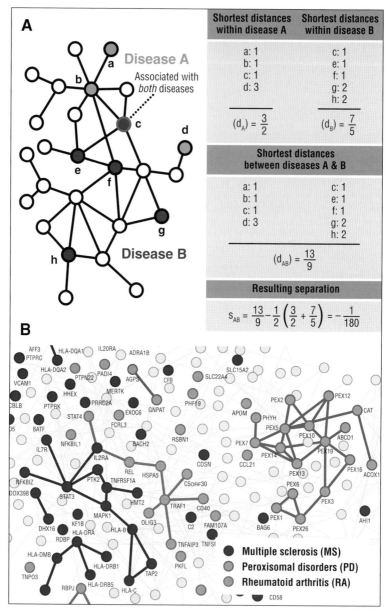

FIGURE 2–5. Network-based separation. A, Illustration of the separation measure s_{AB} for two node sets A (blue) and B (red) with one shared node (c). The tables on the right give the values of the mean shortest distances *within* the sets, $<d_{AA}>$ and $<d_{BB}>$, as well as the distances for all node pairs *between* them, $<d_{AB}>$. Negative values of s_{AB} indicate a topological overlap of the two node sets, whereas positive s_{AB} means that they are topologically separated. In general, s_{AB} is bound by $-d_{max} \leq s_{AB} \leq d_{max}$, where d_{max} denotes the diameter of the network. Since nodes that are shared between sets A and B have $d_{AB} = 0$, the minimal value increases to $-d_{max} + 1$ for sets without common nodes. For sets with at least two nodes, the maximal value is $d_{max} - 1$. B, A subnetwork of the interactome highlighting the network-based relationship between the disease proteins associated with multiple sclerosis, rheumatoid arthritis, and peroxisomal disorders.

Network resilience. Biological systems are constantly exposed to external and internal perturbations. Mutations, for example, may affect the ability of a protein to interact with other proteins. A complete loss of function of the protein removes the respective node from the protein-interaction network, whereas link removal corresponds to the case in which only some of its interactions are lost (Zhong, Simonis, et al. 2009).

Networks in which only a fraction of nodes and/or links are present have been studied extensively in the framework of percolation theory (Callaway, Newman, et al. 2000; Cohen, Erez, et al. 2000; Newman, Strogatz, et al. 2001; Dorogovtsev 2003). Generally, as long as a certain critical fraction of all N nodes (or L links) is present, the network remains globally connected (Figure 2–6). More precisely, it has a giant component, a connected subgraph that contains most nodes. Below this critical fraction, the giant component disappears and the network breaks into small disconnected components. For random failure, when all nodes (links) have the same probability p of being present in the network, the critical probability p_c, at which the giant component vanishes (called the percolation threshold), is as follows (Callaway, Newman, et al. 2000; Cohen, Erez, et al. 2000; Newman, Strogatz, et al. 2001; Dorogovtsev 2003):

$$p_c = \frac{\langle k \rangle}{\langle k^2 \rangle - \langle k \rangle} , \tag{2–8}$$

where $<k>$ and $<k^2>$ denote the first and second moment of the degree distribution $P(k)$. Using the corresponding expressions for the binomial distribution in Eq. (2–3) we find that the percolation threshold for random graphs is

$$p_c^{\text{bino}} = \frac{1}{p(N-2)} . \tag{2–9}$$

It follows from Eq. (2–9) that connected random networks always have a finite threshold p_c^{bino}, that is, if a critical fraction of nodes/links are removed, the network disintegrates.

Enhanced robustness. Surprisingly, this is not always the case for scale-free networks because a scale-free distribution has a diverging second moment $<k^2> \rightarrow \infty$ for $\gamma < 3$, leading to $p_c \rightarrow 0$ in Eq. (2–8). This means that in the limit of very large networks, one needs to remove all nodes/links in order to break the network. Strictly speaking, real networks with a finite number of nodes always

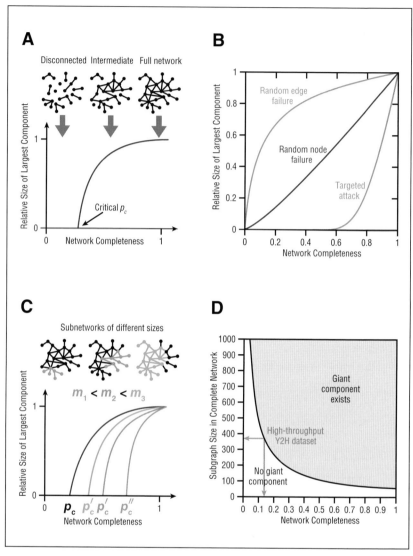

FIGURE 2–6. Percolation theory. A, The behavior of the relative size of the giant connected component as a function of network completeness. Generally, the completeness is given by the product of the observed fractions of all nodes p and all links q. At $pq=1$, all nodes and links are present and the network consists of one single connected component. As more and more nodes/links are missing, the size of the giant component shrinks until it vanishes at the critical completeness p_c. B, Size of the giant component of the inter-actome for three different percolation or failure mechanisms: random failure of nodes/edges and targeted removal of the proteins with the highest degrees. C, We observe a similar behavior when subgraphs of size m are considered instead of the whole network. Generally, the percolation threshold $p_c(m)$ will be larger for smaller subgraphs, that is, smaller subgraphs require a higher completeness in order to be observable. D, The phase diagram shows for every level of network completeness how large a module needs to be in the full network in order to exhibit a giant component in the incomplete one, that is, to be observable. (Y2H = yeast two-hybrid).

have a finite threshold ($p_c > 0$), but its value is negligibly small. For example, for the protein-interaction network discussed above, the threshold is $p_c = 0.01$, so up to 99% of the nodes can be removed before completely fragmenting the network (see Figure 2–6B). Since the vast majority of nodes in scale-free networks have only a few connections, random failure mostly affects such low-degree nodes, which, in turn, have little impact on the overall integrity of the network. Such networks are, therefore, remarkably tolerant against random node removal.

Fragility to attack. This robustness against random failure has also a down side: the networks are particularly vulnerable to a targeted attack that systematically removes the hubs, that is, the nodes in the network with the highest degrees (Albert, Jeong, et al. 2000). The precise fraction of removed hubs under which the network breaks down depends on the details of the degree distribution. For the interactome, we find that removing ~30% of the nodes is sufficient to destroy the network completely (see Figure 2–6B).

Network incompleteness. Percolation theory can also help us understand the implications of the inherent incompleteness of current maps of biological networks. For example, currently available high-throughput human-protein-interaction maps are estimated to cover only around 20% of all true interactions (Venkatesan, Rual, et al. 2009). Using the percolation framework, we can view the current maps as an incomplete sample from the underlying complete network, in which both links and nodes are missing (Stumpf, Wiuf, et al. 2005, 2010; Guimera and Sales-Pardo 2009; Venkatesan, Rual, et al. 2009; Annibale and Coolen 2011). High-throughput interaction maps, as obtained, for example, by yeast two-hybrid (Y2H) assays (Rolland, Tasan, et al. 2014), can be viewed as a uniform subset of the corresponding full interactome: For an unbiased set of proteins, all pairwise interactions have been tested, so the present fraction of all real interactions corresponds to the sensitivity of the experimental protocol. Assuming uniform random sampling, the overall completeness of the obtained network map is given by

$$pq = \text{(fraction of screened proteins) } p \times \text{(sensitivity to detect a link) } q. \qquad (2\text{–}10)$$

In the same way that a whole network can fall apart under random node removal or attack, subgraphs inside a network can become disconnected if network incompleteness exceeds some threshold. Disease modules, for example, are expected to form a connected subgraph within the complete interactome. Yet, within the current datasets, only ~20% of the proteins associated with a given disease are part of the giant component. Figure 2–6C illustrates schematically the percolation curves for subgraphs of different sizes of m. The percolation threshold is inversely proportional to m; that is, smaller subgraphs require a higher network completeness in order to have a giant component. Figure 2–6D shows the minimal subgraph size for which we expect to find a remaining connected component for a given level of network completeness using the Y2H network as input. The yellow arrow indicates the estimated values for the current dataset. We find that the coverage of the current Y2H dataset is still too small to observe significant clustering for the given number of disease-associated genes. Including interactions collected in the literature, however, puts us above the threshold, allowing the systematic identification of multiple disease modules (Menche, Sharma, et al. 2015). We expect that once the ongoing Y2H efforts screen an even larger number of proteins, disease modules can be identified in high-throughput data, as well.

Network-Based Disease Gene Discovery

In addition to missing interactions, we often lack information on important node properties. In particular, for most complex diseases only a fraction of all disease-associated genes are known. As discussed above, disease genes often interact with each other within the same network neighborhood. Building on this observation, and the localization of the disease genes in the same network neighborhood, in recent years a plethora of methods have been developed that exploit the topology of the interactome to infer new disease genes from their connectivity patterns within protein-interaction networks (Tranchevent, Capdevila, et al. 2011). Machine-learning approaches, such as neural networks, support vector machines, or Bayesian networks, typically combine protein-interaction data with other sources of information, such as protein sequence and structure, pathway membership, gene expression, or the genome-wide association study (GWAS) p values (Morrison, Breitling, et al. 2005; Aerts, Lambrechts, et al. 2006; Franke, van Bakel, et al. 2006; Hutz, Kraja, et al. 2008). A number of methods aim to identify possible new disease gene candidates relying solely on the position of known diseases genes in the interactome (Krauthammer, Kaufmann, et al. 2004; George, Liu, et al. 2006; Köhler, Bauer, et al. 2008; Dezso,

Nikolsky, et al. 2009; Vanunu, Magger, et al. 2010; Bailly-Bechet, Borgs, et al. 2011; Erten, Bebek, et al. 2011; Guney and Oliva 2012; Sharma, Menche, et al. 2015). The already known disease genes that serve as input for these methods are commonly referred to as seed genes. In the following, we briefly review the basic network concepts that underlie these node/gene prioritization methods.

Shortest-path approaches. Based on the observation that seed genes tend to interact with each other, several methods consider the intermediate genes along the shortest paths connecting the seed genes as potential disease gene candidates (George, Liu, et al. 2006; Managbanag, Witten, et al. 2008; Dezso, Nikolsky, et al. 2009). Typically, this results in a large number of candidate genes. In order to identify the most promising candidates, the intermediate genes can be ranked, for example, by the number of shortest paths in which they participate (George, Liu, et al. 2006) and their significance (Dezso, Nikolsky, et al. 2009). An approach introduced by Bailly-Bechet, Borgs, et al. (2011) does not consider all shortest paths, but instead identifies a minimal set of intermediate genes that are sufficient to connect all seed genes into a single subgraph, a so-called Steiner tree.

Dynamic approaches. A different approach for identifying likely disease gene candidates is to propagate known disease associations using dynamic models (Krauthammer, Kaufmann, et al. 2004; Köhler, Bauer, et al. 2008; Vanunu, Magger, et al. 2010; Guney and Oliva 2012). In Köhler, Bauer, et al. (2008), for example, the seed genes serve as sources for a diffusion process that can also be formulated in terms of a random walker that wanders from node to node along the links of the network: at every time step of the iterative algorithm, the walker moves to a randomly selected neighbor of its current position. In order to emphasize the local neighborhood around the seed genes, the walker is reset to a randomly chosen seed gene with a given probability r after every move. The frequency with which the nodes in the network are visited converges after many iterations and can be used to rank the corresponding genes. Genes that are visited more often are considered to be "closer" to the seed genes and, therefore, more likely to be relevant to the disease than those visited less often.

Connectivity-based approaches. Several approaches rank candidate genes based on their number of links to seed genes k_s (Erten, Bebek, et al. 2011; Guney and Oliva 2012; Sharma, 2015). Note that k_s

alone is not informative, since hubs (i.e., proteins with many links) are also expected to interact with a large number of seed genes without necessarily implying a disease association. To account for these effects, Sharma, Menche, and colleagues (2015) proposed an algorithm that is based on the significance of k_s. In a network of size N, with s randomly distributed seed genes, the probability that a gene with degree k connects to exactly k_s seed genes is given by the hypergeometric distribution

$$p(X = k_S) = \frac{\dbinom{s}{k_s}\dbinom{N-s}{k-k_s}}{\dbinom{N}{k}}. \tag{2–11}$$

The significance of a given number of connections is, therefore, given by:

$$p\text{-value} = \sum_{n=k_s}^{k} p(X = n), \tag{2–12}$$

which can then be used to iteratively rank all genes in the network (Figure 2–7).

Note that the approaches introduced above can be used for any functional annotation by using suitable protein/gene properties to define seed genes, like pathway membership or differential expression.

Statistical Tools for Network Analysis

In order to assess the statistical significance of a particular network-based finding (e.g., the localization of disease proteins), we need appropriate null models. As many network properties, like the degrees, follow non-Gaussian distributions, we cannot apply standard statistical tests that rely on normality. Network randomization provides a direct way to compare a given measurement with random expectation. Generally, we can randomize the network topology, such as the interaction partners of a particular protein, or randomize the annotation of nodes, like the disease association of proteins. The strategy we apply depends on the statistical feature of the original network we wish to preserve.

Randomizing the Network Topology

Comparison with the random network model. The most basic reference frame is the random network discussed in **Basic Network**

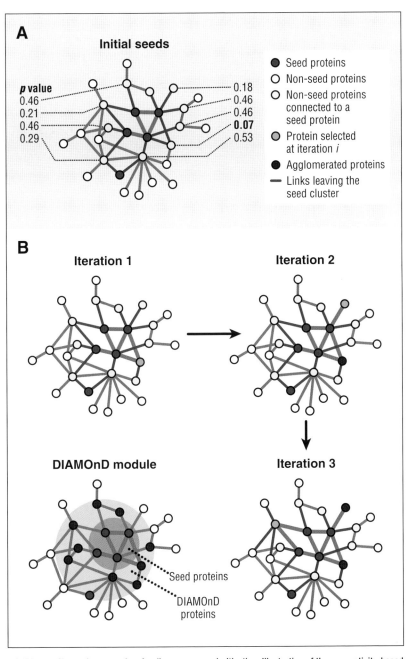

FIGURE 2–7. Network approaches for disease-gene prioritization. Illustration of the connectivity-based DIAMOnD method (Sharma, Menche, et al. 2015) to construct a full disease module from a set of known disease-associated proteins. A, The seed proteins are placed on the interactome. For every neighboring protein a connectivity p value is computed according to Eq. (2-12). B, At each iteration, the protein with the lowest p value is added to the seed cluster. The procedure can be continued until the entire network is selected and added to the module. The order in which the proteins are being pulled in to the module reflects their topological relevance to the disease, resulting in a ranking of all proteins.

Properties. For this approach, we randomize a given network, keeping only the number of nodes N and the number of links L constant. Since many properties of a random network can be calculated analytically, we do not need to perform extensive simulations to achieve this goal. The mean clustering coefficient, for example, is simply given by $<C>=p$. For the completely randomized interactome, this yields $<C>=p=L/L_{max}=0.0016$, in excellent agreement with the value obtained from simulations (Figure 2–8C).

Full randomization does not preserve the degree distribution; hence, hubs will no longer be present in the randomized network. As many network properties depend strongly on the degree distribution and the presence of hubs, this method is not suited for most applications.

Degree-preserving randomization. To maintain the degree distribution of a network, we randomize the interaction partners of the nodes while preserving each node's degree. To implement this method, we can use a switching algorithm (Maslov and Sneppen 2002) (see Figure 2–8A). At each step of the algorithm, two links are selected at random and their endpoints are swapped. For example, the links connecting nodes $n_1 \leftrightarrow n_2$ and $n_3 \leftrightarrow n_4$ are exchanged, resulting in two new interactions $n_1 \leftrightarrow n_3$ and $n_2 \leftrightarrow n_4$, respectively. This rewiring can lead to multiple links between a pair of nodes and self-loops. In networks in which such links are not allowed, the original link pairs are restored. Repeating this process a sufficient number of times leads to a network whose topology is randomized, while the degree distribution remains unchanged. In other words, hubs remain hubs. While there is no precise criterion for the necessary number of switches, empirical results suggest that a good randomization is achieved after $100L$ switching attempts (Milo, Nashtan, et al. 2004).

A more efficient approach is the matching algorithm (see Figure 2–8A), based on the configuration model (Bender and Canfield 1978; Bollobas 1979) used to generate networks with a given degree sequence. The algorithm follows these steps: All links are broken at once and then, iteratively, two "half edges" or "stubs" are chosen at random and connected until all links are restored. As before, this process may produce self-loops and multiple links, in which case the respective stubs are not connected and an alternative pair is selected at random. While this method may introduce bias in the ensemble of the generated net-

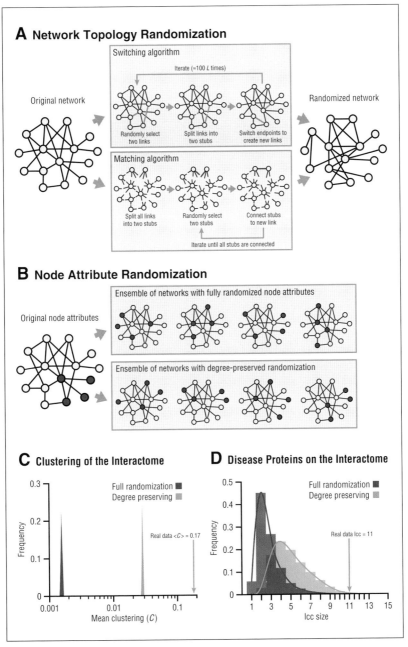

FIGURE 2–8. Network randomization. A, Two algorithms frequently used to randomize the topology of a network while preserving the degrees of the individual nodes. B, Randomizing node attributes, for example, proteins associated with a particular disease with and without preserving the original degrees of the nodes. C, Comparison of the clustering coefficient of the interactome with values obtained by complete randomization and degree-preserving randomization. D, The size of the largest connected component (lcc) of proteins associated with multiple sclerosis in the interactome and compared with the values from randomization according to B.

works, this effect can usually be neglected for large N (Milo, Nashtan, et al. 2004). Figure 2–8C shows the distribution of the mean clustering coefficient obtained from 10,000 randomized versions of the interactome. The mean value $<C>=0.03$ is considerably larger than for the fully randomized network, accounting for the influence of the degree distribution, yet it is still smaller than the real value $<C>=0.17$ for the interactome, indicating that the observed high clustering coefficient could not have emerged by chance.

Randomization can also be designed to preserve other topological features of a network. For example, some algorithms generate randomized networks that preserve the clustering coefficient of the original network (Serrano, Boguna, et al. 2005) or the correlations between the degrees of neighboring nodes (Boguna and Pastor-Satorras 2003; Weber and Porto 2007). In metabolic networks, simple link rewiring would generate biochemically unrealistic reactions. Therefore, we need to use more involved procedures that generate only biochemically valid reactions (Basler, Ebenhoh, et al. 2011; Samal and Martin 2011).

Randomizing Node Properties

Randomization of the network topology is primarily used to identify the impact of the network topology on the system's behavior. To explore the network location of a specific group of nodes, we often need to keep the network fixed and randomize the identity or the location of the nodes. We use this method, for example, when we test whether proteins associated with a particular disease have more connections among themselves than expected by chance.

> **Random label permutation.** The simplest approach is to distribute the node attributes of interest randomly on the network (see Figure 2–8B). For instance, to investigate the connectivity patterns of N_d disease proteins, the same number of proteins are selected randomly from the network, and the quantity of interest is measured for this set of randomized nodes. Repeating this procedure will yield a distribution that can be used as a random control against which the statistical significance of the original quantity can be tested. For example, multiple sclerosis has $N_d=69$ known associated proteins in the interactome, forming a largest connected component of size $S=11$. Figure 2–8D shows the size distribution of the largest connected component for 69 randomly chosen proteins obtained from 10,000 simulations. The mean random expectation is $\langle S_{rand}^{full} \rangle = 2.9$ with a standard deviation $\sigma = 1.4$.

The statistical significance of the observed size can be quantified using its z-score:

$$z\text{-score} = \frac{S - \left\langle S_{rand}^{full} \right\rangle}{\sigma},$$

(2–13)

yielding $z = 5.8$. The empirical p value (i.e., the fraction of all random simulations with $\left\langle S_{rand}^{full} \right\rangle \geq S$, is $p = 0.003$. As z-scores above 1.65, corresponding to a p value under 0.05 for normal distributions, are considered highly significant, we conclude that the connected component for multiple sclerosis could not have emerged by chance, indicating the potential presence of a disease module.

Degree-preserving label permutation. Similar to the randomization of the network topology, we can introduce additional constraints when reshuffling the node labels. One could argue, for example, that the high number of connections among disease proteins is a result of their relatively high degree. To test this hypothesis, we swap the node labels only between nodes of the same or comparable degree (see Figure 2–8B). Yet, we may have very few or even only one node with a particular high degree. It is, therefore, often useful to relax the requirement of an exact match of the degrees for a label swap and, instead, divide the degrees into bins of different degrees and swap the node characteristics within each bin. Figure 2–8D shows the distribution $\left\langle S_{rand}^{degree} \right\rangle$ obtained using such binned degree-preserving randomization. The mean value $\left\langle S_{rand}^{degree} \right\rangle = 5.1$ is increased compared to the full randomization. Yet, the actual value is still significantly higher ($z = 3.1$, empirical p-value $= 0.009$), indicating that the high degree of the disease proteins alone cannot account for the observed large component size.

Perspectives and Further References

In this chapter we discuss only the most frequently used quantities in network science. For a deeper and broader discussion, we refer the reader to the online Network Science textbook (http://barabasi.com/book/network-science) and other reviews (Albert and Barabási 2002; Newman 2003; Dorogovstev, Goltsev, et al. 2008; Newman 2010; Walhout, Vidal, et al. 2013, Buchanan, Caldarelli, et al. 2010). Network science is a very active field of research, with new tools emerging daily. In the following, we highlight a few recent developments that might also provide useful insight for the study of diseases.

> **Layered networks.** As we have seen above, biological systems exhibit different levels of organization, each of which is best described as a separate network (see Figure 2–1). These networks are, however, not independent of each other, but can be considered as *networks of networks*. Such layered or interdependent networks exhibit a number of interesting phenomena, for example, concerning their stability toward perturbations (Buldyrev, Parshani, et al. 2010; Gao, Buldyrev, et al. 2011). The interdependence between different layers of the network can give rise to cascading failure, where the breakdown of a node in one layer propagates throughout all other layers, leading to a global breakdown.

> **Temporal networks.** The networks we have considered here are essentially static in nature—that is, the nodes and their interactions do not change over time. They capture the biochemical skeleton of all interactions that are chemically possible. This is, of course, a simplified view—for example, proteins are not transcribed at all times and molecular interactions may or may not occur depending on internal or external signals. The rapidly evolving field of temporal networks aims to incorporate these dynamic aspects of networks and to explore the impact of this temporality on its structural and dynamic characteristics (Przytycka, Singh, et al. 2010; Holme and Saramaki 2012). Schulz, Pandit, et al. (2013), for example, used time-sequenced expression data of protein-coding genes and miRNAs to construct a dynamic network to predict the most explanatory factors for changes in expression over time.

Conclusion

An important issue in the study of biological networks boils down to a single question: Can we *control* them? In the past few years there have been a series of rigorous results to address network controllability (Liu, Slotine, et al. 2011, 2013). In systems of biochemical reactions, for example, it has been found that by monitoring a few selected nodes one can infer the complete state of the entire system (Liu, Slotine, et al. 2013). These results could have immediate application in the rational design of biomarkers for disease states, as well as in rational drug target(s) selection. The ultimate goal is to control these systems, that is, to drive a cell from a disease state to a healthy state (Liu, Slotine, et al. 2011).

References

Aerts, S., D. Lambrechts, et al. (2006). Gene prioritization through genomic data fusion. Nat Biotechnol **24**(5): 537–44.

Ahn, Y. Y., J. P. Bagrow, et al. (2010). Link communities reveal multiscale complexity in networks. Nature **466**(7307): 761–64.

Albert, R., and A. L. Barabási (2002). Statistical mechanics of complex networks. Rev Mod Phys **74**: 47–97.

Albert, R., H. Jeong, et al. (1999). Internet: diameter of the world-wide web. Nature **401**(6749): 130–31.

Albert, R., H. Jeong, et al. (2000). Error and attack tolerance of complex networks. Nature **406**(6794): 378–82.

Annibale, A., and A. C. Coolen (2011). What you see is not what you get: how sampling affects macroscopic features of biological networks. Interface Focus **1**(6): 836–56.

Ashburner, M., C. A. Ball, et al. (2000). Gene ontology: tool for the unification of biology. The Gene Ontology Consortium. Nat Genet **25**(1): 25–29.

Bailly-Bechet, M., C. Borgs, et al. (2011). Finding undetected protein associations in cell signaling by belief propagation. Proc Natl Acad Sci U S A **108**(2): 882–87.

Barabási, A. L., and R. Albert (1999). Emergence of scaling in random networks. Science **286**(5439): 509–12.

Basler, G., O. Ebenhoh, et al. (2011). Mass-balanced randomization of metabolic networks. Bioinformatics **27**(10): 1397–403.

Bender, E. A. and E. R. Canfield (1978). The asymptotic number of labeled graphs with given degree sequences. J Combinat Theory **24, Series A**(3): 296–307.

Boguna, M., and R. Pastor-Satorras (2003). Class of correlated random networks with hidden variables. Phys Rev E Stat Nonlin Soft Matter Phys **68**(3 Pt 2): 036112.

Bollobas, B. (1979). Random graphs. In: B. Bollobas, Graph Theory. New York: Springer, pp. 123–45.

Buchanan, M., G. Caldarelli, et al., (2010). Networks in Cell Biology. Networks in Cell Biology, by Mark Buchanan, Guido Caldarelli, Paolo De Los Rios, Francesco Rao, Michele Vendruscolo, Cambridge, UK: Cambridge University Press, 2010, p. 1.

Buldyrev, S. V., R. Parshani, et al. (2010). Catastrophic cascade of failures in interdependent networks. Nature **464**(7291): 1025–28.

Callaway, D. S., M. E. Newman, et al. (2000). Network robustness and fragility: percolation on random graphs. Phys Rev Lett **85**(25): 5468–71.

Cohen, R., K. Erez, et al. (2000). Resilience of the internet to random breakdowns. Phys Rev Lett **85**(21): 4626–28.

Cohen, R., and S. Havlin (2003). Scale-free networks are ultrasmall. Phys Rev Lett **90**(5): 058701.

Davidson, E., and M. Levin (2005). Gene regulatory networks. Proc Natl Acad Sci U S A **102**(14): 4935.

Dezso, Z., Y. Nikolsky, et al. (2009). Identifying disease-specific genes based on their topological significance in protein networks. BMC Syst Biol **3**: 36.

Dorogovstev, S. N. (2003). Evolution of Networks: From Biological Nets to the Internet and WWW. New York: Oxford University Press.

Dorogovstev, S. N., A. V. Goltsev, et al. (2008). Critical phenomena in complex networks. Rev Mod Phys **80**(4): 1275–335.

Erdős, P. (1959). On random graphs I. Publ Math Debrecen **6**: 290–97.

Erdős, P., and A. Rényi (1960). On the evolution of random graphs. Publ Math Inst Hung Acad Sci **5**: 17–61.

Erten, S., G. Bebek, et al. (2011). DADA: degree-aware algorithms for network-based disease gene prioritization. BioData Min **4**: 19.

Forster, J., I. Famili, et al. (2003). Genome-scale reconstruction of the Saccharomyces cerevisiae metabolic network. Genome Res **13**(2): 244–53.

Fortunato, S. (2010). Community detection in graphs. Physics Rep **486**(3): 75–174.

Franke, L., H. van Bakel, et al. (2006). Reconstruction of a functional human gene network, with an application for prioritizing positional candidate genes. Am J Hum Genet **78**(6): 1011–25.

Freeman, L. C. (1977). A set of measures of centrality based on betweenness. Sociometry **40**: 35–41.

Gao, J., S. V. Buldyrev, et al. (2011). Networks formed from interdependent networks. Nature Phys **8**(1): 40–48.

George, R. A., J. Y. Liu, et al. (2006). Analysis of protein sequence and interaction data for candidate disease gene prediction. Nucleic Acids Res **34**(19): e130.

Girvan, M., and M. E. Newman (2002). Community structure in social and biological networks. Proc Natl Acad Sci U S A **99**(12): 7821–26.

Goh, K. I., M. E. Cusick, et al. (2007). The human disease network. Proc Natl Acad Sci U S A **104**(21): 8685–90.

Guimera, R., and M. Sales-Pardo (2009). Missing and spurious interactions and the reconstruction of complex networks. Proc Natl Acad Sci U S A **106**(52): 22073–78.

Guney, E., and B. Oliva (2012). Analysis of the robustness of network-based disease-gene prioritization methods reveals redundancy in the human interactome and functional diversity of disease-genes. PLoS One **9**(4): e94686.

Holme, P., and J. Saramaki (2012). Temporal networks. Physics Rep **519**(3): 97–125.

Hutz, J. E., A. T. Kraja, et al. (2008). CANDID: a flexible method for prioritizing candidate genes for complex human traits. Genet Epidemiol **32**(8): 779–90.

Ideker, T., V. Thorsson, et al. (2001). Integrated genomic and proteomic analyses of a systematically perturbed metabolic network. Science **292**(5518): 929–34.

Köhler, S., S. Bauer, et al. (2008). Walking the interactome for prioritization of candidate disease genes. Am J Hum Genet **82**(4): 949–58.

Krauthammer, M., C. A. Kaufmann, et al. (2004). Molecular triangulation: bridging linkage and molecular-network information for identifying candidate genes in Alzheimer's disease. Proc Natl Acad Sci U S A **101**(42): 15148–53.

Liu, Y. Y., J. J. Slotine, et al. (2011). Controllability of complex networks. Nature **473**(7346): 167–73.

Liu, Y. Y., J. J. Slotine, et al. (2013). Observability of complex systems. Proc Natl Acad Sci U S A **110**(7): 2460–65.

Managbanag, J. R., T. M. Witten, et al. (2008). Shortest-path network analysis is a useful approach toward identifying genetic determinants of longevity. PLoS One **3**(11): e3802.

Maslov, S., and K. Sneppen (2002). Specificity and stability in topology of protein networks. Science **296**(5569): 910–13.

Menche, J., A. Sharma, et al. (2015). Disease networks: uncovering disease-disease relationships through the incomplete interactome. Science **347**(6224): 1257601.

Milo, R., N. Nashtan, et al. (2004). On the uniform generation of random graphs with prescribed degree sequences. [arXiv:cond-mat/0312028 [**cond-mat.stat-mech**]

Milo, R., S. Shen-Orr, et al. (2002). Network motifs: simple building blocks of complex networks. Science **298**(5594): 824–27.

Morrison, J. L., R. Breitling, et al. (2005). GeneRank: using search engine technology for the analysis of microarray experiments. BMC Bioinformatics **6**: 233.

Newman, M. E. (2003). The structure and function of complex networks. SIAM Rev **45**(2): 167–256.

Newman, M. E. (2010). Networks: An Introduction. New York: Oxford University Press.

Newman, M. E., S. H. Strogatz, et al. (2001). Random graphs with arbitrary degree distributions and their applications. Phys Rev E Stat Nonlin Soft Matter Phys **64**(2 Pt 2): 026118.

Palla, G., I. Derenyi, et al. (2005). Uncovering the overlapping community structure of complex networks in nature and society. Nature **435**(7043): 814–18.

Przytycka, T. M., M. Singh, et al. (2010). Toward the dynamic interactome: it's about time. Brief Bioinform **11**(1): 15–29.

Ravasz, E., A. L. Somera, et al. (2002). Hierarchical organization of modularity in metabolic networks. Science **297**(5586): 1551–55.

Rolland, T., M. Tasan, et al. (2014). Expansion of the human interactome landscape by a second-generation proteome-wide map. Cell **159**: 1212–26.

Rual, J. F., K. Venkatesan, et al. (2005). Towards a proteome-scale map of the human protein-protein interaction network. Nature **437**(7062): 1173–78.

Samal, A., and O. C. Martin (2011). Randomizing genome-scale metabolic networks. PLoS One **6**(7): e22295.

Schulz, M. H., K. V. Pandit, et al. (2013). Reconstructing dynamic microRNA-regulated interaction networks. Proc Natl Acad Sci U S A **110**(39): 15686–91.

Serrano, M. A., M. Boguna, et al. (2005). Competition and adaptation in an Internet evolution model. Phys Rev Lett **94**(3): 038701.

Sharma, A., J. Menche, et al. (2015). A disease module in the interactome explains disease heterogeneity, drug response and captures novel pathways and genes in asthma. Hum Mol Genet. **24**(11): 3005–20.

Stelling, J., S. Klamt, et al. (2002). Metabolic network structure determines key aspects of functionality and regulation. Nature **420**(6912): 190–93.

Stelzl, U., U. Worm, et al. (2005). A human protein-protein interaction network: a resource for annotating the proteome. Cell **122**(6): 957–68.

Stumpf, M. P., and C. Wiuf (2010). Incomplete and noisy network data as a percolation process. J R Soc Interface 7(51): 1411–19.

Stumpf, M. P., C. Wiuf, et al. (2005). Subnets of scale-free networks are not scale-free: sampling properties of networks. Proc Natl Acad Sci U S A **102**(12): 4221–24.

Tranchevent, L. C., F. B. Capdevila, et al. (2011). A guide to web tools to prioritize candidate genes. Brief Bioinform **12**(1): 22–32.

Vanunu, O., O. Magger, et al. (2010). Associating genes and protein complexes with disease via network propagation. PLoS Comput Biol **6**(1): e1000641.

Venkatesan, K., J. F. Rual, et al. (2009). An empirical framework for binary interactome mapping. Nat Methods **6**(1): 83–90.

Walhout, M., M. Vidal, et al. (2013). Handbook of Systems Biology: Concepts and Insights. Oxford, U.K.: Elsevier.

Wasserman, S., and K. Faust (1994). Social network analysis. Cambridge, U.K.: Cambridge University Press.

Weber, S., and M. Porto (2007). Generation of arbitrarily two-point-correlated random networks. Phys Rev E Stat Nonlin Soft Matter Phys **76**(4 Pt 2): 046111.

Zhong, Q., N. Simonis, et al. (2009). Edgetic perturbation models of human inherited disorders. Mol Syst Biol **5**: 321.

Zhou, X., J. Menche, et al. (2014). Human symptoms-disease network. Nat Commun **5**: 4212.

3

Human Interactomes in Network Medicine

Michael E. Cusick, Benoit Charloteaux, Thomas Rolland,
Michael A. Calderwood, David E. Hill,
and Marc Vidal

Introduction

To accomplish the biological processes needed for organisms to survive, cells act through dynamic complex systems formed by interacting macromolecules. The entire complement of interactions between biomolecules present in a cell constitutes an interactome network. Knowledge of the individual functions of molecular components of cells, including nucleic acids, proteins, and metabolites, is insufficient to model cellular organization without understanding the organization and operation of interactome networks, which can be obtained by mapping them systematically at the scale of the whole proteome.

The full network of biomolecular interactions includes protein–protein, protein–DNA, transcription factor–DNA, and enzyme–substrate interactions. Among these biomolecular interactions, physical interactions between proteins are critical to all biological processes, and these interactions are the focus here. The fundamental challenge is to identify and catalog the protein–protein interactions that can take place among all members of a proteome. From that information, the next challenge is to understand when and where these interactions take place in vivo. Protein–protein interaction maps provide numerous hypotheses to advance focused biological studies, feed into network analyses that lead to the development of dynamic models, and supply the raw material for network medicine investigations, particularly the scaffold models needed to seed investigations of how network perturbations give rise to disease (Vidal, Cusick, et al. 2011) (Figure 3–1).

Multiple approaches exist to map and model protein–protein interactome networks, with the ultimate aim of reaching detailed and informative maps of protein–protein interactions in the cell. In this chapter, we provide an overview of advances in the mapping of the human protein–protein interactome and its implications, particularly with regard to deeper understanding of disease.

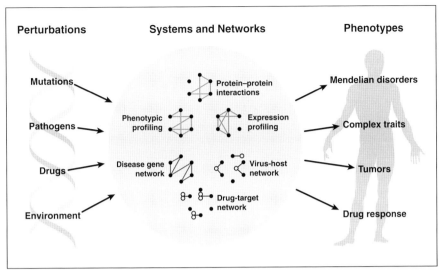

FIGURE 3–1. Understanding diverse perturbations on cellular networks can inform disease phenotypes. Nodes: filled circle = gene/protein, open circle for viral protein, and touching open circles = drug. Edges: physical interactions (Protein interaction, virus-host, and drug-target networks) or functional relationships such as correlated phenotypic profile and coexpression (phenotypic and expression profiling networks, respectively) (Vidal, Cusick, et al. 2011).

Human Protein Interactome Networks

Proteome-Scale Mapping of Interactome Networks

Three fundamentally distinct strategies, which differ greatly in the protein-interaction information they provide, have been used to model human interactome networks at the scale of whole proteomes (Figure 3–2): (1) curation of protein-interaction data from the existing scientific literature, (2) computational predictions of protein interactions based on available orthogonal information, and (3) systematic experimental mapping at proteome scale to identify: (a) co-complex associations or (b) binary interactions.

The vast biomedical literature contains buried within it a tremendous amount of information about protein interactions. Such information can be mined by either direct annotation by trained curators or by computational text-mining methods (Mosca, Pons, et al. 2013), stored in publicly accessible databases (Orchard 2012), and used to produce large interactome-network maps. While the protein-interaction data in such databases have been the source of numerous interactome-network analyses (Peri, Navarro, et al. 2004; Reguly, Breitkreutz, et al. 2006), these maps suffer from both variability in quality and completeness of the curation (Cusick, Yu, et al. 2009; Turinsky, Razick, et al. 2010,

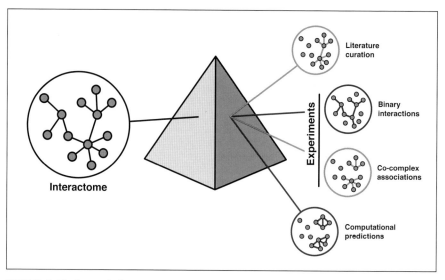

FIGURE 3–2. The three major interactome mapping approaches: curation, experimental (in two forms), and computational as distinct projections of the interactome "prism."

2011). Even more troublesome is inspection bias (also termed study bias or investigational bias), originating from ever deeper investigations of already well-studied proteins, which is widespread in the scientific literature (Yu, Braun, et al. 2008; Das and Yu 2012). Literature-curated interaction maps are comprised of a preponderance of small-scale interaction mapping experiments that can be affected by inspection bias. Such bias complicates the interpretation of global network topological properties (Bertin, Simonis, et al. 2007; Yu, Braun, et al. 2008; Das, Fragoza, et al. 2014; Woodsmith and Stelzl 2014). Also troubling is that production of experimental protein–protein interactions outweighs the manual curation efforts needed to keep up with experimental reports (Baumgartner, Cohen, et al. 2007; Mosca, Pons, et al. 2013). Despite efforts to standardize record keeping between different protein-interaction databases and to reduce duplication of curation effort (Orchard, Kerrien, et al. 2007, 2012; Orchard 2014), and notwithstanding improvements in the accuracy and convenience of automated text mining (Roberts 2006; Gerstein, Seringhaus, et al. 2007), literature mining cannot proceed fast enough to be sustainable long term (Mosca, Pons, et al. 2013). Moreover, it is just as important to know which proteins were tested and did not interact as to know which did interact. With few exceptions, negative results are not reported in the primary literature and hence are not available in curated protein-interaction databases (Trabuco, Betts, et al. 2012; Blohm, Frishman, et al. 2014).

With the dramatic increase in availability of: (1) protein–protein interaction data (Yu, Braun, et al. 2008; Guruharsha, Rual, et al. 2011), (2) functional genomics datasets such as gene co-expression correlations or phenotypic pro-filing (Vidal 2001; Ge, Walhout, et al. 2003), and (3) compilations of specific interaction-mediating protein domains (Yellaboina, Tasneem, et al. 2011), numerous computational prediction tools have been developed to exploit these data to predict protein interactions (Jansen, Yu, et al. 2003; Navlakha and Kingsford 2010; Elefsinioti, Sarac, et al. 2011; Lees, Heriche, et al. 2011; Wass, David, et al. 2011; Gonzalez and Kann 2012; Mosca, Pons, et al. 2013). The most far-reaching of these computational predictions combined structural information from the Protein Data Bank (Berman, Westbrook, et al. 2000) with sequence-based homology models and other functional clues to predict over 25,000 high-quality interactions for human proteins (Zhang, Petrey, et al. 2012). Predicted interactions should be extensively tested experimentally before drawing firm conclusions (Wass, David, et al. 2011; Gonzalez and Kann 2012; Mosca, Pons, et al. 2013). Although computational efforts can mitigate the shortfall of literature-curated efforts (Navlakha and Kingsford 2010; Mosca, Pons, et al. 2013) and involve minimal experimental cost, any computational effort would be restricted by current limited knowledge of biological systems.

The third approach to mapping the interactome at proteome scale consists of experimentally testing systematically for all possible physical protein–protein interactions. Proteome-scale approaches are now feasible because of the availability of genome-scale collections of protein-coding genes, typically in the form of full-length open reading frame (ORF) clones, and of methods for facile manipulation of entire ORF collections (Brasch, Hartley, et al. 2004). Although there are scores of experimental technologies that can detect interactions between proteins (Stynen, Tournu, et al. 2012; Ngounou Wetie, Sokolowska, et al. 2014), only two are feasible at proteome scale: (1) isolation and identification of the protein membership of complexes (co-complex associations) (Gingras, Gstaiger, et al. 2007), and (2) screening of all pairwise combinations for detection of binary physical interactions (Fields and Sternglanz 1994).

Co-complex associations interrogate the protein composition of protein complexes in one or several cell lines. The most common approach uses affinity purification (Figure 3–3) to extract the proteins that associate with the "bait" proteins (Oeffinger 2012), followed by mass spectrometry to identify the proteins associating with the baits (Gingras and Raught 2012; Walzthoeni, Leitner, et al. 2013). Using proteome-scale collections of cloned ORFs, affinity purification followed by mass spectrometry (AP–MS) efforts have been reported for simpler model organisms (Gavin, Aloy, et al. 2006; Krogan, Cagney, et al. 2006). Similar approaches have been reported for human cells (Ewing, Chu, et al. 2007; Sowa,

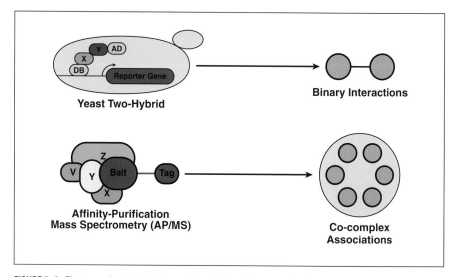

FIGURE 3–3. The two main strategies for experimental interactome mapping. In yeast two-hybrid (Y2H) screening, physical interaction between two hybrid proteins within the nucleus of a yeast cell reconstitutes a transcription factor that activates expression of a selectable reporter gene. Y2H returns binary interactions. In affinity purification followed by mass spectrometry (AP–MS), a protein complex between a tagged bait protein and associated cellular proteins is purified by affinity purification, and the constituents of the complex are identified by mass spectrometry. AP–MS returns co-complex associations.

Bennett, et al. 2009; Huttlin, Ting, et al. 2015), but achieving stable expression of bait proteins is challenging (Dunham, Mullin, et al. 2012). An alternative approach, which sidesteps some of the difficulties inherent in affinity purification, uses chromatographic separation of cell extracts into biochemical fractions that are subsequently analyzed by tandem mass spectrometry (Havugimana, Hart, et al. 2012). Co-complex association maps are composed of indirect, and some direct, binary associations, but the raw association data cannot distinguish the many indirect from the fewer direct associations (Gingras, Gstaiger, et al. 2007). Co-complex datasets can be filtered and enriched for binary interactions by incorporating prior knowledge (Ewing, Chu, et al. 2007; Sowa, Bennett, et al. 2009; Havugimana, Hart, et al. 2012), but such filtering necessarily leads to an inspection bias similar to that which skews literature-derived interactome maps (Yu, Braun, et al. 2008; Das and Yu 2012; Rolland, Taşan, et al. 2014).

For experimental determination of binary interactions between proteins, all possible pairs of proteins are systematically tested to first generate a dataset of all possible biophysical interactions—all interactions that can occur between proteins (Venkatesan, Rual, et al. 2009) (see Glossary). With the human genome containing ~20,000 unique genes, considering only a single isoform of each gene, this equates to ~200 million possible combinations, re-

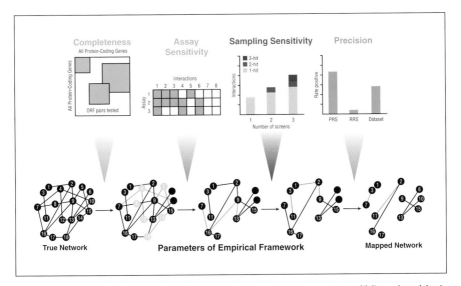

FIGURE 3–4. The empirical framework provides a means to calculate completeness, sensitivity, and precision to estimate the coverage and accuracy of a proteome-scale interactome mapping project. (Reprinted with permission from Venkatesan, Rual, et al. (2009). An empirical framework for binary interactome mapping. Nat Methods 6(1):83–90.)

quiring a robust systematic binary interaction mapping pipeline. To meet this requirement, proteome-scale experimental mapping of binary interactions is carried out today by variants of the original yeast two-hybrid (Y2H) technology (Fields and Song 1989) (Figure 3–3), as this is the only technology currently sufficiently scalable to address the problem (Vidal and Legrain 1999; Braun, Taşan, et al. 2009; Fields 2009). Y2H technologies have undergone numerous upgrades in throughput and reliability (Vidal, Brachmann, et al. 1996; Walhout and Vidal 1999, 2001; Venkatesan, Rual, et al. 2009) and are now able to interrogate hundreds of millions of human protein pairs for binary interactions (Rolland, Taşan, et al. 2014). Following primary mapping by Y2H, orthogonal assays are used, along with positive and random reference sets, to benchmark the quality of the binary dataset. Through an integrated empirical framework (Figure 3–4), the completeness, precision, and sensitivity of binary datasets can be estimated (Venkatesan, Rual, et al. 2009). This framework is now routinely followed for high-throughput binary interactome mapping (Braun 2012; Rajagopala, Sikorski, et al. 2014). Ultimately, given proper attention to controls and quality assurance, large numbers of high-quality, highly reproducible binary biophysical protein interactions can be mapped (Box 3–1) (Hengartner, Ellis, et al. 1992; Hengartner and Horvitz 1994; del Peso, Gonzalez, et al. 1998, 2000; Woo, Jung, et al. 2003; Yan, Gu, et al. 2004; Sonnichsen, Koski, et al. 2005).

Box 3–1. Binary Interactome Mapping Pipeline

A typical binary interactome mapping pipeline consists of four stages.

1. Screening: High-throughput first pass screens by a high-quality implementation of yeast two-hybrid analysis of all available open reading frames (ORFs) in the ORFeome collection at hand (Dreze, Monachello, et al. 2010). Genes encoding potentially interacting ORFs are identified by next-generation sequencing technology (Yu, Tardivo, et al. 2011). The interacting sequence tags (ISTs) so obtained mark the first-pass pairs of interacting proteins.

2. Verification: First-pass pairs are retrieved from the ORFeome collection and tested pairwise by the same implementation of yeast two-hybrid analysis that was used for first-pass screening. Pairwise tests distinguish artifacts, such as spontaneous auto-activators (Walhout and Vidal 1999), from reproducibly verified interacting pairs. Only verified interacting pairs should be released for public access (Orchard 2012). These interactions represent verified interactions, interactions that occur reproducibly between pairs of proteins

3. Validation: Verified interacting pairs are then tested by an orthogonal binary assay with characteristics distinct from Y2H (Braun, Taşan, et al. 2009). Such assays are slower and less economical than Y2H, so they cannot be used as screening assays. Binary assays that have been used for validation include mammalian protein–protein interaction trap (MAPPIT) (Eyckerman, Verhee, et al. 2001), protein complementation assays (Nyfeler, Michnick, et al. 2005), luminescence-based mammalian interactome mapping (LUMIER) (Taipale, Krykbaeva, et al. 2012), nucleic acid programmable protein array (NAPPA) (Ramachandran, Raphael, et al. 2008), co-immunoprecipitation (Li, Armstrong, et al. 2004; Rajagopala, Sikorski, et al. 2014), and *Gaussia princeps* luciferase complementation assay (GPCA) (Neveu, Cassonnet, et al. 2012).

4. Biological function: One way to turn biophysical interactions into biological interactions is to place confidence in the biological relevance of the identified interacting pairs by integrating orthogonal functional data, such as co-expression profiling or phenotypic profiling (Gunsalus, Ge, et al. 2005), into the interactome dataset. The biological function of individual interactions can also be ascertained through small-scale experimental follow-up by independent laboratories interested in hypotheses presented by a particular reported interaction (see, for example, Horgan, Hanscom, et al. 2013). Interactions not functionally confirmed do not necessarily represent false positives, but rather could represent pseudo-interactions, true biophysical interactions that do not occur physiologically or that do occur but have no discernable functional relevance (Landry, Levy, et al. 2013; Venkatesan, Rual, et al. 2009).

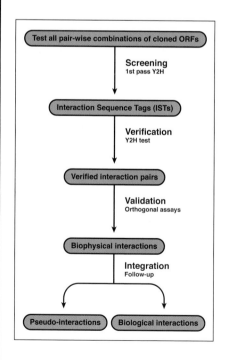

Binary and co-complex screens interrogate vastly different parts of the interactome (Yu, Braun, et al. 2008; Schramm, Jayaswal, et al. 2013). Although this difference may seem obvious (Mosca, Pons, et al. 2013), early analyses of interactome quality did not properly apprehend the differences (Deane, Salwinski, et al. 2002; von Mering, Krause, et al. 2002). Data are often downloaded from an interaction database without due consideration given to the reliability or source of the data (Gillis, Ballouz, et al. 2014). The fundamental distinction between binary protein interactions and co-complex associations, a mix of binary and non-binary interactions, is often overlooked, as protein-interaction databases do not necessarily provide such distinctions, making it difficult to know which interactions to include and which to exclude for a particular investigation (Gillis, Ballouz, et al. 2014).

Rather, third-party users have made attempts to distinguish binary from indirect interactions by defining the methods that have been used to map protein interactions as primarily binary or primarily indirect (Venkatesan, Rual, et al. 2009; Das and Yu 2012). This strategy has obvious deficits in that it annotates the underlying technology and not the actual experiment; moreover, no technique is exclusively binary or exclusively indirect. A binary method may detect an indirect interaction between bait and prey proteins bridged by an endogenous third protein (Fields 2005); the indirect affinity purification technologies include binary interactions among a larger set of indirect interactions (Collins, Kemmeren, et al. 2007). This classify-the-method strategy is operative at least for interaction databases that adhere to the PSI-MI (Proteomics Standards Initiative for Molecular Interactions) initiative, which defines all interaction-detection methods (Kerrien, Orchard, et al. 2007; Isserlin, El-Badrawi, et al. 2011), but unfortunately there are large resources that do not adhere to PSI-MI (Prasad, Goel, et al. 2009; Chatr-aryamontri, Breitkreutz, et al. 2013). The situation might improve, as consolidation of protein-interaction databases with attendant standardization is ongoing (Rid, Strasser, et al. 2013; Orchard, Ammari, et al. 2014).

It is not that one technology provides better or lesser maps of the interactome. The two principal experimental technologies provide complementary, almost orthogonal, views of the protein interactome (Saha, Kaur, et al. 2010; Landry, Levy, et al. 2013; Westermarck, Ivaska, et al. 2013; Rajagopala, Sikorski, et al. 2014). As such, both will be needed to map the totality of protein interactions that carry out cellular functions and are perturbed in human disease. Both Y2H and AP–MS exhibit biases toward or against particular regions of interactome space. AP–MS datasets are heavily biased toward detection of highly expressed proteins and against proteins of low abundance, while Y2H seems to show no bias regarding native protein abundance (Saha, Kaur, et al. 2010) and can readily detect interactions between low-abundance proteins (Rolland, Taşan, et al. 2014). Both technologies seem to be biased against detection of interactions of hydrophobic membrane proteins (Miller, Lo, et al. 2005; Futschik, Chaurasia, et al. 2007; Huang, Jedynak, et al. 2007). Y2H seems to be able to detect transient interactions readily, which are common in signaling pathways (Yu, Braun, et al. 2008; Vinayagam, Stelzl, et al. 2010; Westermarck, Ivaska, et al. 2013), while AP–MS approaches seem to be inherently refractory toward transient interactions and biased toward interactions within stable complexes (Westermarck, Ivaska, et al. 2013). Further biases are being assessed (Wodak, Vlasblom, et al. 2013; Rolland, Taşan, et al. 2014). As the biases of different approaches— literature, computational, or experimental—in mapping protein interactions become appreciated (Futschik, Chaurasia, et al. 2007; Gillis, Ballouz, et al. 2014), strategies toward reaching a complete human interactome map can be suitably adapted.

Progress toward a Reference Human Interactome

Given the efforts being applied to mapping the interactome systematically, there come inescapable questions: How far away is a complete "reference" human interactome map? Is a complete map even within reach? Analogous soul-searching accompanied the Human Genome Project (Naidoo, Pawitan, et al. 2011; Hood and Rowen 2013). To determine how far current interactome maps are from a complete reference map, the goal must first be known, that is, how many distinct interactions comprise the interactome? Estimations of the size of the yeast and human interactomes, the two proteomes with the fullest binary interactome maps, have been made using statistical approaches that determine and evaluate overlaps between interactome datasets (Grigoriev 2003; Sprinzak, Sattath, et al. 2003; Hart, Ramani, et al. 2006; Reguly, Breitkreutz, et al. 2006; Huang, Jedynak, et al. 2007; Stumpf, Thorne, et al. 2008; Sambourg and Thierry-Mieg 2010). Given the biases in interactome mapping among different methods (Yu, Braun, et al. 2008; Saha, Kaur, et al. 2010), biases not accounted for in such statistical estimates of interactome size, these estimates might be focusing on a limited region of the full interactome space, ignoring unexplored regions.

The empirical framework shows that maps generated using a high-quality binary mapping pipeline, such as Y2H, have high precision (at least 80% of reported pairs are true positives) but low sensitivity (~15% of the true interactions were captured in the experiment) (Venkatesan, Rual, et al. 2009; Rajagopala, Sikorski, et al. 2014). Integrating these measures with the fraction of the genome that was tested (completeness), gives an estimate that the human binary interactome might contain ~130,000 ± 30,000 interactions (Venkatesan, Rual, et al. 2009). This estimate indicates that current binary maps of the human interactome

(Rual, Venkatesan, et al. 2005; Stelzl, Worm, et al. 2005; Rolland, Taşan, et al. 2014) contain in aggregate ~10% of the full reference binary interactome. There is, accordingly, a vital need to continue to improve the throughput of current binary mapping pipelines. Development of alternative mapping strategies, beyond Y2H technologies, will also be needed to reach the full binary interactome. No single interaction assay may ever be capable of attaining full sensitivity (Chen, Rajagopala, et al. 2010; Braun 2012; Wodak, Vlasblom, et al. 2013), hence different detection assays covering different subtypes of binary interactions will need to be used to fully elucidate a reference binary interactome map for any organism.

Elements of the empirical framework (Figure 3–4) and screening pipeline (see Box 3–1) developed for binary interactome mapping are being adapted for the other wing of experimental interactome mapping, determination of co-complex associations. Analogous to removal of autoactivators (Dreze, Monachello, et al. 2010), reproducible background contaminants can be cataloged and these likely false positives can be excluded from AP–MS interactome datasets (Tackett, DeGrasse, et al. 2005; Mellacheruvu, Wright, et al. 2013). Efforts have been undertaken to estimate experimental parameters, such as protein abundance, experimental reproducibility, and detection specificity, parameters that can be integrated to estimate experimental precision (Jäger, Cimermancic, et al. 2011). A multiple laboratory consortium has rigorously standardized the AP–MS pipeline (Varjosalo, Sacco, et al. 2013), allowing high reproducibility and increased sensitivity in future mapping efforts (Braun 2013), paralleling efforts to standardize the binary mapping pipeline (Dreze, Monachello, et al. 2010). Sets of high-confidence literature-curated AP–MS associations are being compiled for rigorous comparison to high-throughput datasets (Jäger, Gulbahce, et al. 2010; Braun 2013; Varjosalo, Sacco, et al. 2013), analogous to the efforts to create sets of high-confidence literature-curated binary interactions for the estimation of sensitivity and specificity in the binary empirical framework (Cusick, Yu, et al. 2009; Venkatesan, Rual, et al. 2009). Lastly, probabilistic scoring systems have been derived that can statistically evaluate the quality of each interaction in an AP–MS dataset (Armean, Lilley, et al. 2013), and are used in a way that is analogous to scoring schemes applied to estimate the confidence of binary interactions (Braun, Taşan, et al. 2009; Braun 2012; Hosur, Peng, et al. 2012).

All these efforts to rigorously control the quality and reproducibility of systematic protein-interaction maps have greatly increased confidence in their quality. Small-scale one-off protein-interaction experiments, which constitute the bulk of literature-curated interaction datasets (Peri, Navarro, et al. 2004; Reguly, Breitkreutz, et al. 2006; Lehne and Schlitt 2009), do not apply the same rigor. With few exceptions, the controls applied and the quality assessments are not reported in databases (Huttlin, Ting, et al. 2015). Much as the Human Genome Project could reach completion only once efforts transitioned from small-scale sequencing efforts of uneven and inestimable quality to sequencing consortiums of definable quality and rigor (Hood and Rowen 2013), so too must systematic mapping of the human interactome make a similar transition (Vidal 2006; Varjosalo, Sacco, et al. 2013). And just as with the Human Genome Project, proteome-scale interactome mapping projects do not preclude small-scale focused investigations of biological mechanisms, but rather, stimulate and augment them (Häuser, Ceol, et al. 2014). Reports of an interaction originally detected in a systematic study being validated in a focused experiment are frequent. A functional confirmation of the interaction between Rab11 and GRAB (Horgan, Hanscom, et al. 2013), originally detected systematically (Rual, Venkatesan, et al. 2005), is one such example.

Implications of Inspection Bias

Despite the advancements of systematic experimental pipelines, literature-curated protein-interaction data continue to be the primary data for investigation of focused biological mechanisms. Notwithstanding the variable quality of curated interactions available in public databases (Cusick, Yu, et al. 2009; Lehne and Schlitt 2009; Martha, Liu, et al. 2011), the impact of inspection bias on the ability of literature maps to provide insightful information remains equivocal. The problems posed by inspection bias extend beyond mapping of protein interactions to the development of pharmacological agents and other aspects of modern biomedicine (Edwards, Isserlin, et al. 2011). Essentially the same 10% of the proteome is being investigated today as was being investigated before the announcement of completion of the reference genome sequence (Lander, Linton, et al. 2001; Venter, Adams, et al. 2001), the release of which was expected to stimulate research into new areas. The dial has hardly budged. For protein kinases, choice targets for drug discovery efforts in cancer, most of the ~500 annotated kinases remain uncharacterized, while a handful are targets of many different drugs (Fedorov, Muller, et al. 2010). This bias exists despite the range of mutations and their importance for tumor survival being homogeneously distributed across all known kinases (Grueneberg, Degot, et al. 2008; Fedorov, Muller, et al. 2010) and presumably across other disease-relevant classes of proteins as well. One way forward, at least with regard to interactome mapping, is to continue the transition toward systematic and relatively unbiased experimental interactome mapping (Table 3–1) (Schramm, Jayaswal, et al. 2013; Wodak, Vlasblom, et al. 2013).

With continued advancement of systematic protein-interaction mapping efforts, the expectation is that interactome "deserts," the zones of the interactome

TABLE 3–1. Comparing Experimental Strategies Towards the Complete Interactome. All Are Needed and Are Complementary to One Another.

FEATURE	EXPERIMENTAL BINARY	EXPERIMENTAL CO-COMPLEX	LITERATURE-CURATED
Study type	Discovery-driven	Discovery-driven	Hypothesis-driven
Functional inference	Determinable from network	Determinable from network	Determinable from study design
Inspection bias	Negligible	Moderate	Strong
Expression bias	None	Strong	Strong
Functional bias	Weak	Moderate	Strong
Completeness	Estimable	Somewhat estimable	Not estimable
Reliability	Determinable	Determinable	Indeterminable

space where biomedical researchers simply do not look for interactions owing to the lack of prior knowledge, might eventually become more populated (Rolland, Taşan, et al. 2014). Efforts at mapping protein interactions will continue to be instrumental for furthering biomedical research (Woodsmith and Stelzl 2014).

Interactome Networks and Human Disease

Disease Networks

Identifying individual human genes mutated in disease is critical to understanding disease etiology. Network biology can shed light on the complex relationships between genotype and phenotype in human disease (del Sol, Balling, et al. 2010; Vidal, Cusick, et al. 2011; Furlong 2013). An effective way to identify novel disease genes is to examine the interaction partners of proteins encoded by known disease genes (Oti, Snel, et al. 2006; Gonzalez and Kann 2012).

Focused protein–protein interaction mapping efforts have identified novel interactions among proteins encoded by known disease genes and have also predicted new disease-susceptibility genes. Such efforts reported so far have focused on ataxia (Lim, Hao, et al. 2006; Lim, Crespo-Barreto, et al. 2008), autism (Sakai, Shaw, et al. 2011; Corominas, Yang, et al. 2014), breast cancer (Pujana, Han, et al. 2007; De Nicolo, Parisini, et al. 2009; Taylor, Linding, et al. 2009), Usher syndrome (Reiners, Nagel-Wolfrum, et al. 2006), Huntington disease (Goehler, Lalowski, et al. 2004; Kaltenbach, Romero, et al. 2007), schizophrenia (Camargo, Collura, et al. 2007), Bardet–Biedl syndrome and related ciliopathies (Zaghloul and Katsanis 2009), and Alzheimer disease (Soler-Lopez, Zanzoni, et al. 2011).

Integration of data from network mapping, biochemistry, expression profiling, and genetic variation led to the hypothesis that breast cancer susceptibility could be linked to centrosome dysfunction via perturbation of an interaction between BRCA1 and HMMR (Pujana, Han, et al. 2007; Maxwell, Benitez, et al. 2011). In an interactome subnetwork mapped for spinocerebellar ataxia–associated proteins, most ataxia-causing proteins interact either directly or via shared neighbors, even though the 23 ataxia-causing proteins used as baits had not previously been known to interact with each other (Sakai, Shaw, et al. 2011). In an autism interactome subnetwork, as with the ataxia network, unexpectedly high connectivity between disparate autism disease proteins was discovered, suggesting that convergent molecular pathways underlie autistic phenotypes in distinct syndromes (Corominas, Yang, et al. 2014). Interactome mapping efforts are beginning to decipher the molecular bases of the high genetic heterogeneity exhibited by both of these neurological diseases.

An investigation into Huntington disease identified a large number of proteins that bind to normal and mutant forms of the huntingtin protein, and strikingly, ~45% of these interactors in humans corresponded to genetic modifiers of neurodegeneration in a *Drosophila* model of Huntington disease (Goehler, Lalowski, et al. 2004; Kaltenbach, Romero, et al. 2007; Soler-Lopez, Zanzoni, et al. 2011). Systematic mapping of the interactome of the tandem BRCA1 C-terminal (BRCT) domain, a protein domain resident in many members of DNA damage response pathways, combined experimental binary interaction mapping and co-complex association mapping with reported BRCT interactions from the literature (Woods, Mesquita, et al. 2012). This integrated interactome map led to discovery of two previously unrecognized DNA damage response genes associated with cancer progression.

The common finding among these disease-centric interactome models is the discovery of unexpected relationships between disease genes that initially appeared unrelated. Accordingly, building and analyzing disease-centered networks is a critical step toward the fundamental understanding of underlying disease mechanisms and may also lead to improved predictions of disease survival. For example, the differences observed in the dynamic modularity of interactome hubs (Han, Bertin, et al. 2004) between patients with breast cancer who had a poor prognosis versus those who had a good prognosis led to a prognostic classifier that effectively predicted survival in individual patients (Taylor, Linding, et al. 2009).

Interactome maps have highlighted new candidate disease genes, disease pathways, and disease-modifier genes, but the task of investigating the impact of causal variants on interactome networks is in its infancy. Interactome mapping platforms are being enhanced and expanded to provide mechanistic insights into the consequences of mutations. ATXN1 mutants with an increased polyglutamine repeat led to a protein that preferentially interacts with RBM17, which promotes neurotoxicity, whereas there is reduced interaction of mutant ATXN1 with the capicua protein and reduced neuroprotection (Lim, Crespo-Barreto, et al. 2008). Interactome-based approaches have been developed to help identify disease genes within strongly associated genome-wide association study (GWAS) loci for complex immune-mediated diseases (Rossin, Lage, et al. 2011). Similar approaches are leveraging interactome networks to identify and prioritize candidate disease genes for other human disorders (Oti, Snel, et al. 2006; Navlakha and Kingsford 2010; International Multiple Sclerosis Genetics Consortium 2013).

Network Modules

In the disease-module hypothesis, proteins involved in the same disease have a tendency to interact with each other in a "local neighborhood" of the interactome network (Barabási, Gulbahce, et al. 2011). A disease module is defined as a group of interacting network nodes that ordinarily contribute to a common cellular function and that, when disrupted, lead to disease (Oti and Brunner 2007). If the disease-module hypothesis holds, then human interactome networks can be used to identify novel candidate disease genes, because genes related to specific, or similar, disease phenotypes would tend to locate in a local neighborhood of the network (Menche, Sharma, et al. 2015). The corollary of the disease-module hypothesis is that a disease rarely arises solely because of the alteration of a single gene product. In accord with the disease-module model, proteins involved in the same disease appear to interact with each other preferentially in existing interactome maps (Menche, Sharma, et al. 2015). Given these findings, fuller maps of the human interactome would lead to more accurate maps of modules, which in turn would lead to novel or more complete hypotheses regarding disease-gene candidates (Menche, Sharma, et al. 2015). Investigating disease modularity (Gstaiger and Aebersold 2013) has proven productively informative for multiple diseases, such as ataxias (Lim, Hao, et al. 2006), Fanconi anemia (D'Andrea 2010), chronic obstructive pulmonary disease (McDonald, Mattheisen, et al. 2014), pulmonary arterial hypertension (Parikh, Jin, et al. 2012), breast cancer (Taylor, Linding, et al. 2009), and asthma (Sharma, Menche, et al. 2015).

Bardet–Biedl syndrome (BBS) illustrates the distance that has yet to be traveled in mapping disease modules. BBS is an autosomal recessive, genetically heterogeneous, extraordinarily pleiotropic disorder (Nishimura, Swiderski, et al. 2005; Abu-Safieh, Al-Anazi, et al. 2012). At a minimum, 18 discrete genetic loci have been causally associated with BBS (Katsanis, Beales, et al. 2000; Slavotinek, Stone, et al. 2000). Preliminary interactome mapping of BBS-associated proteins has produced a model in which seven conserved BBS proteins associate into a core complex required for ciliogenesis, with noncore BBS proteins modulating core complex activity and regulation in uncertain ways (Kim, Badano, et al. 2004; Nachury, Loktev, et al. 2007; Oeffner, Moch, et al. 2008). Phenotypic overlaps with Meckel syndrome, Alström syndrome, Joubert syndrome, and McKusick–Kaufman syndrome are unexplained but likely indicate disruption of overlapping disease modules in the interactome (Zaghloul and Katsanis 2009).

Cancer Genes as Hubs

A finding often replicated is that cancer-gene products tend to be highly connected nodes, or hubs, in human interactome-network models (Jonsson and Bates 2006; Sun and Zhao 2010; Xia, Sun, et al. 2011). Cancer genes tend to be exceptionally well studied, and given the inspection bias inherent to literature-curated protein interactions (Edwards, Isserlin, et al. 2011; Das and Yu 2012), there is the nagging worry that topological properties determined solely with literature-derived maps could be severely distorted. To determine whether cancer genes are true hubs, or whether they have more interactions only because they are so well studied, their topological properties are best determined with large systematic binary interactome maps that do not suffer from such bias. There is a significantly higher connectivity of gene products from the Sanger Cancer Gene Census (Futreal, Coin, et al. 2004) in the largest currently available experimental human binary interactome map (Rolland, Taşan, et al. 2014), so cancer proteins are indeed hubs in interactome networks not subject to inspection bias.

Complex Genotype–Phenotype Relationships in Human Disease

Charting the path from genotype to phenotype in human disease is not straightforward. In addition to genetic and environmental modifiers, differences in gene variants can affect how disease genes are expressed and function, and how a disease phenotype manifests. While direct causal relationships between a gene mutation and a disease may seem clear for some disorders (Botstein and Risch 2003), such simple models fail when confronted with confounding genetic heterogeneity commonly observed even for "simple" Mendelian diseases (Scriver and Waters 1999). The situation is more intricate for complex traits, for which the disease states appear to result from multiple perturbations of molecular machines and pathways (Sebat, Levy, et al. 2009). As disease-associated mutations can impinge on health through specific interactome-network perturbations, studying these perturbations can improve the resolution of disease etiology.

Phenotypic Variations Result from Specific Network Perturbations

Many proteins have been found to interact with p53, a central player in the regulation of cell proliferation and apoptosis frequently found mutated in cancers (Vogelstein, Papadopoulos, et al. 2013). The function of p53 is inhibited by the Mdm2 E3 ubiquitin-protein ligase through ubiquitination and subsequent degradation of p53 by the proteasome. In response to ribosomal stress, Mdm2 is in turn inhibited by the ribosomal proteins L5 and L11, resulting in p53 activation and inhibition of c-Myc–induced lymphomagenesis (Macias, Jin, et al. 2010). One allele of Mdm2, bearing a C305F mutation in the zinc-finger domain, encodes a protein unable to interact with L5 and L11, with the outcome of increased tumorigenesis, a single point mutation giving rise to disease by altering specific protein interactions. Wild-type p53 does not bind nardilysin, a metalloendopeptidase involved in the invasiveness of tumor cells, but the R273H point mutant does (Coffill, Muller, et al. 2012). Detection of this gained interaction between nardilysin and p53R273H uncovered a new aspect of p53-driven invasion, and exemplifies cancer-associated missense mutations that alter specific protein interactions (Nishi, Tyagi, et al. 2013).

Mutations in the *FBXW7* gene are often found in human tumors, notably T-cell acute lymphoblastic leukemia (Akhoondi, Sun, et al. 2007; O'Neil, Grim, et al. 2007; Thompson, Buonamici, et al. 2007). The FBXW7 protein is a subunit of the Skp1-Cul1-F box (SCF) ubiquitin ligase complex, which regulates key cellular regulators, especially c-Myc (Crusio, King, et al. 2010). The most commonly found mutation of FBXW7, R465C, precludes FBXW7 binding to c-Myc, thus preventing degradation of c-Myc mediated by the SCF complex (King, Trimarchi, et al. 2013). In cancer cells in which c-Myc is expressed, this inability to degrade c-Myc resulting from loss of FBXW7 binding to c-Myc leads to a dramatic increase in the leukemia-initiating cell population.

What these telling examples relate is that human disorders do not necessarily reflect the absence of the incriminated gene product, as per conventional models of human disease (Botstein and Risch 2003). Often, the disease results from subtler molecular defects that impinge on specific protein–protein interactions (Chakravarti, Clark, et al. 2013).

From Variome to Edgetics

Enhanced comprehension of genotype–phenotype relationships in human disease will require modeling of how disease-causing mutations affect interactome properties (Carter, Hofree, et al. 2013; Yates and Sternberg 2013).

Deleterious mutations associated with disease, constituting the human variome (Cotton, Auerbach, et al. 2008), may cause a wide spectrum of molecular defects in gene products (Laskowski and Thornton 2008). At one end of the

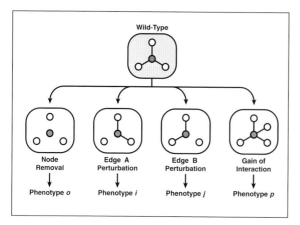

FIGURE 3–5. Classification of different types of edge perturbation as distinct edgotypes leading to distinct phenotypes.

spectrum are nonsense mutations and mutations affecting splicing, which usually truncate the gene product by introducing a premature stop codon into the protein-coding region. Most of these mutations are predicted to result in the absence of any protein product either due to nonsense-mediated messenger (mRNA) decay (Chang, Imam, et al. 2007) or to major protein-folding and stability problems (Studer, Dessailly, et al. 2013).

In network models of the interactome, these truncating mutations can be thought of as the removal of one node along with all of its edges—a node removal (Figure 3–5). Nonconservative missense mutations of amino acids in the protein core that lead to major folding problems, protein aggregation, and premature protein degradation can also be modeled as node removals (Studer, Dessailly, et al. 2013). At the other end of the mutational spectrum are small in-frame indels or missense mutations. These can preserve protein folding, but may modify the active site of an enzyme or affect the binding to another protein or macromolecule. In network models, these mutations, which specifically perturb a single molecular interaction (Figure 3–5), have been labeled as edge-specific or "edgetic" (Dreze, Charloteaux, et al. 2009; Zhong, Simonis, et al. 2009; Charloteaux, Zhong, et al. 2011; Lambert, Ivosev, et al. 2013; Mosca, Tenorio-Laranga, et al. 2015). While investigation of the precise interaction defects associated with point mutations is of course not new, the term *edgetic* promotes a subtle yet meaningful archetype shift from conventional gene-centric approaches toward interaction-centric approaches. Edge perturbing network models, which emphasize consideration of which specific edges are affected by a mutation, complement and extend classic gene-centric models, which ascertain only whether a gene product is present or not present and neglect less overt alterations of a given gene or gene product (Botstein and Risch 2003; Chakravarti, Clark, et al. 2013; Sahni, Yi, et al. 2013).

Two complementary strategies can be pursued to investigate edgetic perturbation models: forward edgetics and reverse edgetics (Charloteaux, Zhong, et al. 2011) (Figure 3–6), analogous to the distinction long made in genetics between classical forward genetics (produce a phenotype then identify the responsible genetic variants) and more modern reverse genetics (create specific mutations in specific proteins then identify the resulting phenotype) (Lehner 2013). Having a set of mutations responsible for particular disease phenotypes (the genotype), the forward edgetics approach endeavors to uncover mechanistic connections from genotype to phenotype by determining the specific interactome-network perturbations that result from these mutations (the edgotype) (Zhong, Simonis, et al. 2009). In reverse edgetics, alleles with specific interaction defects are produced first (the edgotype), then these alleles are reintroduced in vivo in place of or alongside the wild-type allele to investigate the functional relevance of the corresponding interaction (the phenotype) (Dreze, Charloteaux, et al. 2009).

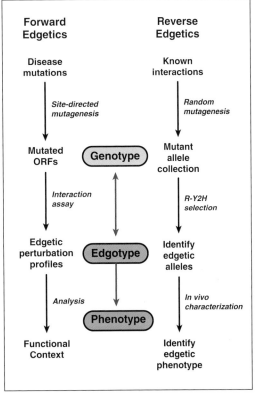

FIGURE 3–6. Forward edgetics and reverse edgetics strategies to explore network perturbations caused by specific mutations.

Edgotyping—Systematic Edgetic Profiling

Direct tests of the edgetics model reported so far are beginning to resolve particular issues of confounding genetic heterogeneity in human disease (Ryan, Cimermancic, et al. 2013; Das, Fragoza, et al. 2014). An intriguing example involves the human senataxin protein, which has a long N-terminal domain common to all senataxin homologs in other species and a C-terminal DNA/RNA helicase domain common to many proteins involved in DNA repair (Bennett, Chen, et al. 2013; Yüce and West 2013). Some mutations in the senataxin N-terminal domain cause autosomal recessive spinocerebellar ataxia (SCAR1), also known as ataxia with oculomotor apraxia (OAO2), whereas other distinct mutations in the same domain cause autosomal dominant amyotrophic lateral sclerosis type 4 (ALS4). The allelic heterogeneity of two distinct neurodegenerative disorders, one recessive and one dominant, echoes edgetic models in which mutations at different interfaces of a protein can cause different diseases through disruption of distinct interactions (Wang, Wei, et al. 2012; Das, Fragoza, et al.

2014). Y2H screens of wild-type (wt) senataxin and SETX-L389S against a brain cDNA library identified about a dozen reproducible interactors. While most of the partners identified interacted with wt, and with the L389S (associated with ALS4) and W305C (associated with OAO2) mutations, one interaction with a peptide encoded by the antisense sequence of BCYRN1 non-coding RNA occurs only with L389S but not wt or W305C. The predicted BCYRN1 gene product has a patch of identity in the uncharacterized predicted protein C14orf178, and when tested C14orf178 also interacts with L389S but not wt senataxin. The edgetic effect of SETX-L389S is replicated with a predicted interacting partner containing a small region of sequence identity (Bennett, Chen, et al. 2013).

To such lone tests of edgetic perturbation models now comes edgetic profiling, or edgotyping, the systematic analysis of many mutations in many disease genes concurrently (Sahni, Yi, et al. 2013, 2015). The first matter to resolve is what fraction of human disease mutations causes perturbations of specific interactions versus major disruptions of the gene product similar to null alleles. That is, what is the proportion of node-removal perturbations versus edgetic perturbations? There are arguments that nearly all missense mutations drastically affect the encoded gene product, resulting in an inactive or absent protein that in a network representation has lost all its edges (Ferrer-Costa, Orozco, et al. 2002; Botstein and Risch 2003; Yue, Li, et al. 2005). In actuality, retention of partly functional proteins that show perturbations of specific protein-binding interfaces (see Figure 3–5) is not exceptional (Schuster-Bockler and Bateman 2008; Zhong, Simonis, et al. 2009; Guo, Wei, et al. 2013; Sahni, Yi, et al. 2015).

Modeling network perturbations induced by mutations in alleles associated with human Mendelian disorders led to an estimate that up to half of the disease-associated mutations examined could potentially encode proteins with edgetic interaction defects (Zhong, Simonis, et al. 2009). The actual proportion of disease-associated missense mutations that are edgetic is indeterminate, likely less than the 50% maximal estimate but still considerable (Schuster-Bockler and Bateman 2008; Zhong, Simonis, et al. 2009; Wang, Wei, et al. 2012; Guo, Wei, et al. 2013; Mosca, Tenorio-Laranga, et al. 2015). A quantitative survey of almost 3000 human mutant ORFs, each harboring a single disease-associated nucleotide change, estimated that most missense disease mutations do not dramatically impact protein structure or protein folding (Sahni, Yi, et al. 2015).

Putative edgetic alleles of the same gene, but associated with different diseases, tend to be located in distinct interaction domains, leading to the hypothesis that they perturb distinct protein–protein interactions (Zhong, Simonis, et al. 2009; Wang, Wei, et al. 2012). An example involves two clinically distinct developmental disorders, ectrodactyly ectodermal dysplasia (EEC) and ankyloblepharon ectodermal dysplasia (AEC), caused by mutations in two separate domains of TP63, one predicted to bind DNA and the other to mediate protein–protein interactions (van Bokhoven and Brunner 2002). Overlaying protein three-dimensional information onto disease-associated mutations indicated that disease-associated in-frame mutations preferentially locate at putative protein-binding sites and that putative edgetic alleles of the same gene, but associated with different diseases, do tend to be located in distinct interaction domains (Wang, Wei, et al. 2012) (Figure 3–7).

Detection of edgetic perturbations is efficacious with binary interaction-detection methods, primarily Y2H assays (Dittmer, Sahni, et al. 2014; Wang, Zhong, et al. 2014), but there is no reason why methods that detect co-complex associations cannot be adapted to detect edgetic perturbations associated with disease. Development of a robust yet sensitive quantitative AP–MS technology, called

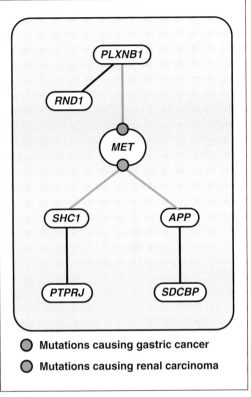

FIGURE 3–7. Mutations in the MET oncogene that cause distinct cancers perturb distinct sets of interactors and disrupt distinct interfaces of the MET protein. (Adapted with permission of the Royal Society of Chemistry from Das, J., R. Fragoza, et al. (2014). Exploring mechanisms of human disease through structurally resolved protein interactome networks. Mol Biosyst 10:9–17.)

AP-SWATH, allowed a first test of differential interactomes between wild-type CDK4 and two CDK4 missense mutations associated with melanoma (Lambert, Ivosev, et al. 2013). Pronounced differences in protein associations between the wild-type and mutant forms of CDK4 were identified, with the mutants showing sharp decreases in association with the INK family of CDK inhibitors, but sharp increases in association with particular chaperone proteins. The response to a potent chaperone inhibitor in clinical testing was sharply different between the mutants and wild-type CDK4, giving therapeutic context to the altered associations. AP-SWATH can now be used to quantify dynamic changes in protein-complex interaction networks resulting from mutations (Collins, Gillet, et al. 2013; Lambert, Ivosev, et al. 2013).

Reverse Edgetics

Reverse engineering presents a potent approach to delineate genotype–phenotype relationships. Y2H assays are an especially potent tool to delineate mutations that perturb specific protein–protein interactions and even to demarcate protein–protein binding sites (Amberg, Basart, et al. 1995; Vidal, Braun, et al. 1996; Inouye, Dhillon, et al. 1997; Shi, Rojas, et al. 2006).

A proof-of-principle demonstration that edgetic perturbation models constitute powerful approaches to investigate complex genotype–phenotype relationships investigated the function of the *Caenorhabditis elegans* anti-apoptotic CED-9 by reverse edgetics (Dreze, Charloteaux, et al. 2009). Binary interactions of CED-9 to four other proteins were mapped by both Y2H and co-affinity purifications. Alleles with interaction defects, ranging from the loss of all four interactions to the specific loss of interaction with a single partner (edgetic), were isolated. Structural analyses substantiated that mutations in edgetic alleles specifically affect protein binding sites, while in vivo characterization of a subset of CED-9 edgetic alleles demonstrated that distinct alleles manifest with distinct phenotypes (Dreze, Charloteaux, et al. 2009). (Box 3–2; Walhout and Vidal 1999; Eyckerman, Verhee, et al. 2001; Li, Armstrong, et al. 2004; Gunsalus, Ge, et al. 2005; Nyfeler, Michnick, et al. 2005; Ramachandran, Raphael, et al. 2008; Braun, Taşan, et al. 2009; Venkatesan, Rual, et al. 2009; Dreze, Monachello, et al. 2010; Yu, Tardivo, et al. 2011; Neveu, Cassonnet, et al. 2012; Orchard, Kerrien, et al. 2012; Taipale, Krykbaeva, et al. 2012; Horgan, Hanscom, et al. 2013; Landry, Levy, et al. 2013; Rajagopala, Sikorski, et al. 2014).

Reverse engineering can also generate proteins with point mutations that do not lose an interaction but that actually have increased affinity for a specific interactor, a gain-of-interaction (see Figure 3–5). Such an edgetic strategy was reported for proliferating-cell nuclear antigen (PCNA), a DNA replication processivity protein that interacts with and holds multiple DNA replication and repair enzymes to the DNA replication fork (Fridman, Palgi, et al. 2010). Many gain-of-interaction point mutations in PCNA actually exhibit more deleterious phenotypes than mutations that lose the binding altogether. Such subtle edgetic perturbations can produce more pronounced effects than conventional genetic perturbations that remove a protein node altogether (Vidal, Cusick, et al. 2011; Carter, Hofree, et al. 2013).

Prospects for Edgetics

With sweeping advancements in genotyping technologies (Altshuler, Gibbs, et al. 2010) and with the phenomenal improvements in genome-sequencing capacity presented by next-generation sequencing (Pareek, Smoczynski, et al. 2011), biomedical research is being deluged with genotypic information (Hood

Box 3–2. A Reverse Edgetics Case Study

Caenorhabditis elegans CED-9

The *C. elegans* apoptosis *ced-9* gene, the homolog of mammalian *BCL2,* was originally identified by the isolation of a dominant allele, *ced-9(n1950),* corresponding to a G169E mutation. This mutation prevents embryonic cells from undergoing programmed cell death, or apoptosis, by precluding the EGL-1-induced dissociation of the CED-9/CED-4 apoptosis effector complex (del Peso, Gonzalez, et al. 1998, 2000; Hengartner and Horvitz 1994). The isolation of this allele, which is now understood to be edgetic (Dreze, Charloteaux, et al. 2009), was followed by identification of four recessive *ced-9* loss-of-function alleles, each of which caused increased apoptosis and embryonic lethality similar to those phenotypes observed when *ced-9* expression is knocked down by RNAi (Hengartner, Ellis, et al. 1992; Sonnichsen, Koski, et al. 2005). Two of these recessive ced-9 alleles are nonsense mutations [*ced-9(n2812)* and *ced-9(n2077)*]; one leads to a disruption of a splice acceptor site [*ced-9(n2161)*]; and the fourth [*ced-9(n1653)*], a Y149N mutation, likely completely destabilizes the structure of CED-9. The impact of all of these four alleles can now be understood to represent a node removal, depleting CED-9 in the cell (Dreze, Charloteaux, et al. 2009).

An updated implementation of reverse yeast two-hybrid, providing cleaner resolution of obtained missense mutations than previous implementations (Inouye, Dhillon, et al. 1997), was used to identify four additional edgetic alleles (Dreze, Charloteaux, et al. 2009). Two (G169E and G169R) recapitulated the original *ced-9(n1950)* allele, one being the identical substitution. Two others (G173D and A183T) were close by in the CED-9 sequence. Analysis of structural models of CED-9, alone or complexed with the BH3 domain of EGL-1 (Woo, Jung, et al. 2003; Yan, Gu, et al. 2004), found that these edgetic mutations specifically disrupted the physical interactions between the two proteins. Gly169 and Gly173 are both in direct contact with EGL-1, and substitution of a glycine with bulkier residues would disrupt the interaction—explaining the edgetic effects—while the nearby A183T mutation disrupts the α-helix in which all edgetic mutations reside and, hence, also disrupts the EGL-1–CED-9 interaction. The path from genotype through edgotype to phenotype is resolved in this case study.

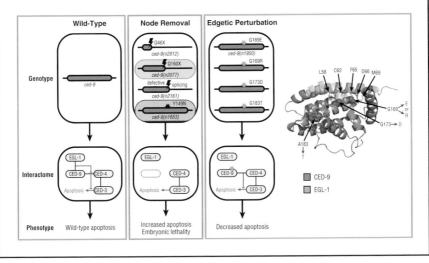

and Rowen 2013). Despite impressive progress, the wealth of information provided by the genomic revolution has not yet been translated into actionable knowledge about disease pathogenesis (Furlong 2013). It is now undeniable that the complexity of genotype–phenotype relationships will not be understood without considering the underlying system. Part of the resolution will hopefully come from the emergence of edgetic perturbation models. With few exceptions (Raj, Rifkin, et al. 2010), large-scale genetic screens have focused on the impact of deleting or overexpressing genes and not grappled with the consequences of allelic variation (Chakravarti, Clark, et al. 2013). Edgetic modeling provides a route to deal more forthrightly with these consequences.

Interactomes and Viral Pathogens

Viruses are obligate parasites of their hosts and as such must usurp host pathways to complete their life cycle. From a network medicine perspective, the diseases associated with viral infection can be attributed to the interaction between viral proteins and host proteins (Davey, Trave, et al. 2011; Vidal, Cusick, et al. 2011). Interactions between viral proteins and the proteins encoded by their host cells were initially studied only on a small scale, one virus protein at a time. Just as with protein–protein interactions in host cells, hundreds of such small-scale viral-host protein interactions were eventually collected in specific curated databases (Chatr-aryamontri, Ceol, et al. 2009) for public download and analysis. Mirroring the progression seen with interactome mapping between cellular proteins, virus–host interactome mapping has now progressed from small-scale to systematic, proteome-scale interrogation of all the proteins encoded by a viral genome or even several viral genomes at once.

Systematic Y2H studies of human virus–host binary protein–protein interactions have been conducted for Epstein–Barr virus (EBV) (Calderwood, Venkatesan, et al. 2007), hepatitis C virus (HCV) (de Chassey, Navratil, et al. 2008), human immunodeficiency virus (HIV) (Konig, Zhou, et al. 2008), vaccinia virus (Zhang, Villa, et al. 2009), influenza virus (Shapira, Gat-Viks, et al. 2009), human T-cell lymphotropic viruses (Simonis, Rual, et al. 2012), and four distinct classes of human tumor viruses (Rozenblatt-Rosen, Deo, et al. 2012). AP–MS technologies have witnessed a similar progression from small-scale (mapping the host interactors of hepatitis B virus multifunctional protein HBx [Zhang, Xie, et al. 2013]) to systematic virus–host co-complex mapping. Systematic virus–host co-complex protein association maps have been reported for HIV (Jäger, Cimermancic, et al. 2011), for viral proteins exhibiting immune-modulating functions from a diverse set of 30 human viruses (Pichlmair, Kandasamy, et al. 2012), for the E6 oncoproteins from 16 different human papillomavirus (HPV) types (White, Kramer, et al. 2012), for all the oncoproteins encoded by four distinct classes of human tumor viruses (Rozenblatt-Rosen, Deo, et al. 2012), and for all hepatitis C proteins (Germain, Chatel-Chaix, et al. 2014).

These systematic proteome-scale screens provide unbiased lists of viral-targeted proteins through which to identify cellular pathways and functions crucial to the viral life cycle. The HCV-host binary interactome map (de Chassey, Navratil, et al. 2008) showed a significant enrichment of HCV target proteins in three known pathways (insulin, TGFβ, Jak-STAT) and one novel pathway (focal adhesion). An influenza–host interactome map (Shapira, Gat-Viks, et al. 2009) demonstrated enrichment in major intracellular pathways, and integration of the physical targets with transcriptional targets of the same influenza proteins showed that not only does influenza virus target multiple components of each pathway, but it also affects the pathway by more than one mechanism.

Host proteins targeted by EBV and HCV proteins tend to be central in the human interactome network (Calderwood, Venkatesan, et al. 2007; de Chassey, Navratil, et al. 2008; Navratil, de Chassey, et al. 2011), suggesting that viral proteins from multiple viral classes preferentially target proteins central in the host interactome (Dyer, Murali, et al. 2008; Garamszegi, Franzosa, et al. 2013). Host proteins directly targeted by HIV proteins predominantly localized in groups of human proteins strongly interconnected in the underlying network (Wuchty, Siwo, et al. 2010). Interacting with highly connected cellular proteins enables a viral protein to manipulate diverse cellular pathways simultaneously and efficiently.

The global landscape of host proteins targeted by proteins from DNA tumor viruses helped to prioritize genes and pathways involved in cancer (Rozenblatt-Rosen, Deo, et al.

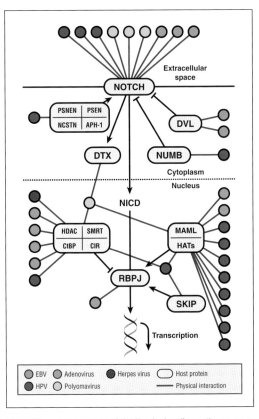

FIGURE 3–8. Components of the Notch signaling pathway, many of which are mutated in numerous distinct cancers, are targeted by multiple viral proteins from distinct viral classes. (Adapted with permission from Rosenblatt-Rosen, O. (2012) Interpreting cancer genomes using systematic host network perturbations by tumor virus proteins. Nature 487:491–95.)

2012). Systematic mapping of the interactions and expression perturbations induced by proteins of four classes of tumor viruses, polyomaviruses, papillomaviruses, adenovirus, and Epstein–Barr virus, produced a list of virally perturbed host genes that showed a significant overlap with known genes in the COSMIC Classic list of cancer-associated genes (Forbes, Bindal, et al. 2011). Integrated analyses of the interactome and transcriptome datasets highlighted pathways that go awry in cancer (Figure 3–8).

Comparison of the host–protein interactions of the E6 oncoproteins found differences in the patterns of observed interactions between the low-risk cutaneous HPV5 and HPV8 strains and the high-risk oncogenic HPV6b, HPV11, HPV16, and HPV18 strains. Analysis of these differential interactions implicated mutations in a Notch pathway component, Mastermind-like 1 (MAML1), in tumorigenesis (Rozenblatt-Rosen, Deo, et al. 2012; White, Kramer, et al. 2012). *MAML1* was independently validated as a cancer-causing gene, confirming the predictive power of systematic interactome mapping in oncogenesis (Brimer, Lyons, et al. 2012; Tan, White, et al. 2012).

Another illustration of systematic virus–host interaction mapping opening a window into disease mechanisms comes from the characterization of the previously unannotated cellular FAM111A protein as a host range restriction factor specifically targeted by the large T antigen of simian virus 40 (SV40) polyomavirus (Fine, Rozenblatt-Rosen, et al. 2012). Shortly thereafter, a set of heterozygous point mutations in FAM111A arising de novo was shown to be a cause of two phenotypically related developmental disorders of unknown molecular etiology, Kenny–Caffey syndrome (KCS) and osteocraniostenosis (OCS) (Unger, Gorna, et al. 2013; Isojima, Doi, et al. 2014). These disease mutations map to the same minimal region of FAM111A that is required for large-T-antigen binding of SV40 (Fine, Rozenblatt-Rosen, et al. 2012). The obvious implication is that pathogenesis in KCS and OCS is due to these mutations disrupting the binding of FAM111A to important cellular proteins that are also targeted by SV40 large T (Alabert, Bukowski-Wills, et al. 2014).

Genes in close network proximity to host proteins targeted by EBV and HPV16 viral proteins showed significantly shifted expression patterns in diseases associated with the viral infection and are significantly closer to genes associated with virally implicated diseases than to genes associated with other diseases (Gulbahce, Yan, et al. 2012), leading to the Local Impact Hypothesis, similar to the local neighborhood hypothesis for disease modules (Barabási, Gulbahce, et al. 2011). Exploitation of the local impact hypothesis to viral disease networks prioritized several diseases as candidate virally implicated diseases based on network topology and on population-based clinical associations between candidate diseases and viral infection. One such prioritization highlighted a novel connection between HPV infection and Fanconi anemia (Gulbahce, Yan, et al. 2012).

Just as with host interactome networks, one substantial benefit of systematic "virhostome" interactome mapping is that the data can be drilled down to individual protein–protein interactions to improve insight into specific aspects of infection and disease. One such example involves the EBV tegument protein encoded by BLRF2, which had been shown to be essential for replication in gamma-herpesviruses, but the mechanism of action remained ill defined. Systematic EBV–host binary interactome mapping showed that human serine–arginine-rich protein kinase 2 (SRPK2) interacts with and phosphorylates an RS motif in the BLRF2 C-terminal region (Duarte, Wang, et al. 2013). Mutation of this RS motif abrogated the ability of BLRF2 to support replication in a gamma-herpesvirus model system, suggesting that phosphorylation by SRPK2 of the BLRF2 RS motif is crucial for viral replication, and presenting a potential therapeutic strategy by which to inhibit gamma-herpesvirus replication.

Variations on a Reference Interactome

Alternatively Spliced Isoforms

Alternative splicing vastly increases proteome diversity, and occurs in nearly all eukaryotes (Kim, Magen, et al. 2007). Transcriptome sequencing in different human and murine tissues shows that nearly all genes exhibit alternative splicing (Pan, Shai, et al. 2008; Wang, Sandberg, et al. 2008). The accumulation of introns, so much more prevalent in mammals (especially in primates) than in metazoans and other eukaryotes, confers an evolutionary advantage by efficiently increasing the number of protein isoforms (Barbosa-Morais, Irimia, et al. 2012) without commensurate increases in the gene count. Alternative splicing affects protein sequence and structure drastically (Lareau, Green, et al. 2004; Talavera, Vogel, et al. 2007) and seems to play critical regulatory roles in development, cell-type differentiation, and regulation of signal-transduction pathways (Gabut, Samavarchi-Tehrani, et al. 2011; Kalsotra and Cooper 2011; Merkin, Russell, et al. 2012), but how alternative splicing contributes to phenotypic complexity remains unclear.

Although the hypothesis that different alternative isoforms can exhibit distinct patterns of protein interactions is well accepted (Davis, Shin, et al. 2012; Dittmer, Sahni, et al. 2014), in current interactome network models, genes are still represented by a single splice isoform, generally the longest isoform. Information about which splice isoform is responsible for an interaction is hardly ever presented (Talavera, Robertson, et al. 2013). Incorporating transcript diversity is critical to generation of biologically relevant networks, which would be more informative than currently available interactome datasets (Davis, Shin, et al. 2012; Schramm, Jayaswal, et al. 2013).

The exact number of different proteins produced by alternatively spliced isoforms from the human genome is not currently determinable (Taneri 2011). Examples in which different alternative spliced isoforms exhibit different functions, arising from differential protein interactions, have been uncovered (Nilsen and Graveley 2010). With neuroligin, a protein involved in synaptogenesis, isoforms that bind only β-neurexins stimulate synapse formation, whereas other isoforms that bind both α- and β-neurexins promote synapse expansion (Boucard, Chubykin, et al. 2005).

One salient example in which alternative splicing affects disease presentation involves Usher syndrome, a genetically heterogeneous, autosomal recessive, pleiotropic disorder. For Usher syndrome an interactome subnetwork has been built around established causative disease genes (Adato, Michel, et al. 2005; Reiners, Nagel-Wolfrum, et al. 2006; van Wijk, van der Zwaag, et al. 2006). Although the Usher syndrome interactome subnetwork has provided many tantalizing clues as to disease etiology, considerably more mapping is needed. Different mutations in cadherin 23 (CDH23/USH1D) cause either syndromic Usher syndrome (deafness associated with retinitis pigmentosa and vestibular dysfunction) or nonsyndromic deafness (Bork, Peters, et al. 2001). The alternative disease outcome appears to result from alternative CDH23 isoforms differentially expressed in the retina and inner ear (Lagziel, Ahmed, et al. 2005; Lagziel, Overlack, et al. 2009; Zaghloul and Katsanis 2010). The disease-associated isoform of lamin A, responsible for Hutchinson–Gilford progeria syndrome, presents a spectrum of interacting proteins vastly different from the interactors of the wild-type isoform (Dittmer, Sahni, et al. 2014).

Tissue-specific exons are enriched in conserved disordered residues and in linear binding motifs (Buljan, Chalancon, et al. 2012; Dinkel, Van Roey, et al. 2014). The types of protein domains selectively removed by alternative splicing at much higher frequencies than average include many well-known protein-interaction domains (Resch, Xing, et al. 2004). These observations taken together are consistent with removal or inclusion of protein–protein interaction domains being a major role of alternative splicing (Resch, Xing, et al. 2004; Davis, Shin, et al. 2012). Differential protein binding by isoforms could potentially allow for tissue-specific protein-interaction networks without increasing the number of genes in the genome. Experimental deletion of tissue-specific exons in several dozen genes, and systematically testing effects of these deletions on known interactions, demonstrated that alternative splicing can turn protein interactions on or off (Ellis, Barrios-Rodiles, et al. 2012). These systematic efforts, combined with a growing body of examples of differential splicing variably affecting specific protein interactions (Jiao, Robison, et al. 2008; Wethkamp, Hanenberg, et al. 2011; Thakar, Votteler, et al. 2012), argue that altering protein interactions could be the primary function of alternative splicing. That most human genes undergo alternative splicing (Pan, Shai, et al. 2008; Wang, Sandberg, et al. 2008) suggests that nearly all human protein–protein interactions may be modulated by alternative splicing (Davis, Shin, et al. 2012).

There is an urgent need for the evolution of technologies to systematically map proteome-wide the interactions of naturally occurring isoforms. Just as the evolution of high-throughput sequencing technologies enabled study of the extent of alternative splicing in the human transcriptome (Modrek and Lee 2002), high-throughput methods are also needed to study the effects of alternative splicing on the interactome network. Systematic cloning of alternatively spliced isoforms for thousands of genes, using reverse-transcription polymerase chain reaction (RT-PCR) on RNA from multiple tissues, is now feasible (Salehi-Ashtiani, Yang, et al. 2008). The complementary technology of RNA-seq can identify thou-

sands of alternatively spliced junctions between exons (Sultan, Schulz, et al. 2008), but it cannot overcome the connectivity problem of determining which alternatively spliced exon is connected linearly to which other exons in any single transcript. Nor does RNA-seq provide cloned open reading frame (ORF) resources suitable for downstream functional assays, particularly protein-interaction mapping.

With resources of cloned alternatively spliced ORFs now in hand, systematic isoform-specific interactome maps are appearing (Corominas, Yang, et al. 2014). Isoform-specific interactome maps will enable a more precise map of the organization of the interactome, blurred in traditional interactome studies by the implicit, and knowingly flawed, assumption that all isoforms of a gene behave identically in the network (Figure 3–9).

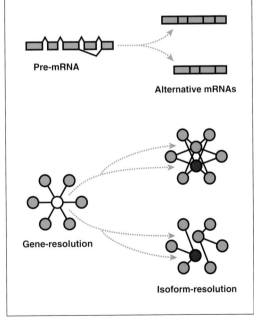

FIGURE 3–9. Alternative inclusion or exclusion of particular exons by alternative splicing gives rise to mRNAs that can produce protein isoforms that are different in structure and presumably in function. In interactome-network maps, different isoforms from the same gene can present identical (upper) or completely different (lower) constellations of interactions.

Domains Involved in Protein Interactions

Proteins interact with other proteins through small regions comprising protein-interaction domains, not through the full protein molecule. There are many conserved protein domains known to specifically mediate protein interactions, and many proteins are composed of multiple such interaction domains that can separately bind to distinct partners (Pawson and Nash 2000, 2003; Aloy and Russell 2005; Han, Batey, et al. 2007; Jadwin, Ogiue-Ikeda, et al. 2012; Westermarck, Ivaska, et al. 2013). Physical interactions between proteins can be grouped into two broad classes: domain–domain interactions and domain–motif interactions (Liddington 2004; Garamszegi, Franzosa, et al. 2013). Domain–domain interactions are more prevalent in stable protein complexes, whereas domain-motif interactions are more prevalent in transient interactions (Fuxreiter, Tompa, et al. 2007; Bader, Kuhner, et al. 2008; Tompa and Fuxreiter 2008). From these observations arise hypotheses that interacting proteins detectable by Y2H, reportedly better able to detect transient interactions than AP–MS (Vinayagam, Stelzl, et al. 2010; Westermarck, Ivaska, et al. 2013), would be enriched in the disordered regions and linear motifs emblematic of domain–motif interactions, whereas interacting proteins detectable by AP–MS would be enriched in domain–domain interactions within stable protein complexes (Westermarck, Ivaska, et al. 2013).

The structures of many domain–motif interaction domains have been solved (Pawson and Nash 2003; Bhattacharyya, Remenyi, et al. 2006; Liu, Engelmann, et al. 2012), providing insight into how cell networks and protein complexes dynamically assemble and disassemble. In interactome-network models, information about the interacting domains is rarely incorporated. Instead, the protein is represented as a uniform node binding to all of its interacting partners concurrently, obscuring the actuality that different regions or domains are physically responsible for the different interactions, at different times or localized in different compartments within a cell.

By comparing which fragments of a protein interact with a given partner, it becomes possible to determine the region of the fragmented protein responsible for that specific interaction (Fields and Sternglanz 1994). In a Y2H screen of multiple fragments of the human Huntington disease protein huntingtin (HTT) diverse interaction partners were identified (Goehler, Lalowski, et al. 2004). One HTT interactor, GIT1, influenced HTT aggregation, the primary pathobiology in Huntington disease progression (Goehler, Lalowski, et al. 2004). Both GIT1 and HTT are large multidomain proteins, but screening multiple fragments of each protein narrowed down the putative interacting regions to the N-terminal region of HTT and the C-terminal region of GIT1 (Goehler, Lalowski, et al. 2004). An interaction critical for the development of Fanconi anemia (D'Andrea

2010) occurs between the FANCA and FANCG proteins. By repeated truncation, the FANCG binding site on FANCA was delineated to an 11 amino acid arginine-rich motif close to the N-terminus, while reciprocally the FANCA binding site on FANCG constituted two lengthy but noncontiguous C-terminal regions of FANCG (Kruyt, Abou-Zahr, et al. 1999). Site-specific alanine mutagenesis was able to delineate the 3 to 4 most critical residues in the 11 amino acid FANCG binding site on FANCA. The FANCA–FANCG interaction is critical for disease progression, as stable transfections of truncation mutants of FANCA lacking the FANCG binding motif rendered the cells sensitive to mitomycin C, a hallmark phenotype of Fanconi anemia (Moldovan and D'Andrea 2009), whereas mutants of FANCA containing an intact FANCG binding motif did not show mitomycin C sensitivity (Kruyt, Abou-Zahr, et al. 1999).

As with other aspects of interactome mapping, technology has advanced to enable mapping of interacting domains systematically at proteome scale. A first systematic experimental mapping of protein-interaction domains used a fragment-based Y2H approach to identify interaction domains for ~700 proteins involved in early embryogenesis in *C. elegans* (Boxem, Maliga, et al. 2008). An average of 40 different bait protein fragments for each tested gene was screened against a library of full-length prey proteins. This systematic "fragmentome" approach identified more interactions than found by screening full-length proteins without increasing the false-positive rate. By mapping the smallest region shared by all fragments for which the interaction was observed, the minimal region of interaction could be determined. Often multiple minimal regions of interaction on a single protein were identified that corresponded to distinct interaction interfaces. Few proteins had minimal regions of interaction that were exclusively full-length, and these proteins were on average quite short in length, suggesting that the entire protein consists of a single globular domain that cannot fold properly when truncated.

Fragmentation for determination of the minimal region of interaction is commonplace because of the ease and convenience of the DNA-based technology underlying Y2H (Figure 3–10) (Boxem, Maliga, et al. 2008; Dreze, Monachello, et al. 2010; Ryan, Cimermancic, et al. 2013). Experimental determinations of the minimal regions of interactions have become almost routine (Mehra, Zahra, et al. 2013). A potential limitation of the fragmentome approach is that protein interactions may be modified conformationally, sterically, or allosterically by the intact protein, effects that would not be detected using only expressed minimal regions of interaction. The other arm of physical interaction mapping, AP–MS technologies, is not amenable for domain mapping, though the next generation of quantitative data acquisition technologies to score-modulated interactions holds promise for quantitative fragmentome mapping eventually

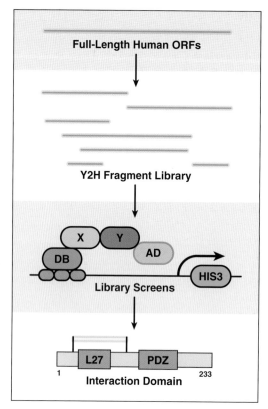

FIGURE 3–10. Fragmented regions of full-length human ORFs can be readily inserted into the Y2H screening pipeline for discernment of protein regions or domains responsible for protein interactions. (Adapted with permission from Waaijers, S., T. Koorman, et al. (2013). Identification of human protein interaction domains using an ORFeome-based yeast two-hybrid fragment library. J Proteome Res 12(7):3181–92.)

(Collins, Gillet, et al. 2013; Lambert, Ivosev, et al. 2013).

The same straightforward technology that underlies fragmentome screens (Boxem, Maliga, et al. 2008; Waaijers, Koorman, et al. 2013) permits domain-centric screens focused on determining the scope of interactions held by a particular protein domain or family of particular biological interest. The domains of interest are cloned and tested for interactions specific to the tested domain. Domain-centric interactome maps reported include those for the SH3 domain, a protein-motif recognition domain found in many signal-transduction proteins (Tong, Drees, et al. 2002; Carducci, Perfetto, et al. 2012; Xin, Gfeller, et al. 2013); the WW domain, a protein-motif recognition domain present in many transcriptional activators (Staub, Dho, et al. 1996; Yagi, Chen, et al. 1999); the PDZ domain, a peptide motif recognition domain involved in diverse cellular processes including cell signaling, protein trafficking, and cell polarity (Belotti, Polanowska, et al. 2013); Polo-box domains involved in phosphorylation of mitotic proteins (Lowery, Clauser, et al. 2007); the nuclear hormone receptor family of transcription factors (Albers, Kranz, et al. 2005); and the tandem BRCT domain present in many DNA damage repair proteins (Woods, Mesquita, et al. 2012). More domain-centric interactomes, which inform upon the biological functions of the tested domain or family, are expected (Jadwin, Ogiue-Ikeda, et al. 2012).

Tissue-Specific or Condition-Specific Interactomes

The interactome networks produced to date are necessarily static interactomes. They describe the interactions that can occur between proteins (biophysical interactions), but within any particular cell or tissue at any particular time, only a subset of the mapped interactions actually functionally occur (biological interactions) (Stelzl and Wanker 2006; Bossi and Lehner 2009; Carvunis, Roth, et al. 2012). What is ultimately desirable are ways by which to generate dynamic condition-specific interactomes (Wilkins and Kummerfeld 2008; Lopes, Schaefer, et al. 2011; Souiai, Becker, et al. 2011; Woodsmith and Stelzl 2014).

Binary interactome mapping methods like Y2H entail induced expression of the pairs of proteins tested for interaction in a yeast cell. Induced expression does not reflect the native expression or the cellular milieu of the physiological interaction. The yeast nucleus in which interactions take place represents a foreign environment for many proteins. Y2H derives true biophysical interactions; whether the interaction might lean towards biological requires additional experimentation. AP–MS associations are often tested in cell lines from the native species, seemingly able to make AP–MS more apt to find biological interactions, but induced expression of the tagged bait and all the rearrangements of cellular structures caused by lysis of the cell makes finding true biological interactions problematic (Oeffinger 2012). The new technology of AP-SWATH might soon enable reliable quantification of temporal changes of protein interaction networks in response to specific conditions (Collins, Gillet, et al. 2013; Lambert, Ivosev, et al. 2013).

Condition-specific interactomes cannot currently be generated experimentally at proteome scale by any technology, although two-hybrid approaches are being developed for conditional expression of a third-party protein, such as a methyltransferase or protein kinase, to probe interactions that are dependent on specific protein modifications (Erce, Abeygunawardena, et al. 2013; Erce, Low, et al. 2013; Grossmann, Benlasfer, et al. 2015). Instead, "virtual" condition-specific interactomes can be obtained by computationally integrating protein-interaction data with gene-expression information (Lopes, Schaefer, et al. 2011; Souiai, Becker, et al. 2011). Two proteins are presumed to interact in a given condition only if the corresponding mRNAs for the two proteins are expressed in this condition. In this manner organ- and cell-type–specific interactome maps can be predicted (Emig and Albrecht 2011; Lopes, Schaefer, et al. 2011). Such condition-specific interactome maps may turn out to be more realistic for interpretation of disease networks, as some disease phenotypes are manifest in certain selected tissues and organs (Furlong 2013). Given current limitations of experimental interaction-detection technologies, true condition-specific interactomes mapped systematically, not just computationally, would seem to be a distant but essential goal.

Tissue-specific expression networks are not the only type of contextual information that can be integrated with interactome networks to provide dynamic resolution. Other types of functional networks that have been integrated with interactome networks include co-expression networks of genes with correlated expression above a set threshold (Stuart, Segal, et al. 2003); phenotypic similarity networks of genes that show correlated phenotypic profiles above a set threshold (Gunsalus, Ge, et al. 2005); and genetic interaction networks, in which edges functionally link genes based on high similarities of genetic interaction profiles (Beltrao, Cagney, et al. 2010; Costanzo, Baryshnikova, et al. 2010).

Conclusion

A reference human interactome map, defined as interactions experimentally profiled for at least one isoform for each annotated human gene, now seems attainable. Milestone releases of fuller interactome maps along the way to a reference interactome have proven beneficial for ongoing efforts aimed at interpreting how network perturbations result in human disease (Menche, Sharma, et al. 2015). Just as was the release of the reference human genome, release of a reference human interactome, although a remarkable achievement, would be just the first step toward deciphering the workings of cellular networks. What would follow are more informative interactome maps spelling out specific isoforms, protein domains, and cellular conditions responsible for specific interactions, entailing perhaps a "1000 interactomes" project akin to the 1000 Genomes Project (1000 Genomes Project Consortium 2012). Although the technologies needed are not yet scaled to carry out a 1000-interactomes project, given anticipated rapid technological advancements, there is every reason to believe that they would be by the time a reference human interactome map is released.

Acknowledgments

Human interactome mapping projects at CCSB are supported by National Human Genome Research Institute (NHGRI) grants U01-HG001715 and RC4-HG006066, by National Institute of General Medical Sciences (NIGMS) grant R01-GM109199, and by a Center of Excellence in Genome Science (CEGS) grant P50-HG004233 from NHGRI.

References

1000 Genomes Project Consortium (2012). An integrated map of genetic variation from 1,092 human genomes. Nature **491**(7422): 56–65.
Abu-Safieh, L., S. Al-Anazi, et al. (2012). In search of triallelism in Bardet-Biedl syndrome. Eur J Hum Genet **20**(4): 420–27.

Adato, A., V. Michel, et al. (2005). Interactions in the network of Usher syndrome type 1 proteins. Hum Mol Genet **14**(3): 347–56.

Akhoondi, S., D. Sun, et al. (2007). FBXW7/hCDC4 is a general tumor suppressor in human cancer. Cancer Res **67**(19): 9006–12.

Alabert, C., J. C. Bukowski-Wills, et al. (2014). Nascent chromatin capture proteomics determines chromatin dynamics during DNA replication and identifies unknown fork components. Nat Cell Biol **16**(3): 281–93.

Albers, M., H. Kranz, et al. (2005). Automated yeast two-hybrid screening for nuclear receptor-interacting proteins. Mol Cell Proteomics **4**(2): 205–13.

Aloy, P., and R. B. Russell (2005). Structure-based systems biology: a zoom lens for the cell. FEBS Lett **579**(8): 1854–58.

Altshuler, D. M., R. A. Gibbs, et al. (2010). Integrating common and rare genetic variation in diverse human populations. Nature **467**(7311): 52–58.

Amberg, D. C., E. Basart, et al. (1995). Defining protein interactions with yeast actin in vivo. Nat Struct Biol **2**(1): 28–35.

Armean, I. M., K. S. Lilley, et al. (2013). Popular computational methods to assess multiprotein complexes derived from label-free affinity purification and mass spectrometry (AP-MS) experiments. Mol Cell Proteomics **12**(1): 1–13.

Bader, S., S. Kuhner, et al. (2008). Interaction networks for systems biology. FEBS Lett **582**(8): 1220–24.

Barabási, A. L., N. Gulbahce, et al. (2011). Network medicine: a network-based approach to human disease. Nat Rev Genet **12**(1): 56–68.

Barbosa-Morais, N. L., M. Irimia, et al. (2012). The evolutionary landscape of alternative splicing in vertebrate species. Science **338**(6114): 1587–93.

Baumgartner, W. A., Jr., K. B. Cohen, et al. (2007). Manual curation is not sufficient for annotation of genomic databases. Bioinformatics **23**(13): i41–48.

Belotti, E., J. Polanowska, et al. (2013). The human PDZome: a gateway to PSD95-disc large-zonula occludens (PDZ)-mediated functions. Mol Cell Proteomics **12**(9): 2587–603.

Beltrao, P., G. Cagney, et al. (2010). Quantitative genetic interactions reveal biological modularity. Cell **141**(5): 739–45.

Bennett, C. L., Y. Chen, et al. (2013). Protein interaction analysis of senataxin and the ALS4 L389S mutant yields insights into senataxin post-translational modification and uncovers mutant-specific binding with a brain cytoplasmic RNA-encoded peptide. PLoS ONE **8**(11): e78837.

Berman, H. M., J. Westbrook, et al. (2000). The Protein Data Bank. Nucleic Acids Res **28**(1): 235–42.

Bertin, N., N. Simonis, et al. (2007). Confirmation of organized modularity in the yeast interactome. PLoS Biol **5**(6): e153.

Bhattacharyya, R. P., A. Remenyi, et al. (2006). Domains, motifs, and scaffolds: the role of modular interactions in the evolution and wiring of cell signaling circuits. Annu Rev Biochem **75**: 655–80.

Blohm, P., G. Frishman, et al. (2014). Negatome 2.0: a database of non-interacting proteins derived by literature mining, manual annotation and protein structure analysis. Nucleic Acids Res **42**(Database issue): D396–400.

Bork, J. M., L. M. Peters, et al. (2001). Usher syndrome 1D and nonsyndromic autosomal recessive deafness DFNB12 are caused by allelic mutations of the novel cadherin-like gene *CDH23*. Am J Hum Genet **68**(1): 26–37.

Bossi, A., and B. Lehner (2009). Tissue specificity and the human protein interaction network. Mol Syst Biol **5**: 260.

Botstein, D., and N. Risch (2003). Discovering genotypes underlying human phenotypes: past successes for mendelian disease, future approaches for complex disease. Nat Genet **33**(Suppl): 228–37.

Boucard, A. A., A. A. Chubykin, et al. (2005). A splice code for trans-synaptic cell adhesion mediated by binding of neuroligin 1 to α- and β-neurexins. Neuron **48**(2): 229–36.

Boxem, M., Z. Maliga, et al. (2008). A protein domain-based interactome network for C. *elegans* early embryogenesis. Cell **134**(3): 534–45.

Brasch, M. A., J. L. Hartley, et al. (2004). ORFeome cloning and systems biology: standard-ized mass production of the parts from the parts-list. Genome Res **14**(10B): 2001–9.

Braun, P. (2012). Interactome mapping for analysis of complex phenotypes: insights from benchmarking binary interaction assays. Proteomics **12**(10): 1499–518.

Braun, P. (2013). Reproducibility restored—on toward the human interactome. Nat Methods **10**(4): 301, 303.

Braun, P., M. Taşan, et al. (2009). An experimentally derived confidence score for binary protein-protein interactions. Nat Methods **6**(1): 91–97.

Brimer, N., C. Lyons, et al. (2012). Cutaneous papillomavirus E6 oncoproteins associate with MAML1 to repress transactivation and NOTCH signaling. Oncogene **31**(43): 4639–46.

Buljan, M., G. Chalancon, et al. (2012). Tissue-specific splicing of disordered segments that embed binding motifs rewires protein interaction networks. Mol Cell **46**(6): 871–83.

Calderwood, M. A., K. Venkatesan, et al. (2007). Epstein-Barr virus and virus human pro-tein interaction maps. Proc Natl Acad Sci USA **104**(18): 7606–11.

Camargo, L. M., V. Collura, et al. (2007). Disrupted in Schizophrenia 1 Interactome: evi-dence for the close connectivity of risk genes and a potential synaptic basis for schizo-phrenia. Mol Psychiatry **12**(1): 74–86.

Carducci, M., L. Perfetto, et al. (2012). The protein interaction network mediated by human SH3 domains. Biotechnol Adv **30**(1): 4–15.

Carter, H., M. Hofree, et al. (2013). Genotype to phenotype via network analysis. Curr Opin Genet Dev **23**(6): 611–21.

Carvunis, A. R., F. P. Roth, et al. (2012). Interactome networks. In: M. Walhout, J. Dekker, and M. Vidal, eds., Handbook of Systems Biology: Concepts and Insights. Waltham, MA: Elsevier–Academic Press, pp. 45–63.

Chakravarti, A., A. G. Clark, et al. (2013). Distilling pathophysiology from complex disease genetics. Cell **155**(1): 21–26.

Chang, Y. F., J. S. Imam, et al. (2007). The nonsense-mediated decay RNA surveillance pathway. Annu Rev Biochem **76**: 51–74.

Charloteaux, B., Q. Zhong, et al. (2011). Protein-protein interactions and networks: forward and reverse edgetics. Methods Mol Biol **759**: 197–213.

Chatr-aryamontri, A., B. J. Breitkreutz, et al. (2013). The BioGRID interaction database: 2013 update. Nucleic Acids Res **41**(Database issue): D816–23.

Chatr-aryamontri, A., A. Ceol, et al. (2009). VirusMINT: a viral protein interaction data-base. Nucleic Acids Res **37**(Database issue): D669–73.

Chen, Y. C., S. V. Rajagopala, et al. (2010). Exhaustive benchmarking of the yeast two-hybrid system. Nat Methods **7**(9): 667–68.

Coffill, C. R., P. A. Muller, et al. (2012). Mutant p53 interactome identifies nardilysin as a p53R273H-specific binding partner that promotes invasion. EMBO Rep **13**(7): 638–44.

Collins, B. C., L. C. Gillet, et al. (2013). Quantifying protein interaction dynamics by SWATH mass spectrometry: application to the 14–3–3 system. Nat Methods **10**(12): 1246–53.

Collins, S. R., P. Kemmeren, et al. (2007). Towards a comprehensive atlas of the physical in-teractome of *Saccharomyces cerevisiae*. Mol Cell Proteomics **6**(3): 439–50.

Corominas, R., X. Yang, et al. (2014). Protein interaction network of alternatively spliced iso-forms from brain links genetic risk factors for autism. Nat Commun **5**: 3650.

Costanzo, M., A. Baryshnikova, et al. (2010). The genetic landscape of a cell. Science **327**(5964): 425–31.

Cotton, R. G., A. D. Auerbach, et al. (2008). The human variome project. Science **322**(5903): 861–62.

Crusio, K. M., B. King, et al. (2010). The ubiquitous nature of cancer: the role of the SCF[Fbw7] complex in development and transformation. Oncogene **29**(35): 4865–73.

Cusick, M. E., H. Yu, et al. (2009). Literature-curated protein interaction datasets. Nat Methods **6**(1): 39–46.

D'Andrea, A. D. (2010). Susceptibility pathways in Fanconi's anemia and breast cancer. N Engl J Med **362**(20): 1909–19.

Das, J., R. Fragoza, et al. (2014). Exploring mechanisms of human disease through structurally resolved protein interactome networks. Mol Biosyst **10**(1): 9–17.

Das, J., and H. Yu (2012). HINT: high-quality protein interactomes and their applications in understanding human disease. BMC Syst Biol **6**: 92.

Davey, N. E., G. Trave, et al. (2011). How viruses hijack cell regulation. Trends Biochem Sci **36**(3): 159–69.

Davis, M. J., C. J. Shin, et al. (2012). Rewiring the dynamic interactome. Mol Biosyst **8**(8): 2054–66.

de Chassey, B., V. Navratil, et al. (2008). Hepatitis C virus infection protein network. Mol Syst Biol **4**: 230.

De Nicolo, A., E. Parisini, et al. (2009). Multimodal assessment of protein functional deficiency supports pathogenicity of BRCA1 p.V1688del. Cancer Res **69**(17): 7030–37.

Deane, C. M., L. Salwinski, et al. (2002). Protein interactions: two methods for assessment of the reliability of high throughput observations. Mol Cell Proteomics **1**(5): 349–56.

del Peso, L., V. M. Gonzalez, et al. (1998). *Caenorhabditis elegans* EGL-1 disrupts the interaction of CED-9 with CED-4 and promotes CED-3 activation. J Biol Chem **273**(50): 33495–500.

del Peso, L., V. M. Gonzalez, et al. (2000). Disruption of the CED-9.CED-4 complex by EGL-1 is a critical step for programmed cell death in *Caenorhabditis elegans*. J Biol Chem **275**(35): 27205–11.

del Sol, A., R. Balling, et al. (2010). Diseases as network perturbations. Curr Opin Biotechnol **21**(4): 566–71.

Dinkel, H., K. Van Roey, et al. (2014). The eukaryotic linear motif resource ELM: 10 years and counting. Nucleic Acids Res **42**(1): D259–66.

Dittmer, T. A., N. Sahni, et al. (2014). Systematic identification of pathological lamin A interactors. Mol Biol Cell **25**(9): 1493–510.

Dreze, M., B. Charloteaux, et al. (2009). 'Edgetic' perturbation of a *C. elegans* BCL-2 ortholog. Nat Methods **6**(11): 843–49.

Dreze, M., D. Monachello, et al. (2010). High-quality binary interactome mapping. Methods Enzymol **470**: 281–315.

Duarte, M., L. Wang, et al. (2013). An RS motif within the Epstein-Barr virus BLRF2 tegument protein is phosphorylated by SRPK2 and is important for viral replication. PLoS ONE **8**(1): e53512.

Dunham, W. H., M. Mullin, et al. (2012). Affinity-purification coupled to mass spectrometry: basic principles and strategies. Proteomics **12**(10): 1576–90.

Dyer, M. D., T. M. Murali, et al. (2008). The landscape of human proteins interacting with viruses and other pathogens. PLoS Pathog **4**(2): e32.

Edwards, A. M., R. Isserlin, et al. (2011). Too many roads not taken. Nature **470**(7333): 163–65.

Elefsinioti, A., O. S. Sarac, et al. (2011). Large-scale de novo prediction of physical protein-protein association. Mol Cell Proteomics **10**(11): M111.010629.

Ellis, J. D., M. Barrios-Rodiles, et al. (2012). Tissue-specific alternative splicing remodels protein-protein interaction networks. Mol Cell **46**(6): 884–92.

Emig, D., and M. Albrecht (2011). Tissue-specific proteins and functional implications. J Proteome Res **10**(4): 1893–903.

Erce, M. A., D. Abeygunawardena, et al. (2013). Interactions affected by arginine methylation in the yeast protein-protein interaction network. Mol Cell Proteomics **12**(11): 3184–98.

Erce, M. A., J. K. Low, et al. (2013). A conditional two-hybrid (C2H) system for the detection of protein-protein interactions that are mediated by post-translational modification. Proteomics **13**(7): 1059–64.

Ewing, R. M., P. Chu, et al. (2007). Large-scale mapping of human protein-protein interactions by mass spectrometry. Mol Syst Biol **3**: 89.

Eyckerman, S., A. Verhee, et al. (2001). Design and application of a cytokine-receptor-based interaction trap. Nat Cell Biol 3(12): 1114–19.

Fedorov, O., S. Muller, et al. (2010). The (un)targeted cancer kinome. Nat Chem Biol 6(3): 166–69.

Ferrer-Costa, C., M. Orozco, et al. (2002). Characterization of disease-associated single amino acid polymorphisms in terms of sequence and structure properties. J Mol Biol 315(4): 771–86.

Fields, S. (2005). High-throughput two-hybrid analysis: The promise and the peril. FEBS J 272(21): 5391–99.

Fields, S. (2009). Interactive learning: lessons from two hybrids over two decades. Proteomics 9(23): 5209–13.

Fields, S., and O. Song (1989). A novel genetic system to detect protein-protein interactions. Nature 340(6230): 245–46.

Fields, S., and R. Sternglanz (1994). The two-hybrid system: an assay for protein-protein interactions. Trends Genet 10(8): 286–92.

Fine, D. A., O. Rozenblatt-Rosen, et al. (2012). Identification of FAM111A as an SV40 host range restriction and adenovirus helper factor. PLoS Pathog 8(10): e1002949.

Forbes, S. A., N. Bindal, et al. (2011). COSMIC: mining complete cancer genomes in the Catalogue of Somatic Mutations in Cancer. Nucleic Acids Res 39(Database issue): D945–50.

Fridman, Y., N. Palgi, et al. (2010). Subtle alterations in PCNA-partner interactions severely impair DNA replication and repair. PLoS Biol 8(10): e1000507.

Furlong, L. I. (2013). Human diseases through the lens of network biology. Trends Genet 29(3): 150–59.

Futreal, P. A., L. Coin, et al. (2004). A census of human cancer genes. Nat Rev Cancer 4(3): 177–83.

Futschik, M. E., G. Chaurasia, et al. (2007). Comparison of human protein-protein interaction maps. Bioinformatics 23(5): 605–11.

Fuxreiter, M., P. Tompa, et al. (2007). Local structural disorder imparts plasticity on linear motifs. Bioinformatics 23(8): 950–56.

Gabut, M., P. Samavarchi-Tehrani, et al. (2011). An alternative splicing switch regulates embryonic stem cell pluripotency and reprogramming. Cell 147(1): 132–46.

Garamszegi, S., E. A. Franzosa, et al. (2013). Signatures of pleiotropy, economy and convergent evolution in a domain-resolved map of human-virus protein-protein interaction networks. PLoS Pathog 9(12): e1003778.

Gavin, A. C., P. Aloy, et al. (2006). Proteome survey reveals modularity of the yeast cell machinery. Nature 440(7084): 631–36.

Ge, H., A. J. Walhout, et al. (2003). Integrating 'omic' information: a bridge between genomics and systems biology. Trends Genet 19(10): 551–60.

Germain, M. A., L. Chatel-Chaix, et al. (2014). Elucidating novel hepatitis C virus-host interactions using combined mass spectrometry and functional genomics approaches. Mol Cell Proteomics 13(1): 184–203.

Gerstein, M., M. Seringhaus, et al. (2007). Structured digital abstract makes text mining easy. Nature 447(7141): 142.

Gillis, J., S. Ballouz, et al. (2014). Bias tradeoffs in the creation and analysis of protein-protein interaction networks. J Proteomics 100: 44–54.

Gingras, A. C., M. Gstaiger, et al. (2007). Analysis of protein complexes using mass spectrometry. Nat Rev Mol Cell Biol 8(8): 645–54.

Gingras, A. C., and B. Raught (2012). Beyond hairballs: the use of quantitative mass spectrometry data to understand protein-protein interactions. FEBS Lett 586(17): 2723–31.

Goehler, H., M. Lalowski, et al. (2004). A protein interaction network links GIT1, an enhancer of Huntingtin aggregation, to Huntington's disease. Mol Cell 15(6): 853–65.

Gonzalez, M. W., and M. G. Kann (2012). Chapter 4: protein interactions and disease. PLoS Comput Biol 8(12): e1002819.

Grigoriev, A. (2003). On the number of protein-protein interactions in the yeast proteome. Nucleic Acids Res 31(14): 4157–61.

Grossmann, A., N. Benlasfer, et al. (2015). Phospho-tyrosine dependent protein–protein interaction network. Mol Syst Biol 11: 794.

Grueneberg, D. A., S. Degot, et al. (2008). Kinase requirements in human cells: I. Comparing kinase requirements across various cell types. Proc Natl Acad Sci USA **105**(43): 16472–77.

Gstaiger, M., and R. Aebersold (2013). Genotype-phenotype relationships in light of a modular protein interaction landscape. Mol Biosyst **9**(6): 1064–67.

Gulbahce, N., H. Yan, et al. (2012). Viral perturbations of host networks reflect disease etiology. PLoS Comput Biol **8**(6): e1002531.

Gunsalus, K. C., H. Ge, et al. (2005). Predictive models of molecular machines involved in *Caenorhabditis elegans* early embryogenesis. Nature **436**(7052): 861–65.

Guo, Y., X. Wei, et al. (2013). Dissecting disease inheritance modes in a three-dimensional protein network challenges the guilt-by-association principle. Am J Hum Genet **93**(1): 78–89.

Guruharsha, K. G., J. F. Rual, et al. (2011). A protein complex network of *Drosophila melanogaster*. Cell **147**(3): 690–703.

Han, J. D., N. Bertin, et al. (2004). Evidence for dynamically organized modularity in the yeast protein-protein interaction network. Nature **430**(6995): 88–93.

Han, J. H., S. Batey, et al. (2007). The folding and evolution of multidomain proteins. Nat Rev Mol Cell Biol **8**(4): 319–30.

Hart, G. T., A. K. Ramani, et al. (2006). How complete are current yeast and human protein-interaction networks? Genome Biol **7**(11): 120.

Häuser, R., A. Ceol, et al. (2014). A second-generation protein-protein interaction network of *Helicobacter pylori*. Mol Cell Proteomics **13**(5): 1318–29.

Havugimana, P. C., G. T. Hart, et al. (2012). A census of human soluble protein complexes. Cell **150**(5): 1068–81.

Hengartner, M. O., R. E. Ellis, et al. (1992). *Caenorhabditis elegans* gene ced-9 protects cells from programmed cell death. Nature **356**(6369): 494–99.

Hengartner, M. O., and H. R. Horvitz (1994). Activation of *C. elegans* cell death protein CED-9 by an amino-acid substitution in a domain conserved in Bcl-2. Nature **369**(6478): 318–20.

Hood, L., and L. Rowen (2013). The human genome project: big science transforms biology and medicine. Genome Med **5**(9): 79.

Horgan, C. P., S. R. Hanscom, et al. (2013). GRAB is a binding partner for the Rab11a and Rab11b GTPases. Biochem Biophys Res Commun **441**(1): 214–19.

Hosur, R., J. Peng, et al. (2012). A computational framework for boosting confidence in high-throughput protein-protein interaction datasets. Genome Biol **13**(8): R76.

Huang, H., B. M. Jedynak, et al. (2007). Where have all the interactions gone? Estimating the coverage of two-hybrid protein interaction maps. PLoS Comput Biol **3**(11): e214.

Huttlin, E. L., L. Ting, et al. (2015). The BioPlex network: a systematic exploration of the human interactome. Cell **162**(2): 425–40.

Inouye, C., N. Dhillon, et al. (1997). Mutational analysis of *STE5* in the yeast *Saccharomyces cerevisiae*: application of a differential interaction trap assay for examining protein-protein interactions. Genetics **147**(2): 479–92.

International Multiple Sclerosis Genetics Consortium (2013). Network-based multiple sclerosis pathway analysis with GWAS data from 15,000 cases and 30,000 controls. Am J Hum Genet **92**(6): 854–65.

Isojima, T., K. Doi, et al. (2014). A recurrent de novo *FAM111A* mutation causes Kenny-Caffey syndrome type 2. J Bone Miner Res **29**(4): 992–98.

Isserlin, R., R. A. El-Badrawi, et al. (2011). The Biomolecular Interaction Network Database in PSI-MI 2.5. Database **2011**: baq037.

Jadwin, J. A., M. Ogiue-Ikeda, et al. (2012). The application of modular protein domains in proteomics. FEBS Lett **586**(17): 2586–96.

Jäger, S., P. Cimermancic, et al. (2011). Global landscape of HIV-human protein complexes. Nature **481**(7381): 365–70.

Jäger, S., N. Gulbahce, et al. (2010). Purification and characterization of HIV-human protein complexes. Methods **53**(1): 13–19.

Jansen, R., H. Yu, et al. (2003). A Bayesian networks approach for predicting protein-protein interactions from genomic data. Science **302**(5644): 449–53.

Jiao, Y., A. J. Robison, et al. (2008). Developmentally regulated alternative splicing of densin modulates protein-protein interaction and subcellular localization. J Neurochem 105(5): 1746–60.

Jonsson, P. F., and P. A. Bates (2006). Global topological features of cancer proteins in the human interactome. Bioinformatics 22(18): 2291–97.

Kalsotra, A., and T. A. Cooper (2011). Functional consequences of developmentally regulated alternative splicing. Nat Rev Genet 12(10): 715–29.

Kaltenbach, L. S., E. Romero, et al. (2007). Huntingtin interacting proteins are genetic modifiers of neurodegeneration. PLoS Genet 3(5): e82

Katsanis, N., P. L. Beales, et al. (2000). Mutations in MKKS cause obesity, retinal dystrophy and renal malformations associated with Bardet-Biedl syndrome. Nat Genet 26(1): 67–70.

Kerrien, S., S. Orchard, et al. (2007). Broadening the horizon—Level 2.5 of the HUPO-PSI format for molecular interactions. BMC Biol 5(1): 44.

Kim, E., A. Magen, et al. (2007). Different levels of alternative splicing among eukaryotes. Nucleic Acids Res 35(1): 125–31.

Kim, J. C., J. L. Badano, et al. (2004). The Bardet-Biedl protein BBS4 targets cargo to the pericentriolar region and is required for microtubule anchoring and cell cycle progression. Nat Genet 36(5): 462–70.

King, B., T. Trimarchi, et al. (2013). The ubiquitin ligase FBXW7 modulates leukemia-initiating cell activity by regulating MYC stability. Cell 153(7): 1552–66.

Konig, R., Y. Zhou, et al. (2008). Global analysis of host-pathogen interactions that regulate early-stage HIV-1 replication. Cell 135(1): 49–60.

Krogan, N. J., G. Cagney, et al. (2006). Global landscape of protein complexes in the yeast Saccharomyces cerevisiae. Nature 440(7084): 637–43.

Kruyt, F. A., F. Abou-Zahr, et al. (1999). Resistance to mitomycin C requires direct interaction between the Fanconi anemia proteins FANCA and FANCG in the nucleus through an arginine-rich domain. J Biol Chem 274(48): 34212–18.

Lagziel, A., Z. M. Ahmed, et al. (2005). Spatiotemporal pattern and isoforms of cadherin 23 in wild type and waltzer mice during inner ear hair cell development. Dev Biol 280(2): 295–306.

Lagziel, A., N. Overlack, et al. (2009). Expression of cadherin 23 isoforms is not conserved: implications for a mouse model of Usher syndrome type 1D. Mol Vis 15: 1843–57.

Lambert, J. P., G. Ivosev, et al. (2013). Mapping differential interactomes by affinity purification coupled with data-independent mass spectrometry acquisition. Nat Methods 10(12): 1239–45.

Lander, E. S., L. M. Linton, et al. (2001). Initial sequencing and analysis of the human genome. Nature 409(6822): 860–921.

Landry, C. R., E. D. Levy, et al. (2013). Extracting insight from noisy cellular networks. Cell 155(5): 983–89.

Lareau, L. F., R. E. Green, et al. (2004). The evolving roles of alternative splicing. Curr Opin Struct Biol 14(3): 273–82.

Laskowski, R. A., and J. M. Thornton (2008). Understanding the molecular machinery of genetics through 3D structures. Nat Rev Genet 9(2): 141–51.

Lees, J. G., J. K. Heriche, et al. (2011). Systematic computational prediction of protein interaction networks. Phys Biol 8(3): 035008.

Lehne, B., and T. Schlitt (2009). Protein-protein interaction databases: keeping up with growing interactomes. Hum Genomics 3(3): 291–97.

Lehner, B. (2013). Genotype to phenotype: lessons from model organisms for human genetics. Nat Rev Genet 14(3): 168–78.

Li, S., C. M. Armstrong, et al. (2004). A map of the interactome network of the metazoan C. elegans. Science 303(5657): 540–43.

Liddington, R. C. (2004). Structural basis of protein-protein interactions. Methods Mol Biol 261: 3–14.

Lim, J., J. Crespo-Barreto, et al. (2008). Opposing effects of polyglutamine expansion on native protein complexes contribute to SCA1. Nature 452(7188): 713–18.

Lim, J., T. Hao, et al. (2006). A protein-protein interaction network for human inherited ataxias and disorders of Purkinje cell degeneration. Cell 125(4): 801–14.

Liu, B. A., B. W. Engelmann, et al. (2012). High-throughput analysis of peptide-binding modules. Proteomics 12(10): 1527–46.

Lopes, T. J., M. Schaefer, et al. (2011). Tissue-specific subnetworks and characteristics of publicly available human protein interaction databases. Bioinformatics 27(17): 2414–21.

Lowery, D. M., K. R. Clauser, et al. (2007). Proteomic screen defines the Polo-box domain interactome and identifies Rock2 as a Plk1 substrate. EMBO J 26(9): 2262–73.

Macias, E., A. Jin, et al. (2010). An ARF-independent c-MYC-activated tumor suppression pathway mediated by ribosomal protein-Mdm2 interaction. Cancer Cell 18(3): 231–43.

Martha, V. S., Z. Liu, et al. (2011). Constructing a robust protein-protein interaction network by integrating multiple public databases. BMC Bioinformatics 12(Suppl 10): S7.

Maxwell, C. A., J. Benitez, et al. (2011). Interplay between BRCA1 and RHAMM regulates epithelial apicobasal polarization and may influence risk of breast cancer. PLoS Biol 9(11): e1001199.

McDonald, M. L., M. Mattheisen, et al. (2014). Beyond GWAS in COPD: probing the landscape between gene-set associations, genome-wide associations and protein-protein interaction networks. Hum Hered 78(3): 131–39.

Mehra, A., A. Zahra, et al. (2013). Mycobacterium tuberculosis type VII secreted effector EsxH targets host ESCRT to impair trafficking. PLoS Pathog 9(10): e1003734.

Mellacheruvu, D., Z. Wright, et al. (2013). The CRAPome: a contaminant repository for affinity purification-mass spectrometry data. Nat Methods 10(8): 730–36.

Menche, J., A. Sharma, et al. (2015). Uncovering disease-disease relationships through the incomplete interactome. Science 347(6224): 1257601.

Merkin, J., C. Russell, et al. (2012). Evolutionary dynamics of gene and isoform regulation in mammalian tissues. Science 338(6114): 1593–99.

Miller, J. P., R. S. Lo, et al. (2005). Large-scale identification of yeast integral membrane protein interactions. Proc Natl Acad Sci USA 102(34): 12123–28.

Modrek, B., and C. Lee (2002). A genomic view of alternative splicing. Nat Genet 30(1): 13–19.

Moldovan, G. L., and A. D. D'Andrea (2009). How the Fanconi anemia pathway guards the genome. Annu Rev Genet 43: 223–49.

Mosca, R., T. Pons, et al. (2013). Towards a detailed atlas of protein-protein interactions. Curr Opin Struct Biol 23(6): 929–40.

Mosca, R., J. Tenorio-Laranga, et al. (2015). dSysMap: exploring the edgetic role of disease mutations. Nat Methods 12(3): 167–68.

Nachury, M. V., A. V. Loktev, et al. (2007). A core complex of BBS proteins cooperates with the GTPase Rab8 to promote ciliary membrane biogenesis. Cell 129(6): 1201–13.

Naidoo, N., Y. Pawitan, et al. (2011). Human genetics and genomics a decade after the release of the draft sequence of the human genome. Hum Genomics 5(6): 577–622.

Navlakha, S., and C. Kingsford (2010). The power of protein interaction networks for associating genes with diseases. Bioinformatics 26(8): 1057–63.

Navratil, V., B. de Chassey, et al. (2011). When the human viral infectome and diseasome networks collide: towards a systems biology platform for the aetiology of human diseases. BMC Syst Biol 5: 13.

Neveu, G., P. Cassonnet, et al. (2012). Comparative analysis of virus-host interactomes with a mammalian high-throughput protein complementation assay based on Gaussia princeps luciferase. Methods 58(4): 349–59.

Ngounou Wetie, A. G., I. Sokolowska, et al. (2014). Protein-protein interactions: switch from classical methods to proteomics and bioinformatics-based approaches. Cell Mol Life Sci 71(2): 205–28.

Nilsen, T. W., and B. R. Graveley (2010). Expansion of the eukaryotic proteome by alternative splicing. Nature 463(7280): 457–63.

Nishi, H., M. Tyagi, et al. (2013). Cancer missense mutations alter binding properties of proteins and their interaction networks. PLoS ONE 8(6): e66273.

Nishimura, D. Y., R. E. Swiderski, et al. (2005). Comparative genomics and gene expression analysis identifies BBS9, a new Bardet-Biedl syndrome gene. Am J Hum Genet **77**(6): 1021–33.

Nyfeler, B., S. W. Michnick, et al. (2005). Capturing protein interactions in the secretory pathway of living cells. Proc Natl Acad Sci USA **102**(18): 6350–55.

O'Neil, J., J. Grim, et al. (2007). FBW7 mutations in leukemic cells mediate NOTCH pathway activation and resistance to γ-secretase inhibitors. J Exp Med **204**(8): 1813–24.

Oeffinger, M. (2012). Two steps forward–one step back: advances in affinity purification mass spectrometry of macromolecular complexes. Proteomics **12**(10): 1591–608.

Oeffner, F., C. Moch, et al. (2008). Novel interaction partners of Bardet-Biedl syndrome proteins. Cell Motil Cytoskeleton **65**(2): 143–55.

Orchard, S. (2012). Molecular interaction databases. Proteomics **12**(10): 1656–62.

Orchard, S. (2014). Data standardization and sharing—the work of the HUPO-PSI. Biochim Biophys Acta **1844**(1 Pt A): 82–87.

Orchard, S., M. Ammari, et al. (2014). The MIntAct project–IntAct as a common curation platform for 11 molecular interaction databases. Nucleic Acids Res **42**(1): D358–63.

Orchard, S., S. Kerrien, et al. (2012). Protein interaction data curation: the International Molecular Exchange (IMEx) consortium. Nat Methods **9**(4): 345–50.

Orchard, S., S. Kerrien, et al. (2007). Submit your interaction data the IMEx way: a step by step guide to trouble-free deposition. Proteomics **7**(S1): 28–34.

Oti, M., and H. G. Brunner (2007). The modular nature of genetic diseases. Clin Genet **71**(1): 1–11.

Oti, M., B. Snel, et al. (2006). Predicting disease genes using protein-protein interactions. J Med Genet **43**(8): 691–98.

Pan, Q., O. Shai, et al. (2008). Deep surveying of alternative splicing complexity in the human transcriptome by high-throughput sequencing. Nat Genet **40**(12): 1413–15.

Pareek, C. S., R. Smoczynski, et al. (2011). Sequencing technologies and genome sequencing. J Appl Genet **52**(4): 413–35.

Parikh, V. N., R. C. Jin, et al. (2012). MicroRNA-21 integrates pathogenic signaling to control pulmonary hypertension: results of a network bioinformatics approach. Circulation **125**(12): 1520–32.

Pawson, T., and P. Nash (2000). Protein-protein interactions define specificity in signal transduction. Genes Dev **14**(9): 1027–47.

Pawson, T., and P. Nash (2003). Assembly of cell regulatory systems through protein interaction domains. Science **300**(5618): 445–52.

Peri, S., J. D. Navarro, et al. (2004). Human protein reference database as a discovery resource for proteomics. Nucleic Acids Res **32**(Database issue): D497–501.

Pichlmair, A., K. Kandasamy, et al. (2012). Viral immune modulators perturb the human molecular network by common and unique strategies. Nature **487**(7408): 486–90.

Prasad, T. S. K., R. Goel, et al. (2009). Human Protein Reference Database—2009 update. Nucleic Acids Res **37**(Database issue): D767–72.

Pujana, M. A., J. D. Han, et al. (2007). Network modeling links breast cancer susceptibility and centrosome dysfunction. Nat Genet **39**(11): 1338–49.

Raj, A., S. A. Rifkin, et al. (2010). Variability in gene expression underlies incomplete penetrance. Nature **463**(7283): 913–18.

Rajagopala, S. V., P. Sikorski, et al. (2014). The binary protein-protein interaction landscape of *Escherichia coli*. Nat Biotechnol **32**(3): 285–90.

Ramachandran, N., J. V. Raphael, et al. (2008). Next-generation high-density self-assembling functional protein arrays. Nat Methods **5**(6): 535–38.

Reguly, T., A. Breitkreutz, et al. (2006). Comprehensive curation and analysis of global interaction networks in *Saccharomyces cerevisiae*. J Biol **5**(4): 11.

Reiners, J., K. Nagel-Wolfrum, et al. (2006). Molecular basis of human Usher syndrome: deciphering the meshes of the Usher protein network provides insights into the pathomechanisms of the Usher disease. Exp Eye Res **83**(1): 97–119.

Resch, A., Y. Xing, et al. (2004). Assessing the impact of alternative splicing on domain interactions in the human proteome. J Proteome Res **3**(1): 76–83.

Rid, R., W. Strasser, et al. (2013). PRIMOS: an integrated database of reassessed protein-protein interactions providing web-based access to *in silico* validation of experimentally derived data. Assay Drug Dev Technol **11**(5): 333–46.

Roberts, P. M. (2006). Mining literature for systems biology. Brief Bioinform **7**(4): 399–406.

Rolland, T., M. Taşan, et al. (2014). A proteome-scale map of the human interactome network. Cell **159**(5): 1012–26.

Rossin, E. J., K. Lage, et al. (2011). Proteins encoded in genomic regions associated with immune-mediated disease physically interact and suggest underlying biology. PLoS Genet **7**(1): e1001273.

Rozenblatt-Rosen, O., R. C. Deo, et al. (2012). Interpreting cancer genomes using systematic host network perturbations by tumour virus proteins. Nature **487**(7408): 491–95.

Rual, J. F., K. Venkatesan, et al. (2005). Towards a proteome-scale map of the human protein-protein interaction network. Nature **437**(7062): 1173–78.

Ryan, C. J., P. Cimermancic, et al. (2013). High-resolution network biology: connecting sequence with function. Nat Rev Genet **14**(12): 865–79.

Saha, S., P. Kaur, et al. (2010). The bait compatibility index: computational bait selection for interaction proteomics experiments. J Proteome Res **9**(10): 4972–81.

Sahni, N., S. Yi, et al. (2013). Edgotype: a fundamental link between genotype and phenotype. Curr Opin Genet Dev **23**(6): 649–57.

Sahni, N., S. Yi, et al. (2015). Widespread interaction perturbations in human genetic disorders. Cell **161**(3): 647–60.

Sakai, Y., C. A. Shaw, et al. (2011). Protein interactome reveals converging molecular pathways among autism disorders. Sci Transl Med **3**(86): 86ra49.

Salehi-Ashtiani, K., X. Yang, et al. (2008). Isoform discovery by targeted cloning, 'deep-well' pooling and parallel sequencing. Nat Methods **5**(7): 597–600.

Sambourg, L., and N. Thierry-Mieg (2010). New insights into protein-protein interaction data lead to increased estimates of the *S. cerevisiae* interactome size. BMC Bioinformatics **11**: 605.

Schramm, S. J., V. Jayaswal, et al. (2013). Molecular interaction networks for the analysis of human disease: utility, limitations, and considerations. Proteomics **13**(23–24): 3393–405.

Schuster-Bockler, B., and A. Bateman (2008). Protein interactions in human genetic diseases. Genome Biol **9**(1): R9.

Scriver, C. R., and P. J. Waters (1999). Monogenic traits are not simple: lessons from phenylketonuria. Trends Genet **15**(7): 267–72.

Sebat, J., D. L. Levy, et al. (2009). Rare structural variants in schizophrenia: one disorder, multiple mutations; one mutation, multiple disorders. Trends Genet **25**(12): 528–35.

Shapira, S. D., I. Gat-Viks, et al. (2009). A physical and regulatory map of host-influenza interactions reveals pathways in H1N1 infection. Cell **139**(7): 1255–67.

Sharma, A., J. Menche, et al. (2015). A disease module in the interactome explains disease heterogeneity, drug response and captures novel pathways and genes in asthma. Hum Mol Genet **24**(11): 3005–20.

Shi, H., R. Rojas, et al. (2006). The retromer subunit Vps26 has an arrestin fold and binds Vps35 through its C-terminal domain. Nat Struct Mol Biol **13**(6): 540–48.

Simonis, N., J. F. Rual, et al. (2012). Host-pathogen interactome mapping for HTLV-1 and -2 retroviruses. Retrovirology **9**(1): 26.

Slavotinek, A. M., E. M. Stone, et al. (2000). Mutations in *MKKS* cause Bardet-Biedl syndrome. Nat Genet **26**(1): 15–16.

Soler-Lopez, M., A. Zanzoni, et al. (2011). Interactome mapping suggests new mechanistic details underlying Alzheimer's disease. Genome Res **21**(3): 364–76.

Sönnichsen, B., L. B. Koski, et al. (2005). Full-genome RNAi profiling of early embryogenesis in *Caenorhabditis elegans*. Nature **434**(7032): 462–69.

Souiai, O., E. Becker, et al. (2011). Functional integrative levels in the human interactome recapitulate organ organization. PLoS ONE **6**(7): e22051.

Sowa, M. E., E. J. Bennett, et al. (2009). Defining the human deubiquitinating enzyme interaction landscape. Cell **138**(2): 389–403.

Sprinzak, E., S. Sattath, et al. (2003). How reliable are experimental protein-protein interaction data? J Mol Biol **327**(5): 919–23.

Staub, O., S. Dho, et al. (1996). WW domains of Nedd4 bind to the proline-rich PY motifs in the epithelial Na⁺ channel deleted in Liddle's syndrome. EMBO J **15**(10): 2371–80.

Stelzl, U., and E. E. Wanker (2006). The value of high quality protein-protein interaction networks for systems biology. Curr Opin Chem Biol **10**(6): 551–58.

Stelzl, U., U. Worm, et al. (2005). A human protein-protein interaction network: a resource for annotating the proteome. Cell **122**(6): 957–68.

Stuart, J. M., E. Segal, et al. (2003). A gene-coexpression network for global discovery of conserved genetic modules. Science **302**(5643): 249–55.

Studer, R. A., B. H. Dessailly, et al. (2013). Residue mutations and their impact on protein structure and function: detecting beneficial and pathogenic changes. Biochem J **449**(3): 581–94.

Stumpf, M. P., T. Thorne, et al. (2008). Estimating the size of the human interactome. Proc Natl Acad Sci USA **105**(19): 6959–64.

Stynen, B., H. Tournu, et al. (2012). Diversity in genetic *in vivo* methods for protein-protein interaction studies: from the yeast two-hybrid system to the mammalian split-luciferase system. Microbiol Mol Biol Rev **76**(2): 331–82.

Sultan, M., M. H. Schulz, et al. (2008). A global view of gene activity and alternative splicing by deep sequencing of the human transcriptome. Science **321**(5891): 956–60.

Sun, J., and Z. Zhao (2010). A comparative study of cancer proteins in the human protein-protein interaction network. BMC Genomics **11**(Suppl 3): S5.

Tackett, A. J., J. A. DeGrasse, et al. (2005). I-DIRT, a general method for distinguishing between specific and nonspecific protein interactions. J Proteome Res **4**(5): 1752–56.

Taipale, M., I. Krykbaeva, et al. (2012). Quantitative analysis of HSP90-client interactions reveals principles of substrate recognition. Cell **150**(5): 987–1001.

Talavera, D., D. L. Robertson, et al. (2013). Alternative splicing and protein interaction data sets. Nat Biotechnol **31**(4): 292–93.

Talavera, D., C. Vogel, et al. (2007). The (in)dependence of alternative splicing and gene duplication. PLoS Comput Biol **3**(3): e33.

Tan, M. J., E. A. White, et al. (2012). Cutaneous β-human papillomavirus E6 proteins bind Mastermind-like coactivators and repress Notch signaling. Proc Natl Acad Sci USA **109**(23): 1473–80.

Taneri, B. (2011). Alternatively spliced transcript isoforms within human and mouse transcriptomes. OMICS Res **1**(1): 1–5.

Taylor, I. W., R. Linding, et al. (2009). Dynamic modularity in protein interaction networks predicts breast cancer outcome. Nat Biotechnol **27**(2): 199–204.

Thakar, K., I. Votteler, et al. (2012). Interaction of HRP-2 isoforms with HDGF: chromatin binding of a specific heteromer. FEBS J **279**(5): 737–51.

Thompson, B. J., S. Buonamici, et al. (2007). The SCF^FBW7 ubiquitin ligase complex as a tumor suppressor in T cell leukemia. J Exp Med **204**(8): 1825–35.

Tompa, P., and M. Fuxreiter (2008). Fuzzy complexes: polymorphism and structural disorder in protein-protein interactions. Trends Biochem Sci **33**(1): 2–8.

Tong, A. H., B. Drees, et al. (2002). A combined experimental and computational strategy to define protein interaction networks for peptide recognition modules. Science **295**(5553): 321–24.

Trabuco, L. G., M. J. Betts, et al. (2012). Negative protein-protein interaction datasets derived from large-scale two-hybrid experiments. Methods **58**(4): 343–48.

Turinsky, A. L., S. Razick, et al. (2010). Literature curation of protein interactions: measuring agreement across major public databases. Database **2010**: baq026.

Turinsky, A. L., S. Razick, et al. (2011). Interaction databases on the same page. Nat Biotechnol **29**(5): 391–93.

Unger, S., M. W. Gorna, et al. (2013). *FAM111A* mutations result in hypoparathyroidism and impaired skeletal development. Am J Hum Genet **92**(6): 990–95.

van Bokhoven, H., and H. G. Brunner (2002). Splitting p63. Am J Hum Genet **71**(1): 1–13.

van Wijk, E., B. van der Zwaag, et al. (2006). The DFNB31 gene product whirlin connects to the Usher protein network in the cochlea and retina by direct association with USH2A and VLGR1. Hum Mol Genet **15**(5): 751–65.

Varjosalo, M., R. Sacco, et al. (2013). Interlaboratory reproducibility of large-scale human protein-complex analysis by standardized AP-MS. Nat Methods **10**(4): 307–14.

Venkatesan, K., J. F. Rual, et al. (2009). An empirical framework for binary interactome mapping. Nat Methods **6**(1): 83–90.

Venter, J. C., M. D. Adams, et al. (2001). The sequence of the human genome. Science **291**(5507): 1304–51.

Vidal, M. (2001). A biological atlas of functional maps. Cell **104**(3): 333–39.

Vidal, M. (2006). Time for a human interactome project? The Scientist **3**: 47–51.

Vidal, M., R. K. Brachmann, et al. (1996). Reverse two-hybrid and one-hybrid systems to detect dissociation of protein-protein and DNA-protein interactions. Proc Natl Acad Sci USA **93**(19): 10315–20.

Vidal, M., P. Braun, et al. (1996). Genetic characterization of a mammalian protein-protein interaction domain by using a yeast reverse two-hybrid system. Proc Natl Acad Sci USA **93**(19): 10321–26.

Vidal, M., M. E. Cusick, et al. (2011). Interactome networks and human disease. Cell **144**(6): 986–98.

Vidal, M., and P. Legrain (1999). Yeast forward and reverse 'n'-hybrid systems. Nucleic Acids Res **27**(4): 919–29.

Vinayagam, A., U. Stelzl, et al. (2010). Repeated two-hybrid screening detects transient protein-protein interactions. Theor Chem Acct **126**(3–6): 613–19.

Vogelstein, B., N. Papadopoulos, et al. (2013). Cancer genome landscapes. Science **339**(6127): 1546–58.

von Mering, C., R. Krause, et al. (2002). Comparative assessment of large-scale data sets of protein-protein interactions. Nature **417**(6887): 399–403.

Waaijers, S., T. Koorman, et al. (2013). Identification of human protein interaction domains using an ORFeome-based yeast two-hybrid fragment library. J Proteome Res **12**(7): 3181–92.

Walhout, A. J., and M. Vidal (1999). A genetic strategy to eliminate self-activator baits prior to high-throughput yeast two-hybrid screens. Genome Res **9**(11): 1128–34.

Walhout, A. J., and M. Vidal (2001). High-throughput yeast two-hybrid assays for large-scale protein interaction mapping. Methods **24**(3): 297–306.

Walzthoeni, T., A. Leitner, et al. (2013). Mass spectrometry supported determination of protein complex structure. Curr Opin Struct Biol **23**(2): 252–60.

Wang, E. T., R. Sandberg, et al. (2008). Alternative isoform regulation in human tissue transcriptomes. Nature **456**(7221): 470–76.

Wang, W., Q. Zhong, et al. (2014). Mutations that disrupt PHOXB interaction with the neuronal calcium sensor HPCAL1 impede cellular differentiation in neuroblastoma. Oncogene **33**(25): 3316–24.

Wang, X., X. Wei, et al. (2012). Three-dimensional reconstruction of protein networks provides insight into human genetic disease. Nat Biotechnol **30**(2): 159–64.

Wass, M. N., A. David, et al. (2011). Challenges for the prediction of macromolecular interactions. Curr Opin Struct Biol **21**(3): 382–90.

Westermarck, J., J. Ivaska, et al. (2013). Identification of protein interactions involved in cellular signaling. Mol Cell Proteomics **12**(7): 1752–63.

Wethkamp, N., H. Hanenberg, et al. (2011). Daxx-β and Daxx-γ, two novel splice variants of the transcriptional co-repressor Daxx. J Biol Chem **286**(22): 19576–88.

White, E. A., R. E. Kramer, et al. (2012). Comprehensive analysis of host cellular interactions with human papillomavirus E6 proteins identifies new E6 binding partners and reflects viral diversity. J Virol **86**(24): 13174–86.

Wilkins, M. R., and S. K. Kummerfeld (2008). Sticking together? Falling apart? Exploring the dynamics of the interactome. Trends Biochem Sci **33**(5): 195–200.

Wodak, S. J., J. Vlasblom, et al. (2013). Protein-protein interaction networks: the puzzling riches. Curr Opin Struct Biol 23(6): 941–53.

Woo, J. S., J. S. Jung, et al. (2003). Unique structural features of a BCL-2 family protein CED-9 and biophysical characterization of CED-9/EGL-1 interactions. Cell Death Differ 10(12): 1310–19.

Woods, N. T., R. D. Mesquita, et al. (2012). Charting the landscape of tandem BRCT domain-mediated protein interactions. Sci Signal 5(242): rs6.

Woodsmith, J., and U. Stelzl (2014). Studying post-translational modifications with protein interaction networks. Curr Opin Struct Biol 24(1): 34–44.

Wuchty, S., G. Siwo, et al. (2010). Viral organization of human proteins. PLoS ONE 5(8): e11796.

Xia, J., J. Sun, et al. (2011). Do cancer proteins really interact strongly in the human protein-protein interaction network? Comput Biol Chem 35(3): 121–25.

Xin, X., D. Gfeller, et al. (2013). SH3 interactome conserves general function over specific form. Mol Syst Biol 9: 652.

Yagi, R., L. F. Chen, et al. (1999). A WW domain-containing yes-associated protein (YAP) is a novel transcriptional co-activator. EMBO J 18(9): 2551–62.

Yan, N., L. Gu, et al. (2004). Structural, biochemical, and functional analyses of CED-9 recognition by the proapoptotic proteins EGL-1 and CED-4. Mol Cell 15(6): 999–1006.

Yates, C. M., and M. J. Sternberg (2013). The effects of non-synonymous single nucleotide polymorphisms (nsSNPs) on protein-protein interactions. J Mol Biol 425(21): 3949–63.

Yellaboina, S., A. Tasneem, et al. (2011). DOMINE: a comprehensive collection of known and predicted domain-domain interactions. Nucleic Acids Res 39(Database issue): D730–5.

Yu, H., P. Braun, et al. (2008). High quality binary protein interaction map of the yeast interactome network. Science 322(5898): 104–10.

Yu, H., L. Tardivo, et al. (2011). Next-generation sequencing to generate interactome datasets. Nat Methods 8(6): 478–80.

Yüce, O., and S. C. West (2013). Senataxin, defective in the neurodegenerative disorder ataxia with oculomotor apraxia 2, lies at the interface of transcription and the DNA damage response. Mol Cell Biol 33(2): 406–17.

Yue, P., Z. Li, et al. (2005). Loss of protein structure stability as a major causative factor in monogenic disease. J Mol Biol 353(2): 459–73.

Zaghloul, N. A., and N. Katsanis (2010). Functional modules, mutational load and human genetic disease. Trends Genet 26(4): 168–76.

Zaghloul, N. A., and N. Katsanis (2009). Mechanistic insights into Bardet-Biedl syndrome, a model ciliopathy. J Clin Invest 119(3): 428–37.

Zhang, L., N. Y. Villa, et al. (2009). Analysis of vaccinia virus-host protein-protein interactions: validations of yeast two-hybrid screenings. J Proteome Res 8(9): 4311–18.

Zhang, Q. C., D. Petrey, et al. (2012). Structure-based prediction of protein-protein interactions on a genome-wide scale. Nature 490(7421): 556–60.

Zhang, T., N. Xie, et al. (2013). An integrated proteomics and bioinformatics analyses of hepatitis B virus X interacting proteins and identification of a novel interactor apoA-I. J Proteomics 84: 92–105.

Zhong, Q., N. Simonis, et al. (2009). Edgetic perturbation models of human inherited disorders. Mol Syst Biol 5: 321.

4

Social Networks in Human Disease

DOUGLAS A. LUKE AND MARTIN W. SCHOEN

Introduction

Medicine has long sought to explain the origins of human disease processes through physical or social relationships. Hippocrates was one of the first to describe malaria in the Western world, and he attributed the characteristic quartan fever to the swamps outside of Athens and the fumes that came from them (Cunha and Cunha 2008), thereby explaining the Italian name for the disease "mal'aria," or bad air. In a famous illustration from public health, John Snow created a map of cholera cases in Soho, London, demonstrating how the cause of a particular ailment could be ascertained through the detailed investigation of disease and geographic locations. Mapping the cases of cholera suggested a causal mechanism involving the Broad Street water pump. Snow helped create the modern discipline of epidemiology with his disease-investigation techniques, and he was able to solve a mystery of infection transmission and prevent further outbreaks of cholera.

Modern medicine has continued to advance the techniques of disease attribution, partly through adding a social component to disease mapping. One of the best-known examples of a social network in human disease comes from the early years of the human immunodeficiency virus–acquired immune deficiency syndrome (HIV–AIDS) crisis. As a result of case-identification efforts of the Centers for Disease Control and Prevention (CDC), a network map was created in 1984 that described the spread of AIDS through a social-contact network (Auerbach et al. 1984) (Figure 4–1). This social network analysis and graphic were highly informative; they helped define the social nature of the disease and suggested the mechanism of transmission and the associated risk factors for the acquisition of HIV.

Just as Snow's map of disease around a water pump described a physical context for the transmission of cholera, the CDC's "Patient 0" network map describes a social context for the transmission of HIV. The network structure of the initial AIDS epidemic emerged in the early 1980s after 19 patients in southern California were diagnosed with AIDS and were interviewed to ascertain their sexual partners. From the original interviews, 21 other patients were identified

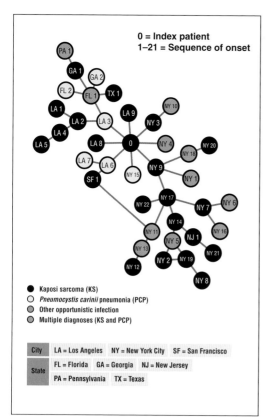

FIGURE 4–1. Sexual and disease status network of 40 men with HIV–AIDS. (Reprinted with permission from Luke, D. A., and K. A. Stamatakis (2012). Systems science methods in public health: dynamics, networks, and agents. *Annu Rev Public Health* **33**:357–76.)

who lived in San Francisco, New York, and other areas across the country. The health and disease status of these contacts was assessed to see whether they had a similar constellation of symptoms that could have been a result of AIDS. In a time when little was known about HIV, this study that described a social network was pivotal in understanding the spread of the virus and the risk factors for the disease.

After the first network map appeared, more formal social network methods were used to analyze the data to help ascertain the source(s) and spread of HIV (Klovdahl 1985). Network analysis verified what was starting to be understood by researchers across the globe: that HIV was transmitted via sexual and blood contact, and some of the risk factors for transmission needed to be reevaluated (Potterat et al. 1999). This network example from HIV–AIDS research is illustrative of the general theme of this chapter: social network analysis has become an important tool in studying and intervening in a wide variety of human infectious and chronic diseases (Friedman and Aral 2001; Luke and Harris 2007).

A Conceptual Model Linking Social Networks and Human Disease

The bulk of the other chapters in this volume outline network concepts that explain disease "under the skin." They explore how the biology of human disease may be understood through the networked structures and processes among genes, proteins, cells, and microbes. This chapter, by contrast, is concerned with how "above the skin" social networks are implicated in human disease.

Social networks connect people as well as groups, organizations, and political entities. Social processes and structures emerge from the friendship, kinship, contact, resource-exchange, and information-exchange ties between people. These social processes and structures influence human behavior and health, including human disease. These social ties also provide vectors for the transmission of disease and disease agents. Although disease has always been seen as responsive to social conditions and forces, only recently has medicine started looking for specific network mechanisms that can explain particular patterns of disease progression and prevention.

The conceptual challenge for social networks in medicine has been how best to link the social to the physical determinants of disease. What are the direct or indirect causal mechanisms that link network structures and processes to disease transmission, onset, progress, and outcomes? Berkman and colleagues (2000) have provided one of the more useful and detailed conceptual models that shows how the social and physical relate to one another to affect human health and disease. Figure 4–2 presents a slightly adapted version of their original model.

Berkman's model has at least three important features. First, the model is ecological and clearly positions social networks between the broader macrosocial environment and the narrower micro-level of psychosocial processes. This positioning suggests how network characteristics such as density, actor location, and local network clustering may mediate the influence of the broader environment on disease processes. For example, during times of social upheaval, communities may be more susceptible to infectious disease outbreaks (Weiss and McMichael 2004). Disease transmission may be slowed in a community that is characterized by isolated network components with low reachability, as compared with a tightly connected community network with high reachability.

Second, the model outlines plausible causal mechanisms whereby specific network characteristics may influence psychosocial processes. For example, the density of friendship ties in an adolescent network, along with the frequency of reciprocated ties, may influence the amount of social support that adolescents receive. High density and reciprocity make it easier for social support to flow through the network. Another example is that networks with more multiplexity (different types of coexisting network ties) may make it more likely that health information flows through both word of mouth and professional communication networks.

Finally, the model shows how social networks influence human disease through various behavioral, psychological, and physiological pathways. This pathway paradigm is the critical part of the model for understanding how the social is connected to the physical. Consider an adolescent network that exhibits disassortative mixing regarding smoking status, which means that many teens who smoke are connected to many teens who do not smoke. This particular

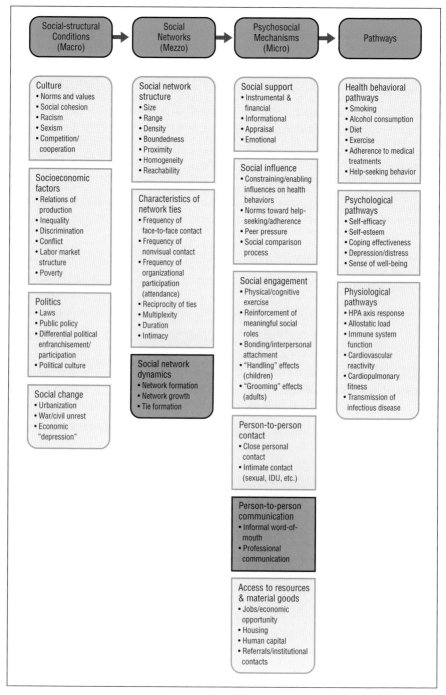

FIGURE 4–2. Conceptual model linking social networks and human disease. (Adapted with permission from Berkman, L. F., T. Glass, et al. (2000). From social integration to health: Durkheim in the new millennium. Soc Sci Med 51(6): 843–57. © 2000 Elsevier Science Ltd.). HPA, hypothalamic–pituitary–adrenal; IDU, intravenous drug use.

network structure may lead to a greater amount of peer pressure, which in turn, may lead to increased smoking over time throughout the network. This example reflects how network structures may lead to behavioral patterns linked to chronic disease. The model also makes clear that networks influence infectious disease processes. In fact, a wide variety of research has linked social isolation to a variety of disease-relevant physiological responses, including cardiovascular reactivity, endocrine response, and suppressed immune function (Uchino et al. 1996).

We have adapted Berkman's original model in two ways. First, we have added several concepts to the model that reflect current research on social networks and links to disease. In addition to network structures and network tie characteristics that may be linked to psychosocial mechanisms and behavioral pathways, we have added a box that includes network dynamics. The implication is that not only static network characteristics may be important influences on disease, but also dynamic processes such as tie formation and network growth may be important predictors of disease. We have also added a new box (under Psychosocial Mechanisms) that identifies person-to-person communication networks as an important process separate from social support. This additional element reflects current understanding of the importance of health communication in professional and nonprofessional (sometimes called word-of-mouth) networks (Albrecht and Goldsmith 2003; Allsop et al. 2007).

Figure 4–3 shows the second way that we have adapted Berkman's model by highlighting the importance of dynamic feedback loops and by emphasizing how network interventions may prevent disease processes. It is important to understand that even though the model is ecological, it is not linear. In particular, disease processes and health outcomes influence earlier parts of the model (as reflected by the feedback loops). For example, we know that patients with cancer and those with other diseases and other health conditions have smaller social networks or become more isolated within their networks (Sapp et al. 2003). Furthermore, if we understand that networks can influence human disease, then it follows that we can design disease treatments and interventions that account for network information. There are two types of network-relevant disease interventions, marked as 1 and 2 in Figure 4–3. First, we can design interventions that work directly on the networks themselves to prevent the occurrence of disease or reduce its impact. Second, we can use network information to inform or enhance more traditional disease interventions.

In the rest of this chapter, we dissect this model and explore how social networks are related to two broad types of human disease: infectious diseases and chronic diseases. We will next discuss how disease interventions can work by influencing social networks or be enhanced using network information. Finally,

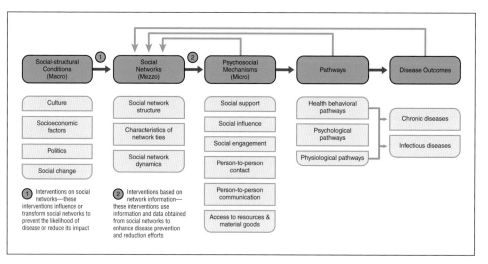

FIGURE 4–3. Dynamic conceptual model illustrating network feedback loops and network-specific disease interventions.

we will consider some methodological issues of network analysis, and consider some of the most significant new network methods and study designs, which hold promise for reducing disease and promoting health.

Social Networks and Infectious Diseases: Social Aspects of Disease Transmission

Human relationships are essential to the spread of disease. Social aspects of disease transmission have been well studied in infectious diseases because of the relative ease of defining affected and unaffected individuals in a population. As opposed to chronic diseases or their risk factors such as smoking and obesity, the ability to determine a specific source of a disease allows for explicit tracking of the transmission among individuals and the isolation of social variables that influence the spread of illness. Epidemiologists and infectious disease specialists have been using the principal elements of social network analysis to control the spread of infection for some time. Contact-tracing efforts during outbreaks of disease have used simple network analytic techniques since the 1970s (McElroy et al. 2003; Wasserman and Galaskiewicz 1994). Similar to the example of AIDS described earlier, ascertainment of the close contacts of anyone affected by disease can help to define an illness in order to understand its spread. This type of epidemiologic investigation can be enhanced by using concepts from social network analysis that describe the relationships among contacts and who may be more susceptible and have a higher likelihood of spreading disease

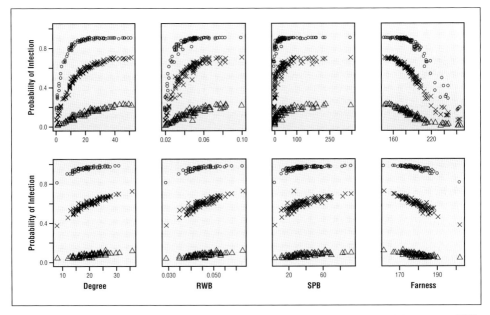

FIGURE 4–4. Relationship between node degree, random-walk betweenness (RWB), shortest-path betweenness (SPB), and farness and the probability of infection during 500 simulations in the small-world (top) and random (bottom) networks, with low (triangles), medium (crosses), and high (circles) levels of infectivity. (Reprinted with permission from Oxford University Press from Christley, R. M., G. L. Pinchbeck, et al. (2005). Infection in social networks: using network analysis to identify high-risk individuals. Am J Epidemiol **162**(10): 1024–31.)

based on the structure of their relationships (Wasserman and Galaskiewicz 1994).

Traditional epidemic models of infectious disease such as the SIR (Susceptible-Infected-Recovered) model and others function well when there are relatively clear mechanisms of transmission, infectivity, and outcomes (Hethcote 2000). These models are particularly useful for predicting the life course of an epidemic: when it started, how long it will last, and how many people will be affected by it. However, most of the research using epidemiological models with three categories: susceptible, infected, and recovered (SIR models) assumes random mixing within a population; that is, social structure is ignored.

Recent empirical and computational modeling studies have begun to demonstrate the need for and advantages of incorporating network information into epidemiological models (Keeling and Eames 2005). Instead of a traditional epidemic outbreak curve, diagramming the network growth of the spread of infection is more revealing of the underlying disease process (Read et al. 2008). Figure 4–4 is a more specific example, presenting the results of simulations showing how dramatically network structural characteristics affect the probability of infection (Christley et al. 2005). By adding social-network variables and random graph modeling, improved models can be created that optimize control of epidemics (Dimitrov et al. 2010).

This work extends to understanding and controlling large-scale global pandemics. In recent years, network information derived from global airline transportation data as well as intranational and international commuting patterns have been used to develop accurate models of infectious disease outbreaks (Hufnagel et al. 2004; Balcan et al. 2009). These network models allow for accurate real-time forecasting of global infectious diseases such as H1N1 (Tizzoni et al. 2012) and severe acute respiratory syndrome (SARS) (Brockmann and Helbing 2013), as well as helping to design surveillance systems for foodborne illnesses (Convertino and Hedberg 2014). It is no longer a radical idea to understand infectious diseases as being driven by social and relational processes, and network analysis is a primary tool for understanding those relationships.

Influenza, Tuberculosis, and Airborne Viruses

Social networks are comprised of interpersonal ties that form a pipeline to structure contagious flows (Borgatti and Halgin 2011). Influenza, tuberculosis, and other respiratory pathogens are prototypical infectious diseases and have ignited interest in using social network tools for describing and controlling disease transmission (Mossong et al. 2008). In the past 20 years, the avian flu, SARS, and swine flu epidemics have given social scientists examples of and opportunities to use social network analysis to define further transmission of disease. In Singapore in 2003, the Singapore Ministry of Health and the World Health Organization investigated 205 patients with SARS and their contacts using contact tracing and other surveillance systems. Interestingly, 5 patients accounted for the transmission of 103 infections (CDC 2003). These highly infectious individuals transmit disease in the settings of hospitals, conference centers, and other places of social congregation and can create "super spread events," in which entire populations can be infected, as occurred with SARS (Riley et al. 2003) and Legionnaire's disease (Fraser et al. 1977). Using the SARS data, Lipsitch and colleagues (2003) modeled the growth of the epidemic by estimating the number of transmissions per case in the acute phase of the outbreak and found that every patient with SARS would infect three others in populations that have not instituted control measures.

In order to control the spread of a respiratory or other easily transmissible virus, contact isolation and quarantine strategies are often employed, which can also be informed by social-network information (Riley et al. 2003). While indi-

viduals with more diverse social networks may have more resistance to respiratory viruses (Cohen et al. 1997), contact surveys show that young children and
adolescents carry the highest incidence of respiratory virus susceptibility (Mossong et al. 2008). Until treatments can be devised and vaccines can be developed,
social isolation and distancing are often the most effective methods of preventing
mass infection. These network interventions can be more successfully targeted
at those who have an increased likelihood of spreading the disease or have higher
levels of social contact, such as teenagers and children (Glass et al. 2006). By
closing schools, meeting places, and transportation centers, the spread of viruses
can be diminished, which is essential for the initial stages of any epidemic. Social network simulation models show the efficacy of antiviral agents, vaccines,
and quarantine strategies in interrupting influenza transmission (Longini et al.
2005) and give information about the management of the national stockpile of
antiviral medications (Dimitrov et al. 2011).

Sexually Transmitted Diseases, HIV–AIDS, and Intravenous Drugs

Social network analysis can provide a more detailed description of diseases
when transmission depends significantly on human behavior (Krause et al.
2007). Contact mapping and subsequent network description in sexually transmitted diseases (STDs) can help to determine risks for acquisition and methods
of intervention. In 1996, researchers at the CDC studied an outbreak of syphilis
among a group of adolescents in the Atlanta area (Rothenberg et al. 1998).
Ninety-nine people were interviewed to create a network of 203 pairs. It was
found that a group of young girls who periodically had sexual interactions with
different groups of older boys were instrumental in propagating the outbreak.
After extensive interviewing, network techniques showed that those with syphilis
had higher scores of betweenness centrality and relationship microstructures,
with network cliques playing a large role in transmission. This study and others
show how social-network data can highlight risks for disease acquisition and
highlight potential targets for medical or psychosocial intervention.

Infections that are spread via sexual contact or intravenous (IV) drug use
have a significant social component. As evidenced by the AIDS network created
from the Patient 0 network map (see Figure 4–1), the connections and relationships among people determine the risk of transmission of certain diseases. Social network analysis can be combined with geographic data to help decipher
the spread of disease among connected persons (Wylie et al. 2005). Members of
large social networks with increased density display higher rates of injection

drug use and other risky behaviors (Latkin et al. 1995). It is thought that the increased density and frequency of interaction create a supportive social environment for risky behaviors.

The propagation of disease and the possibility that a disease will remain endemic and resistant to eradication can depend highly on the social network. By comparing sexual networks in Winnipeg, Manitoba, and Colorado Springs, Colorado, researchers found that smaller, peripheral networks that were poorly connected to the general population were responsible for the ongoing maintenance of infection. In contrast, the larger, denser networks were responsible for the steep rise in incidence when exposures to STDs did occur (Jolly et al. 2001). In order to affect the social components of the transmission of STDs, interventions such as group educational sessions with IV drug users can be helpful in changing behavior (Latkin et al. 1996). By asking drug users to recruit fellow network members for education, needle sharing can be reduced and can limit the risk to individuals at a lower cost than other interventions (Broadhead et al. 1998). As social-network data and methods have developed and evolved, network analyses and interventions have played a more prominent role in the study and treatment of infectious and behavioral diseases (Valente 2012).

Social Networks and Chronic Diseases: Network Influences on Disease Prevention

Cancer and Heart Disease

Historically, one of the most consistent network findings in chronic disease has been the association of social isolation and integration with mortality. Starting with the Alameda County study (Berkman and Syme 1979), a long series of large-scale population studies have identified social isolation as a significant general predictor of higher morbidity and mortality from ischemic heart disease, cancer, as well as other chronic conditions such as respiratory diseases (Berkman 1995). Most of these studies relied on simple self-reported measures of personal social network size and degree of social support received; thus, they have little to say about specific causal mechanisms linking social-network structures to disease outcomes. In addition to general social support, larger social network size (as well as being married) has been shown to be associated with greater cancer survival rates (Pinquart and Duberstein 2010).

Although we still do not know much about the precise mechanisms that link social network characteristics to the risks for developing cancer and heart disease, research over the past 20 years has started to shed light on two particular pathways: the link between social isolation and chronic disease survival, and the relationship between network characteristics and risk-reduction strategies such as cancer screening. Reynolds and Kaplan (1990), with their analyses of the Alameda County study data, were among the first to show that social isolation affects cancer survival rates, but not cancer incidence rates. Since then, a number of studies have confirmed the positive benefits on survival of chronic diseases of social integration (Berkman et al. 2000; Pinquart et al. 2010). These effects are often quite large. Kroenke and colleagues (2006), in their analyses of Nurses' Health Study data, found that women who were socially isolated were more than two times as likely to die from breast cancer than socially integrated women. Another analysis from the Nurses' Health Study looked more broadly at health-related quality of life; Michael and colleagues (2002) found that socially isolated women had significantly lower quality-of-life measures after a breast cancer diagnosis and reported that these effects were more important than tumor size or treatment characteristics. Most of these studies used quite general measures of network characteristics, often not more than the size of a person's social network. One exception is a study by Villingshoj and colleagues (2006), which included measures of frequency of social-network contacts. Clearly, more studies are needed that move beyond simple network size counts as predictors of chronic disease survival.

The second prominent line of research has focused on the role of social networks in risk-reduction strategies for chronic diseases such as cancer screening, genetic testing, and health communications. Almost 20 years ago, Allen and colleagues (1999) showed that social norms (perceptions that screening was normative among one's peers), but not simple measures of network size, were predictive of breast cancer screening among women. Using more varied network measures that included both network size and contact frequency, Suarez (1994) showed that older Mexican-American women with stronger social networks were more likely to get Pap smears and mammograms. More recently, Koehly and colleagues (2003) showed that family social-network characteristics are predictive of the likelihood that two family members will talk to one another about genetic testing for hereditary colorectal cancer.

Smoking

In terms of chronic disease risk factors, social network analysis has been used most frequently to study smoking, tobacco use, and tobacco control. Network analysis has been used primarily to address two broad sets of tobacco-control questions: How do social networks influence individual tobacco use? How are community, state, national, and international tobacco-control systems structured? Although it has long been known that there are strong peer and family influences on smoking behavior, much of the early empirical work on the social influences on smoking ignored the relational aspect, focusing instead on general social support, familial characteristics, or psychological processes (Biglan et al. 1995; Duncan et al. 1995). Smoking behavior, especially smoking initiation, is, however, inherently relational and has a network aspect. Almost all people who start smoking do so before they are 18, and when they start they typically get their first cigarettes from a friend or family member (Kandel and Logan 1984; Flay et al. 1994).

Network analysis has been a very powerful approach to studying social and relational influences on smoking behavior. Ennett and Bauman (1993) were among the first to apply this strategy, showing that adolescents who were more isolated from their peers were more likely to smoke. Isolates were identified as having little or no interaction with peers, and had higher odds of being a current smoker. Clique members, or groups of adolescents who spend more time with each other than with others, and liaisons, who interact with others but not a specific group, both had lower smoking rates. One possible explanation for these effects is that young persons may become exposed to the norms of different groups, any of which may support misuse (Ennett and Bauman 1993; Valente et al. 2004).

Other network studies have shown that having a best friend who smoked positively influenced outsiders to smoke, but did not show the same influence with those who were part of a friendship group (Aloise-Young et al. 1994). Another study confirmed that there is an accumulation of risk takers in isolated positions and that individuals in isolated positions drifted toward risk-taking groups, while clique members shifted from non–risk-taking behaviors to risk-taking behaviors over time (Pearson and West 2003).

More recent network studies of tobacco use have started to use more sophisticated methods that allow testing of richer structural and causal hypotheses. For example, Alexander and colleagues (2001) conducted an important study that demonstrated that an interaction between social-network characteristics and school context influenced the likelihood of smoking. Specifically, they found that popular students (defined in network terms) were more likely to smoke in schools with high smoking prevalence and less likely to smoke in schools with low smoking prevalence. Another complex interaction of social environment and network position was found by Ennett and colleagues (2008). They identified an interaction between the number of friends who smoked and the betweenness centrality of the adolescent on the smoking involvement of that adolescent. Essentially, teens who were more centrally positioned in their friendship networks were less likely to be involved in smoking even when they had more friends who smoked. They proposed the interpretation that teens with higher social status (i.e., greater centrality) may have more resources to help withstand the influence of friends who smoke. Scientists are also starting to identify potential specific network causal mechanisms for smoking behavior. For example, Lakon and colleagues (2010) suggest that networks influence smoking by structuring flows of emotional support.

Obesity and Physical Activity

At first glance, it is less clear how obesity and physical activity may be influenced by social networks as compared to smoking and infectious disease. Smoking is a much more specific behavior that can be modeled through social relationships, and smoking initiation is often triggered by an exchange of cigarettes within family or peer networks. However, in an influential network study using data from the Framingham study, Christakis and Fowler (2007) suggested that obesity is "contagious"—participants in the Framingham study were shown to be 57% more likely to become obese if they had a friend who became obese within a certain time period. Although there have been some methodological critiques of this work (Cohen-Cole and Fletcher 2008; Lyons 2011), its visibility has helped propel further work elucidating the social-network mechanisms that may influence obesity (and other chronic disease risk factors).

For example, we know that physical activity behavior is often socially shared (e.g., sports in high school) and that this behavior can directly or indirectly affect weight status. Valente and colleagues (2009) pursued this line in their study of friendship-network influence on obesity of adolescents. They found that friendship ties were significantly more likely to occur between teenagers who were of the same weight, as compared with those of different weights. Using more sophisticated exponential random graph model (ERGM) analysis of the much larger National Longitudinal Study of Adolescent Health, Schaefer and Simpkins (2014) found that nonoverweight adolescents (as measured by body-mass index [BMI]) tended to avoid forming friendship ties with overweight peers. Although it is challenging to study network effects *on* obesity, it is somewhat easier to assess how networks influence the behavioral risk factors *for* obesity, viz., physical activity and diet. For example, adolescents who report spending more time with friends in physical activity are more likely themselves to be physically active (Voorhees et al. 2005). At the other end of the age spectrum, adults in their 70s who have more social ties show less functional decline and greater physical activity (Unger et al. 1999). In general, physical activity and exercise to reduce obesity can be enhanced via social networks—for example, participating in a car-pool social network has been shown to predict exercise adherence (Gillett 1988).

Theoretical Challenge: Disentangling Social Selection and Social Influence

One of the most consistent characteristics of social networks is that of homophily—the tendency for individuals (or other social actors) to be connected to similar others. Thus comes the saying "birds of a feather flock together" (McPherson et al. 2001). This is no less true when we study social networks and human disease. For example, adolescent smokers are more likely to be friends with other smokers (Flay et al. 1994; Kandel 1985; Kandel and Logan 1984). The challenge has been to disentangle two different social processes that may explain the homophily pattern: (1) social selection, in which network members select partners who are similar to themselves; and (2) social influence, in which the behavior of network partners exerts influence on an actor and the behaviors become more similar over time (Figure 4–5). The difference between social selection and influence on theoretical grounds is relatively clear; the challenge has been finding appropriate statistical and study design methods that can disentangle these effects that dynamically co-occur in evolving networks (Steglich et al. 2010).

Over the years, scientists have studied the association of peer influence and social selection with smoking, drinking, and substance use. Valente and colleagues (2004) frame this as a "chicken or the egg" argument; that is, does friendship grouping precede or follow substance use? A number of early studies have suggested that selection plays a larger role in similarity between friends than influence (Urberg 1998; Aloise-Young et al. 1994). Ennett and Baumann found that it was neither the chicken nor the egg; both peer-group selection and influence within the peer group after selection affected behavior (Ennett and Baumann 1993; Kandel 1985). However, these earlier studies were limited by the statistical methods available at the time. Just in the past decade, new statistical approaches for modeling network ties and structures have been developed that allow the valid determination of the unique contributions of selection and influence on homophily (Luke et al. 2010; Steglich et al. 2010; Harris 2013). Using these new modeling techniques (ERGMs), Mercken and colleagues (2010) have shown that both selection and influence are important processes that shape adolescent smoking behavior. Similarly, Schaefer and

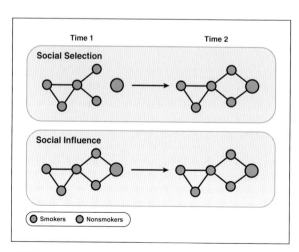

FIGURE 4–5. Two causal mechanisms that can explain network homophily: social selection and social influence.

colleagues have identified selection and influence processes operating on obesity-related behavior (physical activity and BMI) among friendship networks (Simpkins et al. 2012). With these new statistical tools, we will be able to continue to unravel how selection and influence shape the similarities seen in human disease social networks.

Using Social Networks to Enhance Disease Interventions

In the previous sections we have outlined how social network structures and processes are related to the transmission of infectious diseases, as well as the likelihood of experiencing chronic diseases and their associated health outcomes. Given the connection between networks and diseases, it then follows that we should be able to design disease interventions and treatments that promote health and reduce disease either by influencing social networks directly (see note 1 in Figure 4–3), or by using network information to design a more effective intervention (see note 2 in Figure 4–3).

Type 1—Intervening with Social Networks to Reduce Risk of Disease and Promote Health Outcomes.

As Figure 4–3 suggests, network structures and processes are implicated in a variety of psychosocial mechanisms as well as behavioral and biological pathways, which, in turn, influence disease outcomes. Interventions can take advantage of this effect, either by working directly to influence network characteristics or by using the social network itself as the setting for the treatment. Probably the best example of this is how Alcoholics Anonymous (AA) (and other similar self-help groups) reduces substance use partly by influencing the social networks of its members (Copello et al. 2002; Groh et al. 2008). A number of studies have shown that network characteristics (particularly network size and network support for abstinence) mediate the relationship between AA attendance and drinking severity or abstinence (Kaskutas et al. 2002). A more recent study by Kelly and colleagues (2011) reveals one mechanism that may explain this relationship; namely, that members of AA are likely to go through a transition during which they exchange pro-drinking members of their social networks for those who are pro-abstinence. In their study they found that outpatient AA members who attended meetings less than one time per week increased pro-abstinence network ties by 1.5% and reduced pro-drinking ties by 22%. The effects were stronger the more often they attended AA meetings—for those who attended more than three times per week, pro-abstinence ties increased by 15% and pro-drinking ties decreased by 52%.

Centola (2010, 2011) has illustrated the utility of intervening with a social net-work with a pair of computational modeling experiments that show that health behaviors spread more quickly across a social network when that network becomes more clustered and more homophilous. In one of the few empirical studies that has actually attempted to change network characteristics in order to influence disease-related processes, Valente and colleagues (2007) demon-strated that network coalition training reduced the density in the coalition net-works, which, in turn, increased adoption of evidence-based substance abuse prevention practices.

The more common approach for intervention studies is to use complete net-works as the setting for an intervention, rather than delivering treatment or in-tervention to isolated individuals. Valente and colleagues (2007) showed that a network peer-led substance abuse prevention program accelerates peer influence on substance use, in both positive and negative directions. These types of network-delivered disease interventions have also been developed for AIDS pre-vention (Broadhead et al. 1998; Latkin et al. 1996; Heckathorn et al. 1999) and breast cancer screening (Eng 1993).

Type 2—Using Network Information to Develop More Effective Disease Interventions and Treatments.

As Valente has pointed out in two excellent reviews, network data can be used to improve the implementation and effectiveness of disease-related treatment programs (Valente et al. 2004; Valente 2012). For example, consider the pattern of face-to-face contact observed on a hospital pediatric ward (Figure 4–6). This network-contact map reveals an important behavioral fact that should be con-sidered when developing an intervention (e.g., to reduce infectious transmission rates)—viz., that nurses play a more critical interactional role than other staff, including physicians. Network characteristics can reveal important information about social and organizational systems that can directly inform development of disease treatments (Luke and Stamatakis 2012).

The most common way to use network information to enhance interventions is by identifying social-network opinion leaders (Valente et al. 2004). Guided by diffusion of innovations theory (Rogers 2003), these studies recognize that opinion leaders occupy central positions in existing social networks and that the reach, speed, and effectiveness of traditional health interventions can be enhanced by knowing who these opinion leaders are. Other network informa-tion, however, can be used to shape program planning and implementation. For example, systematic planning for pandemic preparedness has been informed by a variety of network studies and models (Dimitrov et al. 2011).

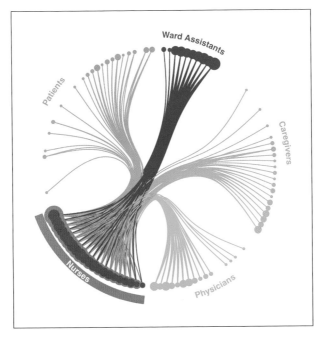

FIGURE 4–6. Face-to-face contact network on a pediatric hospital ward. (Original graphic by Jan Willem Tulp. Based on Matson, J. (2012) RFID tags track possible outbreak pathways in the hospital: Patterns of personal contact in a hospital reveal true pathways of transmission. Sci Am 307, issue 5, with permission from the original artist). http://www.scientificamerican.com/article /rfid-tags-track-possible-outbreak-pathways-in-hospital/

Future Directions for Network Analysis Research on Human Diseases

Social networks are important determinants of both infectious and chronic diseases. The interrelationships of social connections and human disease are complicated, but are being studied in a wide variety of ways. Large epidemiological population surveys, randomized clinical trials, observational studies, and even computational simulations are all being used to uncover potential network causal mechanisms and to design more effective disease treatments and interventions.

Network analysis studies of human disease have gone through three stages. The earliest stage, which accounts for most of the research, is made up of studies that have collected simple data on basic network characteristics such as overall size (Allen et al. 1999). These studies have been useful for first suggesting that social isolation is an important health risk and that social support mitigates a number of disease processes and outcomes. However, the reliance on self-reported data as well as egocentric network designs means that it is impossible to identify specific network structural and process explanations for disease outcomes.

That is, it is difficult, if not impossible, to understand the role of most of the network indicators presented in column 2 of Figure 4–3, such as reciprocity or reachability.

The second stage of network disease studies is characterized by research that focuses on whole networks (as opposed to egocentric networks) and uses more sophisticated network visualization and descriptive methods. These studies are able to identify much more specific network-related causal mechanisms, such as an interaction between network centrality and school social norms in predicting the likelihood of smoking among adolescents (Alexander et al. 2001). This stage of network research has been supported by the rapid development of new social network analysis methods, the availability of easy-to-use network analysis software, and the greater visibility of network science that has occurred over the past 30 years (Prell 2012).

Finally, we are just now entering the third stage of network disease research. Here, studies move beyond viewing networks as static structures and use modern social network modeling and computational modeling techniques to explore network dynamics and how networks are part of larger, complex systems (Luke and Stamatakis 2012). Examples of this work include developing statistical models of dissemination of evidence-based tobacco-control guidelines (Luke et al. 2013), developing dynamic models of alcohol use and friendship networks (Burk et al. 2012), and using social-network information to help develop computational models of the obesity (Bahr et al. 2009) and influenza (Mossong et al. 2008) epidemics.

Conclusion

Although we have made great advances in understanding human disease through a social-network lens, we are still only scratching the surface. Figure 4–7 underscores this point; it presents a count of the types of network-analysis methods used in 76 empirical studies that were reviewed for this chapter. While not a comprehensive, systematic review of a homogeneous research discipline, the figure gives a snapshot of the sorts of network methods that have been used over about 25 years to establish the evidence base for the role of social networks in human disease. What we can see from this review is that basic network visualization and descriptive methods are commonly used in these studies. However, more advanced descriptive methods are relatively rare. For example, multiple networks are examined in less than 15% of the studies, and multiple types of ties (i.e., multiplexity) were examined in just 5% of the papers. Furthermore, we are just starting to realize the incredible potential of modern statistical and dynamic modeling of networks.

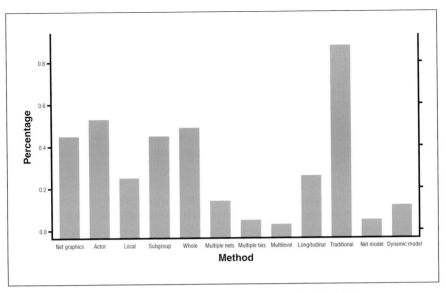

FIGURE 4–7. Types of network analysis methods used in 76 disease-related empirical studies.

Our ability to understand, treat, and prevent human disease is based on a broad and deep evidence base constructed by geneticists, physiologists, clinicians, epidemiologists, and scores of other basic science, medical, and social science disciplines. As this chapter has demonstrated, social networks can influence disease processes. At the same time, knowledge of social networks can be used to design and implement effective disease treatments and prevention strategies. With new advances in network science and computational network modeling, social network analysis will continue to be a critical tool in the study of human disease and in the ultimate success of the discipline of network medicine.

References

Albrecht, Terrance L., and Daena J. Goldsmith (2003). Social support, social networks, and health. In: T. L. Thompson, A. Dorsey, K. I. Miller, and R. Parrott, eds., Handbook of Health Communication. New York Lawrence Erlbaum, pp. 263–84.

Alexander, C., M. Piazza, et al. (2001). Peers, schools, and adolescent cigarette smoking. J Adolesc Health 29(1): 22–30.

Allen, J. D., G. Sorensen, et al. (1999). The relationship between social network characteristics and breast cancer screening practices among employed women. Ann Behav Med 21(3): 193–200.

Allsop, D. T., B. R. Bassett, et al. (2007). Word-of-mouth research: principles and applications. J Advertis Res 47(4): 398.

Aloise-Young, P. A., J. W. Graham, et al. (1994). Peer influence on smoking initiation during early adolescence: a comparison of group members and group outsiders. J Appl Psychol 79(2): 281–87.

Auerbach, D. M., W. W. Darrow, et al. (1984). Cluster of cases of the acquired immune deficiency syndrome: patients linked by sexual contact. Am J Med 76(3): 487–92.

Bahr, D. B., R. C. Browning, et al. (2009). Exploiting social networks to mitigate the obesity epidemic. Obesity (Silver Spring) 17(4): 723–28.

Balcan, D., Hu, H., et al. (2009). Seasonal transmission potential and activity peaks of the new influenze A(H1N1): a Monte Carlo likelihood analysis based on human mobility. BMC Med 7(45).

Berkman, L. F. (1995). The role of social relations in health promotion. Psychosom Med 57(3): 245–54.

Berkman, L. F., T. Glass, et al. (2000). From social integration to health: Durkheim in the new millennium. Soc Sci Med 51(6): 843–57.

Berkman, L. F., and S. L. Syme. (1979). Social networks, host resistance, and mortality: a nine-year follow-up study of Alameda County residents. Am J Epidemiol 109(2): 186–204.

Biglan, A., T. E. Duncan, et al. (1995). Peer and parental influences on adolescent tobacco use. J Behav Med 18(4): 315–30.

Borgatti, S. P., and D. S. Halgin (2011). On network theory. Organ Sci 22(5): 1168–81.

Broadhead, R. S., D. D. Heckathorn, et al. (1998). Harnessing peer networks as an instrument for AIDS prevention: results from a peer-driven intervention. Public Health Rep 113(Suppl 1): 42–57.

Brockmann, D., and D. Helbing (2013). The hidden geometry of complex, network-driven contagion phenomena. Science 342: 1337–42.

Burk, W. J., H. van der Vorst, et al. (2012). Alcohol use and friendship dynamics: selection and socialization in early-, middle-, and late-adolescent peer networks. J Stud Alcohol Drugs 73(1): 89–98.

CDC (2003). Severe acute respiratory syndrome—Singapore, 2003. MMWR Morb Mortal Wkly Rep 52(18): 405–11.

Centola, D. (2010). The spread of behavior in an online social network experiment. Science 329(5996):1194–97.

Centola, D. (2011). An experimental study of homophily in the adoption of health behavior. Science 334(6060): 1269–72.

Christakis, N. A., and J. H. Fowler (2007). The spread of obesity in a large social network over 32 years. N Engl J Med 357(4): 370–79.

Christley, R. M., G. L. Pinchbeck, et al. (2005). Infection in social networks: using network analysis to identify high-risk individuals. Am J Epidemiol 162(10): 1024–31.

Cohen, S., W. J. Doyle, et al. (1997). Social ties and susceptibility to the common cold. JAMA 27 (24): 1940–44.

Cohen-Cole, E., and J. M. Fletcher (2008). Is obesity contagious? Social networks vs. environmental factors in the obesity epidemic. J Health Econ 27(5): 1382–87.

Convertino, M., and C. Hedberg (2014). Optimal surveillance system design for outbreak source detection maximization: a VoI model. Proceedings of the 7th International Congress on Environmental Modeling and Software, San Diego, CA.

Copello, A., J. Orfor, and the Ukatt Research Team. United Kingdom Alcohol Treatment Trial. (2002). Social behaviour and network therapy basic principles and early experiences. Addict Behav 27(3): 345–66.

Cunha, C. B., and B. A. Cunha (2008). Brief history of the clinical diagnosis of malaria: from Hippocrates to Osler. J Vector Borne Dis 45(3): 194–99.

Dimitrov, N., and L.A. Meyers (2010). Mathematical approaches to infectious disease prediction and control. In: J. J. Hasenbein, ed., TutORials in Operations Research: Risk and Optimization in an Uncertain World, vol. 7, pp. 1–25 (http://pubsonline.informs.org/doi /book/10.1287/educ.1100).

Dimitrov, N. B., S. Goll, et al. (2011). Optimizing tactics for use of the U.S. antiviral strategic national stockpile for pandemic influenza. PLoS One 6(1): e16094.

Duncan, T. E., E. Tildesley, et al. (1995). The consistency of family and peer influences on the development of substance use in adolescence. Addiction 90(12): 1647–60.

Eng, E. (1993). The Save our Sisters Project: a social network strategy for reaching rural black women. Cancer 72(3 Suppl): 1071–77.

Ennett, S. T., and K. E. Bauman (1993). Peer group structure and adolescent cigarette smoking: a social network analysis. J Health Soc Behav **34**(3): 226–36.

Ennett, S. T., R. Faris, et al. (2008). Peer smoking, other peer attributes, and adolescent cigarette smoking: a social network analysis. Prev Sci **9**(2):88–98.

Flay, B. R., F. B. Hu, et al. (1994). Differential influence of parental smoking and friends' smoking on adolescent initiation and escalation of smoking. J Health Soc Behav **35**(3): 248–65.

Fraser, D. W., T. R. Tsai, et al. (1977). Legionnaires' disease: description of an epidemic of pneumonia. N Engl J Med **297**(22): 1189–97.

Friedman, S. R., and S. Aral (2001). Social networks, risk-potential networks, health, and disease. J Urban Health **78**(3): 411–18.

Gillett, P. A. (1988). Self-reported factors influencing exercise adherence in overweight women. Nurs Res **37**(1): 25–29.

Glass, R. J., L. M. Glass, et al. (2006). Targeted social distancing design for pandemic influenza. Emerg Infect Dis **12**(11): 1671–81.

Groh, D. R., L. A. Jason, et al. (2008). Social network variables in alcoholics anonymous: a literature review. Clin Psychol Rev **28**(3): 430–50.

Harris, J. K. (2013). An Introduction to Exponential Random Graph Modeling, Quantitative Applications in the Social Sciences. Thousand Oaks, CA: SAGE.

Heckathorn, Douglas D., et al. (1999). AIDS and social networks: HIV prevention through network mobilization. Sociol Focus **32**(2): 159–79.

Hethcote, H. W. (2000). The mathematics of infectious diseases. SIAM Rev **42**(4): 599–653.

Hufnagel, L., Brockmann, D., et al. (2004). Forecast and control of epidemics in a globalized world. Proc Natl Acad Sci U S A **101**(42): 15124–29.

Jolly, A. M., S. Q. Muth, et al. (2001). Sexual networks and sexually transmitted infections: a tale of two cities. J Urban Health **78**(3): 433–45.

Kandel, D. B. (1985). On processes of peer influences in adolescent drug use: a developmental perspective. Adv Alcohol Subst Abuse **4**(3–4): 139–63.

Kandel, D. B., and J. A. Logan (1984). Patterns of drug use from adolescence to young adulthood. I. Periods of risk for initiation, continued use, and discontinuation. Am J Public Health **74**(7): 660–66.

Kaskutas, L. A., J. Bond, et al. (2002). Social networks as mediators of the effect of Alcoholics Anonymous. Addiction **97**(7): 891–900.

Keeling, M. J., and K. T. Eames (2005). Networks and epidemic models. J R Soc Interface **2**(4): 295–307.

Kelly, J. F., R. L. Stout, et al. (2011). The role of Alcoholics Anonymous in mobilizing adaptive social network changes: a prospective lagged mediational analysis. Drug Alcohol Depend **114**(2–3): 119–26.

Klovdahl, A. S. (1985). Social networks and the spread of infectious diseases: the AIDS example. Soc Sci Med **21**(11): 1203–16.

Koehly, L. M., S. K. Peterson, et al. (2003). A social network analysis of communication about hereditary nonpolyposis colorectal cancer genetic testing and family functioning. Cancer Epidemiol Biomarker Prev **12**(4): 304–13.

Krause, J., D. P. Croft, et al. (2007). Social network theory in the behavioural sciences: potential applications. Behav Ecol Sociobiol **62**: 15–27.

Kroenke, C. H., L. D. Kubzansky, et al. (2006). Social networks, social support, and survival after breast cancer diagnosis. J Clin Oncol **24**(7): 1105–11.

Lakon, C. M., J. R. Hipp, et al. (2010). The social context of adolescent smoking: a systems perspective. Am J Public Health **100**(7):1218–28.

Latkin, C. A., W. Mandell, et al. (1996). The long-term outcome of a personal network-oriented HIV prevention intervention for injection drug users: the SAFE Study. Am J Community Psychol **24**(3): 341–64.

Latkin, C., W. Mandell, et al. (1995). Using social network analysis to study patterns of drug-use among urban drug-users at high-risk for HIV AIDS. Drug and Alcohol Depend **38**(1): 1–9.

Lipsitch, M., T. Cohen, et al. (2003). Transmission dynamics and control of severe acute respiratory syndrome. Science 300(5627): 1966–70.

Longini, I. M., Jr., A. Nizam, et al. (2005). Containing pandemic influenza at the source. Science 309(5737): 1083–87.

Luke, D. A., and J. K. Harris (2007). Network analysis in public health: history, methods, and applications. Annu Rev Public Health 28: 69–93.

Luke, D. A., J. K. Harris, et al. (2010). Systems analysis of collaboration in 5 national tobacco control networks. Am J Public Health 100(7):1290–97.

Luke, D. A., and K. A. Stamatakis (2012). Systems science methods in public health: dynamics, networks, and agents. Annu Rev Public Health 33: 357–76.

Luke, D. A., L. M. Wald, et al. (2013). Network influences on dissemination of evidence-based guidelines in state tobacco control programs. Health Educ Behav 40(1 Suppl): 33S–42S.

Lyons, R. (2011). The spread of evidence-poor medicine via flawed social-network analysis. Statistics, Politics, and Policy 2(1) (http://www.bepress.com/spp/vol2/iss1/2).

Matson, J. (2012) RFID tags track possible outbreak pathways in the hospital: Patterns of personal contact in a hospital reveal true pathways of transmission. Sci Am 307(5). http://www.scientificamerican.com/article/rfid-tags-track-possible-outbreak-pathways-in-hospital/

McElroy, P. D., R. B. Rothenberg, et al. (2003). A network-informed approach to investigating a tuberculosis outbreak: implications for enhancing contact investigations. Int J Tuberc Lung Dis 7(12 Suppl 3): S486–93.

McPherson, M., L. Smith-Lovin, et al. (2001). Birds of a feather: homophily in social networks. Annu Rev Sociol 27: 415–44.

Mercken, L., T. A. Snijders, et al. (2010). Smoking-based selection and influence in gender-segregated friendship networks: a social network analysis of adolescent smoking. Addiction 105(7):1280–89.

Michael, Y. L., L. F. Berkman, et al. (2002). Social networks and health-related quality of life in breast cancer survivors: a prospective study. J Psychosom Res 52(5): 285–93.

Mossong, J., N. Hens, et al. (2008). Social contacts and mixing patterns relevant to the spread of infectious diseases. PLoS Med 5(3): e74.

Pearson, M., and P. West (2003). Drifting smoke rings. Connections 25(2): 59–76.

Pinquart, M., and P. R. Duberstein (2010). Associations of social networks with cancer mortality: a meta-analysis. Crit Rev Oncol Hematol 75(2): 122–37.

Potterat, J. J., R. B. Rothenberg, et al. (1999). Network structural dynamics and infectious disease propagation. Int J STD AIDS 10(3): 182–85.

Prell, Christina. (2012). Social Network Analysis: History, Theory & Methodology. Thousand Oaks, CA: SAGE.

Read, J. M., K. T. Eames, et al. (2008). Dynamic social networks and the implications for the spread of infectious disease. J R Soc Interface 5(26): 1001–7.

Reynolds, P., and G. A. Kaplan (1990). Social connections and risk for cancer: prospective evidence from the Alameda County Study. Behav Med 16(3): 101–10.

Riley, S., C. Fraser, et al. (2003). Transmission dynamics of the etiological agent of SARS in Hong Kong: impact of public health interventions. Science 300(5627): 1961–66.

Rogers, E. M. (2003). Diffusion of innovations. 5th ed. New York: Free Press.

Rothenberg, R. B., C. Sterk, et al. (1998). Using social network and ethnographic tools to evaluate syphilis transmission. Sex Transm Dis 25(3): 154–60.

Sapp, A. L., A. Trentham-Dietz, et al. (2003). Social networks and quality of life among female long-term colorectal cancer survivors. Cancer 98(8): 1749–58.

Schaefer, D. R., and Simpkins, S. D. (2014). Using social network analysis to clarify the role of obesity in selection of adolescent friends. Am J Public Health 104: 1223–29.

Simpkins, S. D., Schaefer, D. R., et al. (2012). Adolescent friendships, BMI, and physical activity: untangling selection and influence through longitudinal social network analysis. J Res Adolesc 23(3): 537–49.

Steglich, C., T. A. B. Snijders, et al. (2010). Dynamic networks and behavior: separating selection from influence. Sociol Methodol 4 (1): 329–93.

Suarez, L. (1994). Effects of social networks on cancer-screening behavior of older Mexican-American women. J Natl Cancer Inst **86**(10): 775–79.

Tizzoni, M., Bajardi, P., et al. (2012). Real-time numerical forecast of global epidemic spreading: case study of 2009 A/H1N1pdm. BMC Med **10:** 165.

Uchino, B. N., J. T. Cacioppo, et al. (1996). The relationship between social support and physiological processes: a review with emphasis on underlying mechanisms and implications for health. Psychol Bull **119**(3): 488–531.

Unger, J. B., G. McAvay, et al. (1999). Variation in the impact of social network characteristics on physical functioning in elderly persons: MacArthur studies of successful aging. J Gerontol B Psychol Sci Soc Sci **54**(5):S245–51.

Urberg, K. A., S. M Degirmencioglu,, et al (1998). Adolescent friendship selection and termination: The role of similarity. Journal of Social and Personal Relationships **15**(5) : 703–10.

Valente, T. W. (2012). Network interventions. Science **337**(6090): 49–53.

Valente, T. W., C. P. Chou, et al. (2007). Community coalitions as a system: effects of network change on adoption of evidence-based substance abuse prevention. Am J Public Health **97**(5): 880–86.

Valente, T. W., K. Fujimoto, et al. (2009). Adolescent affiliations and adiposity: a social network analysis of friendships and obesity. J Adolesc Health **45**(2):202–4.

Valente, T. W., A. Ritt-Olson, et al. (2007). Peer acceleration: effects of a social network tailored substance abuse prevention program among high-risk adolescents. Addiction **102**(11): 1804–15.

Valente, T. W., P. Gallaher, et al. (2004). Using social networks to understand and prevent aubstance use: a transdisciplinary perspective. Subst Use Misuse **39**(10–12): 1685–1712.

Villingshoj, M., L. Ross, et al. (2006). Does marital status and altered contact with the social network predict colorectal cancer survival? Eur J Cancer **42**(17): 3022–27.

Voorhees, C. C., D. Murray, et al. (2005). The role of peer social network factors and physical activity in adolescent girls. Am J Health Behav **29**(2): 183–90.

Wasserman, S., and J. Galaskiewicz (1994). Advances in Social Network Analysis: Research in the Social and Behavioral Sciences. Thousand Oaks, CA: SAGE.

Weiss, R. A., and A. J. McMichael (2004). Social and environmental risk factors in the emergence of infectious diseases. Nat Med **10**(12 Suppl): S70–6.

Wylie, J. L., T. Cabral, et al. (2005(. Identification of networks of sexually transmitted infection: a molecular, geographic, and social network analysis. J Infect Dis **191**(6): 899–906.

5

Phenotype, Pathophenotype, and Endo(patho)phenotype in Network Medicine

CALUM A. MACRAE

Introduction

Disease has long been classified as a series of phenomenological clusters (symptoms, signs and objective data) associated with discrete outcomes (Jones 1868). Indeed, until remarkably recently, physicians have been defined not so much by their limited capacity to heal, but, rather, by their ability to synthesize myriad symptoms and signs into cohesive syndromes, or patterns of symptoms and signs (Osler 1892; Talbott 1961). In the small number of conditions for which effective interventions were available, the response to specific therapies also became part of these disease archetypes. The recognition of these patterns allowed physicians to anticipate distinctive natural histories and to help patients adapt to the subsequent morbidities or mortality, largely without any mechanistic insights. The didactic transmission of these archetypal patterns has formed the core of medical education for decades (Talbott 1961).

In many instances, these clinical observations are highly predictive of specific outcomes, but not surprisingly, such associations are most readily recognizable and most robust when the timeline between the onset of the syndrome and the specific outcome is short and when binary observations facilitate agreement between independent observers (Jones 1868). Even in extreme examples, such as an epidemic infectious disease with high case fatality rates, the strength of an association and its systematic recognition were for centuries dependent on temporal and geographic clustering rather than on any mechanistic understanding of the underlying correlation (e.g., characteristic lymphadenopathy and the Black Death of epidemic bubonic plague). Major opportunities for pattern recognition that encompass potential cause and effect occur in a limited number of other contexts, such as birth, death, and uniform acute exposure to environmental agents, or through familial resemblance (Jones 1868; Mayr 1982). While many phenomena were initially attributed to supernatural causes, each of these observational settings eventually spawned a rigorous science (Jones 1868; Mayr 1982).

With the advent of the discipline of epidemiology, the scope of medical phenomenology changed dramatically. Systematic documentation of demographic data, often for economic reasons, led to increasingly sophisticated correlations, which identified exogenous exposures such as cholera or benzene (Pott 1775; Snow 1855). Several large effect-size correlations between external agents and specific diseases were identified and generated empiric public health measures with substantial improvements in human health (Doll and Peto 1976). Despite these early successes, there are many constraints on the traditional epidemiological approach, including historical biases in the data types collected, the resolution of observational tools, and the tempo of longitudinal data collection (Hill 1965; Taubes 1995). There is an ongoing tension between increasing study size and decreasing resolution of observation that sets limits on the biological effects that are detectable. Furthermore, the inability to make causal inferences without controlled interventions has led some to question the relevance of purely correlative science (Hill 1965; Taubes 1995; Ioannidis 2005). Interventional studies have been similarly constrained as modest treatment effect sizes have driven the growth of clinical trials to test tens of thousands of subjects with the anticipated effects on cost and resolution.

There is a recognition that specific tradeoffs in the interest of increasing study size have resulted in the aggregation of large numbers of etiologically distinct entities (on the basis of superficial resemblance) in both epidemiological investigation and clinical trials, in turn leading to the dilution of relationships between cause (or intervention) and effect. Diminishing returns from epidemiology and from large-scale clinical trials, combined with the burgeoning fields of genetics and genomics, have driven the emergence of the reductionist concepts of individualized medicine (Gonzaga-Jauregui, Lupski, et al. 2012; Chen and Snyder 2013). In this construct, care is rooted in the molecular definition of distinct disease mechanisms and the administration of etiology-specific therapies with precisely predicted efficacy and safety. The implementation of this concept has been slowed by the realization that reductionist science has not proven predictive with the rigor necessary even for contemporary clinical decision making (Janssens, Ioannidis, et al. 2011). Similarly, current approaches to drug discovery are not readily able to generate mechanism-specific therapies on a scale and at a cost compatible with truly personalized or precision medicine (Trusheim, Burgess, et al. 2011). Reductionism applied to testing a single overarching hypothesis is the driving force for many of the largest studies. However, despite the successes of modern molecular medicine, it is becoming obvious that as large-scale data begin to emerge in biology, our capacity to test each hypothesis iteratively is rapidly reaching impracticality.

In contrast, the goal of network medicine is a quantitative, holistic understanding of human biology in heath and disease (Barabási, Gulbahce, et al. 2011). While there have been numerous efforts to define rigorous mathematical models of very specific biological events, the completion of the human genome project (and parallel projects for other genomes) has highlighted advantages of global descriptions in biological frameworks (Jones 1868; Ganesh, Zakai, et al. 2009; Bansal, Harismendy, et al. 2010; Abecasis, Auton, et al. 2012; Anonymous 2012a,b; Garnaas, Cutting, et al. 2012; Gerstein 2012). Network science approaches the problems of medicine through comprehensive descriptions of the components of an entire system, their quantitative relationships, and their combined response to specific perturbations. While global strategies are often viewed as hypothesis generating, with the derivation of rigorous models that capture the empiric relationships among large numbers of components, truly emergent properties can be predicted that would not be accessible through traditional linear pathway models. With ever more comprehensive and quantitative descriptions of the inputs and outputs in human biology, it will be feasible to develop rigorous network models, ranging from molecular to population scale, and capable of quantitative predictions for health and disease (Barabási, Gulbahce, et al. 2011). These new integrative models of biology are anticipated to transform our ability not only to assign prognoses, but also to discern fundamental mechanisms and to specify therapies that effectively restore the pathological network to a physiological state, rather than simply counter one disruption with another (Loscalzo, Kohane, et al. 2007; Hansen and Iyengar 2013).

At the core of the tensions between reductionism and holism in medicine lies the biological complexity of the phenomena themselves and the relatively rudimentary tools that we use for observation and modeling. These two complementary scientific philosophies reconcile around the specific processes they each propose to describe, with many of the distinctions between the two perspectives eliminated when phenomena are considered at the appropriate scale and resolution (Popper 1959; Mayr 1982). In practical terms, realization of the vision of network medicine demands observational outputs that can describe precisely the network state under a broad range of conditions and across a broad range of scales (Wolf, Karev, et al. 2002; Barabási, Gulbahce, et al. 2011; Hansen and Iyengar 2013). No longer can we rely on serendipity, history, or existing tools to define this universe of outcomes. This chapter describes the ways in which the biological outputs of a genome and its environment (an operating definition of a phenotype) define our understanding of health and disease. It will also highlight ways in which more systematic approaches to phenotypes and phenotyping will be necessary if we are to achieve the advances in medicine that network approaches promise.

What Is a Phenotype?

Classification by careful observation of patterns of association has proven remarkably powerful. Even in ancient times, there were well-recognized empiric solutions to several conditions that had been serendipitously discovered in different cultures across the globe (Jones 1868). However, the systematic observation initiated during the Enlightenment combined with the technologies that emerged during this fertile period revolutionized our understanding of the human state (Osler 1892; Dolan and Holmes 1984). Definitive catalogs of human anatomy, physiology, and pathophysiology were assembled for the first time. While the overarching classification schemes used to define health and disease were in essence those accessible to the naked eye, it was still possible to make substantial advances in the correlation of particular structural or functional observations with discrete outcomes (Leshchiner, Alexa, et al. 2012).

Many of the phenomenological clusters that were defined during this period had remarkable specificity for particular etiologies. For example, the combination of a lobar pneumonia, endocarditis, and meningitis was almost pathognomonic of pneumococcal sepsis (Osler 1892). However, the specificity of these clinical findings is highly conditioned by geographic location, the local prevalence of the organism and its biological tropisms, the temporal nature of the presentation, as well as the nutritional state of the host, to name but a few of the relevant variables (Osler 1892; Talbott 1961). These findings are rarely seen in the antibiotic-modified pneumococcal illnesses of today, while other less common infections may result in identical syndromes in the immunocompromised. The refining role of temporal clustering in the identification of a causal association is also clear in syphilis, in which the primary infection generates syndromes with excellent discriminant power for etiology when compared to the "great imitator" that is tertiary or quaternary treponemal infection (Osler 1892; Kumar, Alibhai, et al. 2011). These diagnostic dilemmas have not been fully resolved, despite our ability to detect molecular components of the treponeme, simply because the diagnosis is not often considered (Scythes and Jones 2013).

The fundamental power of clustering is often quite obvious in the shared inheritance and environmental exposures of familial disease, and it was in the discipline of genetics that the formal concept of *phenotype* first arose. Early assumptions of a single mechanism as the driver of familial resemblance were especially powerful when combined with delineation of the transmission of specific traits. Careful observation is required to discriminate shared environmental exposures from shared genetics, and even in the era of modern genomics these two etiological threads may be closely associated, especially in infectious diseases, in which multiple genomes may be transmitted in parallel within a family (Williams-Blangero, Criscione, et al. 2012; Brestoff and Artis 2013). In individual kindreds, it is feasible to study at-risk individuals at increased resolution with proportionate changes in the discriminatory power of any recognized pattern. The frameworks of observation and quantitative analysis that family studies permit have defined strategies for correlating all biological observations to the point at which "all that is not genotype is now considered phenotype" (Lalouel, Rao, et al. 1983). How did this framework emerge, and what are the insights that the tools of genetics can offer for network science?

Genotype, Phenotype, and Endophenotype

A physical basis for transmitted familial resemblance was not established until the discovery of deoxyribonucleic acid (DNA) and the empiric demonstration of trait transfer by cloned nucleic acid sequences. However, the concept of phenotype emerged many years prior to this from the quantitative study of the transmitted traits themselves (Mahner and Kary 1997). Mathematical approaches to genetics, initially used in crop science, led to the realization that even the rigorous quantitative definition of observed characteristics did not describe features with distinct causal bases (Falconer 1960; Churchill 1974). For example, two discrete populations displaying partially overlapping binomial distributions of a given character, such as seed dimensions, could readily be combined to generate a single population, itself described by a simple binomial distribution. Thus, the mathematical description of a trait offered no insight into its biological unity (Churchill 1974). Moving beyond this realization required the addition of transmissibility, first expressed in the concept of the *pure line*, in which individuals were defined by the average characteristics of their own offspring (Churchill 1974). Subsequent breeding of these "pure" lines established beyond doubt that even in the absence of any selection pressure, the transmitted trait characteristic was constant in the offspring, suggesting some stable physical basis for the trait: an intrinsic genotypic difference (Figure 5–1). To this day phenotyping by offspring remains the most rigorous form of study for heritable traits (Falconer 1960; Lynch and Walsh 1998; Gonzaga-Jauregui, Lupski, et al. 2012). Thus, in its earliest definition, phenotype was the quantitative description of a transmitted trait, and it was made explicit that in itself phenotype had no bearing on the underlying biology.

Once DNA was established as the physical basis for inheritance, it became feasible to relate trait characteristics in the individual to the genotype of that individual (Collins 1992). In these early studies, phenotype became defined as the unique representation or "revelation" of the underlying genotype (Mahner and Kary 1997). This framework has persisted to the current day, as the notion developed that all observable attributes of an organism other than the fixed genotypic state are part of the phenotype. Once genome sequencing had defined the comprehensive static genetic code for an organism, all downstream consequences were readily aggregated in the definition of phenotype. Only in recent years, as the dynamism of the individual genome during development and beyond has been recognized (Poduri, Evrony, et al. 2013) and organismal phenotypes have been discovered that represent the integrated output of multiple genomes (e.g., via host–microbiome interactions), have these distinctions again become blurred (Wang, Klipfell, et al. 2011; Brestoff and Artis 2013).

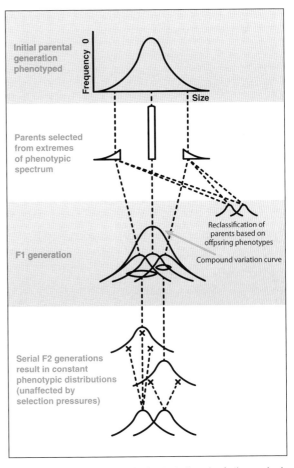

FIGURE 5–1. Phenotyping by offspring tests the role of other randomly segregating alleles. The original definitions of heritability are deeply enshrined in the concept of phenotype. A quantitative trait might rationally be defined as heritable only if it were reproducibly transmissible in successive matings independent of any selection. A parental trait can be robustly established as the mean phenotype in the offspring.

Importantly, for genetics and for network medicine alike, the addition of a specified perturbation has a powerful effect on the resolution of underlying biological unity (Churchill 1974). In classic genetics, the perturbation may include study of a trait on discrete genetic backgrounds where the phenotypic output of a specific variant may be attenuated by other segregating alleles (Poduri, Evrony, et al. 2013). However, any number of other stressors may act to add an additional dimension to any phenotype. Indeed, many of the major problems with etiologic heterogeneity might be resolved if phenotype definitions incorporated dynamic responses to standardized challenges or objective transmission likelihoods. While the tension between population and individual definitions of phenotype has continued, the practical application of careful phenotyping within disease kindreds combined with modern genotyping has allowed the remarkable successes of positional cloning (Lander and Botstein 1989; Collins 1992). In the mid-1980s, it became possible to map even subjective binary traits to a unique genomic location and to clone the underlying physical mutations that are both sufficient and necessary to cause the phenotype (Gusella, Wexler, et al. 1983). In this context, the statistical cost of misphenotyping even a single individual in a pedigree is all too apparent, and one or two erroneous phenotypes have prevented the cloning of many disease genes (Bates, MacDonald, et al. 1991). Notably, family studies of virtually every Mendelian disorder have also concluded that, even in the setting of very large single gene-effect sizes, the final outcome of a given genotype is usually so diverse within even a single extended kindred (pleiotropy) that deterministic prediction based purely on genotype remains elusive (Shimizu, Moss, et al. 2009; Watkins, Hendricks, et al. 2009).

The limited predictive utility of major effect-size genes suggests that the observed phenotypes are strongly modified by other genes or by nongenetic factors. Indeed, the primary phenotype that is transmitted may be an underlying diathesis such as susceptibility to some unmeasured environmental challenge or interaction with cosegregating common alleles. This more uniform underlying trait, or endophenotype, may be more penetrant than the final disease, yet also more difficult to detect without the requisite tools (Figure 5–2). A central argument for changing the approach to phenotyping is our inability to rigorously attribute the factors determining penetrance or pleiotropy without systematic studies of the heritability of each component of the phenotype and measurement of the relevant environmental contributions.

Among the benefits of network science is the feasibility of employing specific network modules and module states as endophenotypes. These modules would capture a much broader range of phenotypic elements across multiple states (e.g., health and disease), thus offering a less biased and more quantitative revelation of the underlying genotypes (Barabási, Gulbahce, et al. 2011). Is there any evidence that such approaches to phenotype would aid in our understanding of the mechanisms of disease?

Few, if any, human traits have been studied at the resolution necessary to define their genetic basis in a comprehensive manner. Where formal studies of the genetic architecture of a trait have been undertaken, they have been remarkably informative (Lalouel, Rao, et al. 1983). Systematic kin-cohort studies and the investigation of large kindreds led not only to the identification of unsuspected heritability in Hirschsprung disease, a disorder of colonic innervation, but also, in conjunction with genetic model organisms, have enabled dissection of the interactions of several genes to cause less penetrant and more pleiotropic forms

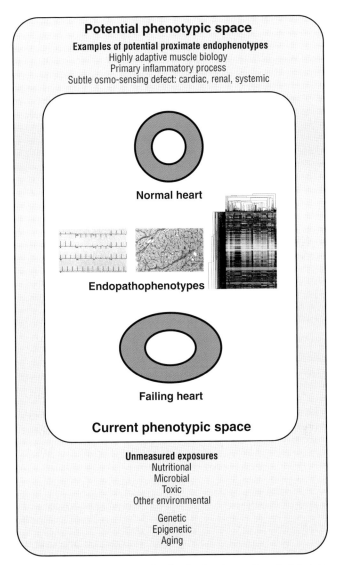

FIGURE 5–2. Endophenotypes and endopathophenotypes. Current clinical assessment is dominated by the detection of end-stage diagnostic syndromes that have evolved from simple bedside examination or serendipitous observation—illustrated here using heart failure as a paradigm. While traditional clinical or pathological tools in some circumstances may offer endopathophenotypes that discriminate distinctive disease subsets, in most settings, this is not the result of any systematic endeavor. Modern genomic techniques are emerging as useful tools in resolving current relatively crude clinical syndromes, but until we are able to define preclinical or even prepathological endophenotypes, the predictive goals of modern medicine are unlikely to be realized. This will require much more systematic exploration of phenotypic space and similar approaches to the definition of a vast range of stimuli that are currently unmeasured.

of the trait (Badner, Sieber, et al. 1990). This remains one of the few examples in which unraveling complex interactions among multiple genes and environment has proven feasible in humans, and highlights the mechanistic rigor that is possible when a quantitative understanding of a gene network and its interactions with the environment is achieved.

As noted above, robustness to genetic variance is rarely, if ever, assessed for human traits, but even in genetic animal models, where inbred murine strains and costly husbandry restrict what is practical, there are few examples of genetic challenge as a perturbation. When mutations have been modeled on discrete genetic backgrounds, the chasm between our classification of phenotypes and the rigorous biological output of even a single variant is often all too apparent. In one early example, the effects of RXR alpha null alleles on different genetic backgrounds were evident in completely different organ systems; to date, there is no mechanistic understanding of the discrepancies between these experiments (Kastner, Grondona, et al. 1994; Sucov, Dyson, et al. 1994).

The downstream implications of the original concepts of genotype and phenotype have become more obvious as genetics has approached smaller effect sizes at a population level. Transmissibility and effect size offer constraints that render causality accessible, but it has also become evident that quantitative traits, such as those one might exploit in network medicine, are not immediately tractable in a single dimension. Precise analysis of quantitative traits, including the meticulous mapping of such phenotypes in closed genetic populations, has shed further light on the nature of the phenotypes themselves (Lynch and Walsh 1998).

The successful initial mapping of trait variance to specific quantitative trait loci (QTLs) for many different phenotypes in mouse crosses has not led to large numbers of cloned genes. Subsequent breeding demonstrates the loss of heritability or the absence of genotypic difference (Rikke and Johnson 1998; Talbot, Nicod, et al. 1999). Several mechanisms may underlie these observations. For example, there may be unanticipated synthetic interactions between unlinked loci that emerge only under very particular combinations of other genotypes. Some of this lack of observed transmissibility undoubtedly reflects epigenetic differences among murine strains, but perhaps more importantly, a substantial proportion is a consequence of restricted dimensionality of the traits themselves. For any given quantitative trait, while the effects of individual alleles may contribute evenly to the normal distribution across that trait, the presence or absence of specific alleles may be discernible through distinctive effects on other orthogonal traits between alleles. Even within a given quantitative trait subsumed in a single binomial distribution, there may be distinctive phenotypic contributions from different loci that are accessible to higher-resolution phenotyping technologies. For example, while height may behave as a single trait, a particular gene may contribute to changes in the dimensions of only specific skeletal segments (Robinson, Arteaga-Solis, et al. 2006; Lanktree, Guo et al. 2011; Durand and Rappold 2013). These observations underscore the complexity of the possible relationships between genotype and phenotype. Selection pressures may be acting across a much broader phenotypic spectrum than that arbitrarily defined by the phenotyper (Kemper, Visscher, et al. 2012). In concert with empiric data from more tractable model organisms, these concepts have led to more holistic approaches to phenotype (Manolio, Collins, et al. 2009; Morozova, Goldman, et al. 2012).

The inescapable conclusion is that many genetic determinants of phenotypes are undetected by modern investigation, not as a result of any limits of genotyping, but rather as a result of the limitations of phenotyping (MacRae and Vasan 2011). The core concepts of phenotype incorporated within transmission likelihoods include not just a superficial resemblance in one baseline state, but, rather, a much more robust quantitative set of parameters observed in the context of specific genetic or environmental challenges (Kemper, Visscher, et al. 2012; Morozova, Goldman, et al. 2012).

Without the relevant phenotypic assay or without the necessary stimulus to generate a particular dynamic phenotypic response, the major alleles may simply be silent. These phenotypic phenomena likely account for a significant proportion of the "hidden" heritability inferred in many modern human genetic studies (Manolio, Collins, et al. 2009; Eichler, Flint, et al. 2010).

Prediction of all of the possible outcomes of a given genotype at a single locus is unlikely to be feasible without a comprehensive description of the full genotypic context, and even then prediction will be dependent on a similarly nuanced knowledge of the phenotypic consequences of all conceivable gene–gene interactions across the genome. Deconvoluting interactions on such a scale, and in the setting of high rates of de novo variation, is currently inconceivable without a holistic probabilistic framework such as network medicine. For most important phenotypes, the correlation between genotype and phenotype is already known to be far from deterministic. More sophisticated models that incorporate genes of differing effect size, environmental factors, and stochastic components will have to be developed.

As the concept of phenotype has evolved, in particular in model organisms and then in human genetics, the distinction between individual and population genetics is coming full circle. Extended phenotypes that reflect the composite characteristics of the organism in its wider context, and include responses to environment and interactions with commensal organisms, are now being studied, further reinforcing the concept that all that is not genotype is phenotype. The advent of whole-exome or whole-genome sequencing independently supports these observations with the documentation of significant numbers of bona fide morbid mutations in phenotype-negative individuals in the general population (Bick, Flannick, et al. 2012; Flannick, Beer et al. 2013). If nothing else, these data force us to reconsider the deterministic implications of specific sequence variants, and to reevaluate the particular phenotypes we have associated with these variants (Seidman and Seidman 2001). Without massively parallel data on phenotype as well as genotype, it will be challenging to deconvolute whole-genome variation (MacArthur, Balasubramanian, et al. 2012). Before we can address these challenges, we must first change the scale of phenotyping.

Pathophenotypes and Endopathophenotypes

There are several considerations that apply in particular to pathophenotypes and to endopathophenotypes, the disease correlates of the phenotypes and endophenotypes outlined above. Human disease characterization is, for many biological processes, the highest-resolution phenotyping that exists. Much of the technological innovation that has taken place in biology has been driven by the incentives of clinical medicine, in which we often imagine that the resolution of our diagnoses can barely be improved. Pathophenotypes, however, are likely more heterogeneous than the basal physiological traits, simply as a result of the range of mechanisms by which normal biology may be perturbed. Gain-of-function alleles in disease genes and novel signals from environmental exposures contribute substantially to the pathophysiological repertoire. Endopathophenotypes are currently defined, not so much by their heterogeneities, but, rather, by the shared commonalities crossing multiple different etiologies. These pathophenotypes may represent upstream, and potentially targetable, components of the clinical disorder, or final common pathways that serve only to mask the distinctive underlying disease mechanisms (Barabási, Gulbahce, et al. 2011).

The genetic concept of *gain of function* has particular resonance in network medicine. Not only the state of a network, but also the patterns of connectivity (physical, chemical, genetic, or other) between different genes or gene products may differ dramatically in the setting of a mutation or an environmental challenge (Tewari, Hu, et al. 2004; Loscalzo, Kohane, et al. 2007). Thus, the very structure of any biological network that exists in health may have been replaced by a distinctive network, composed of discrete genes and proteins, as a result of changes in the affinity of pairs of molecules, based only on modifications of individual nucleic acid or protein residues (Temporini, Calleri, et al. 2008; Park, Williams, et al. 2012). Furthermore, the selection pressures operating to define the connectivity of a baseline physiological network may affect a very different function of that network or component modules in disease. A comprehensive picture of any network must include its behavior under a relevant set of distinctive conditions—ideally across diverse time scales (Barabási and Bonabeau 2003; Lim, Hao, et al. 2006; Goh, Cusick. et al. 2007; Loscalzo, Kohane, et al. 2007). Even if the network components or their connectivity has not been disrupted, pathophenotypes or endopathophenotypes may operate in parts of the dynamic range discrete from the physiological state. Here again, the central role of a defined stimulus to elicit (and organize) a measured response can be appreciated. Without a series of calibrated stimulus–response pairs that traverse the different network states from organogenesis to adulthood or from a timescale of microseconds to decades, it may be difficult even to detect an abnormal disease network. Given these conclusions, the scope of network medicine looms large even compared with whole genomes and again suggests that new ways of capturing phenotypic data across multiple scales will be necessary for the execution of a network medicine vision (Barabási and Albert 1999; Jeong, Tombor, et al. 2000; Barabási, Gulbahce, et al. 2011).

Phenocopies

For each and every phenotype there are so-called phenocopies or "indistinguishable" biological outcomes that do not share the same underlying genotype (Goldin, Cox, et al. 1984; Badner, Sieber, et al. 1990). Phenocopies obviously not only exhibit distinct genotypes, but also may encompass a wide range of downstream natural histories and so dilute any genetic or mechanistic investigation (Keating and Sanguinetti 2001). There is a fundamental relationship between the resolution of phenotyping and the probability of phenocopies that has been observed in numerous genetic studies. Indeed, many of the most robust common disease phenotypes may simply represent endpoints that are most readily detectable, inflating the prevalence of phenocopies (Risch 2000). Most common disease entities are defined by anatomic classification schemes based on autopsy studies (Seidman and Seidman 2001) or clinical correlations dating to the eighteenth century (e.g., glycosuria), and subjected to increasingly refined measurement only over the past few decades. The concept of increased dimensionality in phenotyping that is incorporated in network approaches may improve the resolution of any trait and thereby reduce the likelihood of a mechanistically unrelated phenocopy.

Notably, these attributes of common disease may also explain the shared alleles seen across multiple phenotypes in recent genome-wide association studies (Cross-Disorder Group of the Psychiatric Genomics Consortium, Lee. et al.

2013). While there may be discrete etiologies for specific disorders, the focus of medicine over the past few decades has been on lumping or aggregating numbers of cases for epidemiology or for clinical trials. In this setting, the sharing of final common pathways such as inflammation or fibrosis may be the basis for rigorous studies of the mechanisms of these endopathophenotypic modules across multiple disease syndromes (Goh, Cusick, et al. 2007; Loscalzo, Kohane, et al. 2007).

Environment

The silence of many pharmacologic response alleles without drug challenge is an excellent example of how many traits may simply be undetectable without the correct assay or without the correct conditioning variable (Roden, Altman, et al. 2006; Peterson and MacRae 2012). While drugs are usually readily recognized as contributors to specific phenotypes, be they beneficial or adverse, the nature and timing of most environmental stimuli are not known. Microbiological challenges can be systematically defined in an unbiased and quantitative manner directly through microbial genomics (Brestoff and Artis 2013), but there are, as yet, no generic tools for the detection of other environmental factors. A wide range of small molecules is now accessible to mass spectrometry–based metabolomics techniques (Raamsdonk, Teusink, et al. 2001), but the universe of potential environmental molecules is many orders of magnitude larger. Perhaps the most readily measured environmental contributors to disease are diet, exercise, and other self-administered "perturbations" such as tobacco and alcohol (Deo, Hunter, et al. 2010; Masel and Trotter 2010; Wang, Klipfell, et al. 2011; Jones, Park, et al. 2012). Standardized questionnaires in epidemiological studies have demonstrated that these exposures have major effects on numerous health outcomes, but quantitation of such environmental factors across time is not routinely performed in clinical care. The same technologies that are being exploited to improve the collection of phenotypic data must be adapted to begin to record the exposome at a similar level of resolution (Jones, Park, et al. 2012). For example, the availability of granular personal GPS datasets from smart phones might accelerate the correlation of measured, rather than estimated, exposures to a broad range of environmental chemicals. Importantly, objectively measured shared exposures represent exactly the robust and relevant perturbations that are needed to characterize network dynamics. Ultimately, the collection and analysis of "big data" on metrics such as nutritional or other purchase data, personal habits, travel, and other exposures, will be a core component of network approaches to understanding human biology (Praneenararat, Takagi, et al. 2012).

More Global Approaches to Phenotypes: Phenomics

Despite the emphasis on phenotype and phenotyping resolution in the early science of genetics, the field has been dominated by genotyping technologies for some time. It is only in the past few years, as comprehensive genotyping has become feasible on an individual scale, that a more systematic approach to the study of phenotype has been seen as an area for investment (Freimer and Sabatti 2003).

Perhaps the most generalizable insight from the genomics revolution has been the utility of comprehensive and unbiased approaches in biology. The universality of genomic sequence and its immediate facilitation of translation between different species has led to parallel approaches for other molecular classes, including proteomics, lipidomics, and metabolomics (Woolfe, Goodson, et al. 2005; Boja, Hiltke, et al. 2010). There remains a massive universe of "non-omic" information that must be captured if unbiased approaches are to be extended to all phenotyping. An important goal for network medicine will be to redefine the tools for capturing variation in the phenome in a way in which the information content can be maximized.

No other organism is capable of being phenotyped with the granularity that is feasible in humans. Many phenotypes that incorporate higher cognitive faculties are inconceivable or not present in other organisms. Self-report alone defines a phenotypic universe that cannot be accessed in any other species and often exceeds the sensitivity of current objective technologies. Our ability to discern subtleties in our own physiological performance is remarkable, although it is also prone to subjective errors. It is no coincidence that psychiatry has been one of the few areas in which phenotyping has been systematically addressed (Freimer and Sabatti 2003).

The considerable overlap present in traditional psychiatric diagnoses stimulated the development of a consensus set of diagnostic criteria enshrined in the *Diagnostic and Statistical Manual* (DSM) by the American Psychiatric Association in 1952 (American Psychiatric Association 2013; Solovieff, Cotsapas, et al. 2013). This complex set of definitions is built on the general strategy of breaking an individual disorder down into a series of nonoverlapping dimensions. These traits themselves have been refined iteratively on their performance in studies of natural history, genetics, and therapies, and the DSM is now in its fifth iteration. What have we learned from this approach and can we discern specific lessons for phenotypes of the future in network medicine?

Perhaps the most salient lessons from psychiatric phenotyping are encompassed in two of the earliest insights. First, the recognition that subjective assessments, no matter how well defined, curated, and promulgated, do not offer the resolution that is necessary to comprehend the underlying biological defects (Bilder, Sabb, et al. 2009; American Psychiatric Association 2013; Cross-Disorder Group of the Psychiatric Genomics Consortium, Lee, et al. 2013). This shortcoming may reflect the fact that there are unmeasured diatheses with very comparable downstream outcomes, but there is also evidence from the field that it is likely a result of the lack of specificity of what in the early twentieth century appeared to be quite specific clinical observations. For example, it is now evident that there is merit in including apparently orthogonal neurological traits, such as response latency or regional metabolic differences detectable with modern functional magnetic resonance imaging (fMRI) techniques, into the definition or characterization of psychiatric syndromes, as these features allow more mechanistically faithful clustering of clinical observations. Conceptually, this validation of individual phenotypic dimensions as truly independent is an important component of defining phenotypes not on the basis of one apparently pathognomonic element, but, rather, on the basis of unique modules of multiple traits with distinctive modular responses to defined perturbations.

Parallel work in the common variant genetics of psychiatric disease has revealed a large number of loci that are shared across apparently very different phenotypes (Cross-Disorder Group of the Psychiatric Genomics Consortium, Lee, et al. 2013; Solovieff, Cotsapas, et al. 2013). While this has been interpreted as evidence of a shared etiology, in the context of the known high heritability of many of the underlying disorders, it is likely to represent a downstream endo-pathophenotype that modulates much more generic neuropsychiatric outputs such as tuning contributions to the core disease modules. Ultimately, these insights have led the psychiatric community to drive toward more global approaches to phenotype firmly based in quantitative objective metrics. It is clear that as biology enters a more quantitative and holistic era, a rigorous reappraisal of all phenotypes will be required.

Next-Generation Phenotypes for Network Medicine

Together these observations on the origins, evolution, and limitations of the phenotype concept argue for a much more comprehensive approach, one that documents the fundamental genetic molecular and cellular architecture of physiological and pathophysiological traits, not only under baseline conditions, but also in response to a range of empirically tested perturbations. A consensus is emerging that such a phenotyping project is necessary, as holistic network concepts of biology and disease are being defined (Bilder, Sabb, et al. 2009). This last section of this chapter will outline some of the basic principles that might inform these converging frameworks at a time when genetics, genomics, and other tools are being deployed in the clinical arena.

When compared with the finite scope of the genome, the enormity of measuring the phenome is all too apparent. The development of panels of quantitative (patho)phenotypes that cross traditional organ-based domains is closely aligned with efforts to understand human biology at a network level, where myriad influences can be objectively weighted and their (quantitative) interactions modeled (Freimer and Sabatti 2003). As phenotyping resolution reaches a molecular scale in the context of functional networks or "disease modules," it is clear that specific causal genes or environmental factors are not necessary to derive "diagnostic" feature sets with distinctive outcomes or therapeutic responses (Ostrowski and Wyrwicz 2009; Antonucci, Atzori, et al. 2010; Boja, Hiltke, et al. 2010). Nevertheless, the generalizability of this core tenet of network medicine remains unproven. Numerous examples exist in functional genomics, where downsampling enables a substantial proportion of the information content to be captured using only a fraction of the features accessible through a given technique (Peck, Crawford, et al. 2006). Such downsampling requires empiric validation, although theoretically the representation of independent orthogonal phenotypic components may form the basis for a rational strategy. It is possible to prioritize elements for assay based on existing knowledge, focusing on representation of existing metabolic networks or organismal RNA features (known modules), as has been accomplished in metabolomics and metagenomics, respectively (Lewis, Farrell, et al. 2010; Sharon and Banfield 2013).

New diagnostic tools to discriminate homogeneous disease subsets and to identify causally related, more penetrant endophenotypes are urgently required (Cannon, Gasperoni, et al. 2001; Freimer and Sabatti 2003; Cannon 2005; Singer 2005). "Unbiased" phenotypes are emerging as an efficient tool for network building in model organisms, but large-scale application in human disease has not been undertaken (Walhout, Reboul, et al. 2002; Ge, Walhout, et al. 2003; Rual, Ceron, et al. 2004). Even the most rigorous genetic studies can be confounded by phenotypes in which affection status can be defined only by rare events or by responses to particular stimuli. Here the concept of an underlying diathesis toward the phenotype is often used, but in the absence of systematic approaches to define the full scope of such a diathesis, many of the alleles that might affect such a trait are simply inaccessible (Morozova, Goldman, et al. 2012). As outlined above, obvious examples include drug-response phenotypes or environmental exposures (Roden, Altman, et al. 2006). Systematic approaches to detection and quantitation of the exposome will be required to make any inferences regarding the relevant biological networks.

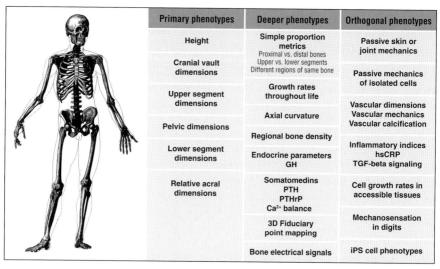

	Primary phenotypes	Deeper phenotypes	Orthogonal phenotypes
	Height	Simple proportion metrics Proximal vs. distal bones Upper vs. lower segments Different regions of same bone	Passive skin or joint mechanics
	Cranial vault dimensions		Passive mechanics of isolated cells
	Upper segment dimensions	Growth rates throughout life	Vascular dimensions Vascular mechanics Vascular calcification
	Pelvic dimensions	Axial curvature	
		Regional bone density	
	Lower segment dimensions	Endocrine parameters GH	Inflammatory indices hsCRP TGF-beta signaling
	Relative acral dimensions	Somatomedins PTH PTHrP Ca²⁺ balance	Cell growth rates in accessible tissues
		3D Fiduciary point mapping	Mechanosensation in digits
		Bone electrical signals	iPS cell phenotypes

FIGURE 5–3. Improving phenotypic resolution. In many instances, simply changing the resolution of a phenotype might dramatically improve our understanding of the pathophysiology of disease. A simple trait such as height might be deconvoluted into multiple constituent traits, each with distinctive genetic and environmental contributors. This could be achieved through "deeper" phenotyping in areas known to be biologically related to the primary trait or by considering other orthogonal phenotypes that might be influenced in parallel by the distinctive subsets of biology responsible for the integrated whole. GH, growth hormone; hsCRp, high sensitivity C-reactive protein; iPS, induced pluripotent stem cells; PTH, parathyroid hormone; PTHrP, parathyroid hormone related peptide; TGF, transforming growth factor.

Another prevalent influence in modern phenotyping is the failure to collect orthogonal data with any meaningful granularity as a result of clinical subspecialization (Figure 5–3). Functional genomics has begun to break down the boundaries between disease silos in ways that emphasize how poorly our current organ-specific disease frameworks represent the primary pathobiology. For example, elegant metabolomic data from population cohorts demonstrate abnormalities of amino acid metabolism in those who will go on to develop overt diabetes over a decade prior to any detectable abnormality of glucose handling (Wang, Larson, et al. 2011). Using the same technology to extend the phenotypic assessment of the response to an oral glucose challenge resulted in the identification of orthogonal pathways with the potential to redefine the entire scope of diabetes as a disease entity (Ho, Larson, et al. 2013). Ex vivo cell profiling has also revealed distinctive responses to small molecule perturbations in subsets of those with Mendelian forms of diabetes (Shaw, Blodgett, et al. 2011). Ultimately, there is only limited recognition of specific phenotypes outside narrowly defined regions of expertise, and, as a result, there is always a tendency to try to reduce complexity to make it more manageable by the clinician. Together these emerging examples highlight a profound discordance between the limited dimensionality of even the most modern clinical phenotypes and the biologic heterogeneity of the very diseases for which these current phenotypes are the effective gold standard.

At its core, *diagnosis* is an understanding of disease mechanism or a constellation of clinical phenotypic features that associate with a particular outcome or a response to a specific therapy. Despite the success of today's molecular technologies and other emerging sensors, there remains a fundamental need for highly sensitive phenotyping techniques that capture the underlying pathobiology at different scales, for example at the level of the organelle, cell, or tissue (Figure 5–4). With innovation in this arena, functional abnormalities might be detectable at a stage where downstream final common pathways are not yet activated and when more robust etiologic discrimination is feasible. These inferences have stimulated efforts to begin to improve the granularity of human clinical phenotyping (Freimer and Sabatti 2003; Robinson and Mundlos 2010; Bendall and Nolan 2012), to broaden the scope of phenotyping assays, and to develop more global, digital approaches to phenotype classification in order to reduce the biases from traditional nosology (Oti and Brunner 2007; Oti, Huynen, et al. 2009; Robinson and Mundlos 2010).

The ideal phenotypes for network medicine are beginning to be imagined, not only in the ivory towers of academic medicine, but also in laboratories where digital devices are being developed, in online data warehouses, and within lay organizations such as the "quantified self" movement. What are the fundamental characteristics that will define the phenotypic measures that will accelerate the implementation of network medicine? One lesson from functional genomics would appear to be that we should avoid excessive determinism during the discovery phase. Data types that we may not imagine as contributory, such as keystroke data on a computer or driving behavior, may represent sophisticated integrators of different neurologic circuits or transcription factor outputs (described by cellular or molecular networks, respectively). The most successful next-generation phenotypes will likely emphasize several core attributes, while reevaluating, extending, or complementing existing technologies. A suite of digital clinical measurements that reproducibly captures information in multiple dimensions, across different spatial and temporal scales will be vital for network science. To ensure maximum fidelity, linear response characteristics across several log orders to empirically defined stimuli will be vital, at the very least over a range of physiologically relevant responses. The stimuli themselves will represent essential metadata, and ideally will also facilitate rapid translation across different cellular and animal models, allowing anchoring of phenotype in the same way that sequence homology anchors genotype. These empirically derived stimulus–response pairs will have to be mapped onto existing disease ontologies in a wave of new clinical investigation. Ultimately, as innovative personal

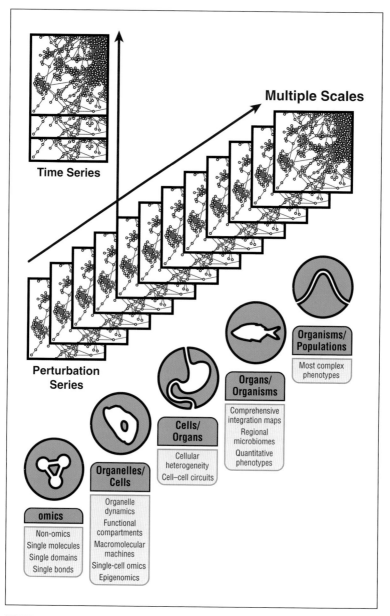

FIGURE 5–4. The changing scales of network phenotypes. Comprehensive multiscale phenotyping will be critical to build the networks necessary to describe complex disease biology. At
present, the relatively unbiased phenotyping required for network analysis is available only at one
or two levels across the necessary spectrum. Text in grey area illustrates the obvious phenotypic
components that are not routinely collected at each scale, but are already known to be central to
the pathophysiology of most diseases.

and ambient technologies emerge, many of these strategies will move beyond the domain of disease classification to the active documentation and mainte- nance of wellness. In this process, it will be possible to refine endophenotypes, pathophenotypes, and endopathophenotypes progressively toward a series of ever more specific core elements, ideally opening the door to the definition of *generalizable biologic rules.*

In the first instance, the addition of even a limited number of superficial orthogonal phenotypes may suffice to resolve underlying heterogeneity (Garver, Holcomb, et al. 2000; Cannon, Gasperoni, et al. 2001; Cannon 2005; Anttila, Kallela, et al. 2006). In other cases, only directed application of profiling technologies, such as cytokine profiling, cellular profiling, or metabolomics, will uncover the discrete subsets (Weckwerth and Morgenthal 2005; Shaw, Westly, et al. 2008). Many transformative phenotypes might be imagined for downstream integrative studies, but the feasibility of translation to and from model systems is likely to be a critical attribute for the empiric definition of ge- netic architecture and for pathway entry or exploration (Lee 2008; MacRae and Vasan 2011). Reassessment of existing technologies outside the constraints of cur- rent nosology using techniques such as machine vision and machine learning will offer early insights. Innovative phenotyping tools, standardized perturba- tions, and vast electronic health records integrating institutional and personal data will allow the generation and validation of in silico network models capable of predictive utility (Barabási, Gulbahce, et al. 2011). To accelerate this process, much greater rigor and standardization of electronic health records will be necessary. Importantly, these innovations in phenotyping will parallel the most disruptive period in the reinvention of clinical care delivery in centuries (Lee 2008).

A Novel Minimal Clinical Dataset

A final implication of the more global approach to phenotype that network bi- ology demands is a need for vastly larger datasets than those we have previously collected. For rigorous analytics that might facilitate the early detection of de- viations from health, the prediction of disease, and the enabling of real-time monitoring, we will need to collect a standardized multidimensional dataset on vast numbers of individuals across their lifespan. To undertake this analysis at the necessary scale will require the definition of a novel minimal phenotyping dataset for modern medicine, paralleling the standard "history and physical" of the past two centuries (Osler 1892; Leshchiner, Alexa, et al. 2012). This dataset must incor- porate new smart ontologies for self-reported data, definitive imaging series at high resolution (with no exposure risk), functional genomics, novel digital in-patient or outpatient technologies, and personal data on a scale that has to date only been imagined for commercial transactions or transnational security.

Conclusion

Medicine will need to train a generation of generalists, capable of reconciling the deterministic approaches of recent decades with the holistic integrative strategies of network medicine. Physicians and the data-collection networks to which they will have access will measure dynamic pathway responses to objective genomic and environmental perturbations. Perhaps the most daunting hurdle to be overcome in this transformation is the change in scale of the data that clinicians must manage, understand, and act on. These challenges will mandate that physicians have access to the requisite skills to develop network analytics, as well as innovative methods of data display, knowledge management, and real-time education to allow all providers to practice network medicine. Through more universal approaches to phenotype, and the unbiased analysis of such phenotypes, the ultimate goal of a mechanistic understanding of the differences between clinical entities will be attained, but even before such insights are realized, probabilistic diagnoses will be feasible.

References

Abecasis, G. R., A. Auton, et al. (2012). An integrated map of genetic variation from 1,092 human genomes. Nature **491**(7422): 56–65.

Anonymous (2012a). Cracking ENCODE. Lancet **380**(9846): 950.

Anonymous (2012b). Decoding ENCODE. Nat Chem Biol **8**(11): 871.

Antonucci, R., L. Atzori, et al. (2010). Metabolomics: the new clinical chemistry for person-alized neonatal medicine. Minerva Pediatr **62**(3 Suppl 1): 145–48.

Anttila, V., M. Kallela, et al. (2006). Trait components provide tools to dissect the genetic susceptibility of migraine. Am J Hum Genet **79**(1): 85–99.

American Psychiatric Association (2013). Diagnostic and Statistical Manual of Mental Disorders, 5th ed. Washington, DC: Author.

Badner, J. A., W. K. Sieber, et al. (1990). A genetic study of Hirschsprung disease. Am J Hum Genet **46**(3): 568–80.

Bansal, V., O. Harismendy, et al. (2010). Accurate detection and genotyping of SNPs utilizing population sequencing data. Genome Res **20**(4): 537–45.

Barabási, A. L., and R. Albert (1999). Emergence of scaling in random networks. Science **286**(5439): 509–12.

Barabási, A. L., and E. Bonabeau (2003). Scale-free networks. Sci Am **288**(5): 60–69.

Barabási, A. L., N. Gulbahce, et al. (2011). Network medicine: a network-based approach to human disease. Nat Rev Genet **12**(1): 56–68.

Bates, G. P., M. E. MacDonald, et al. (1991). Defined physical limits of the Huntington disease gene candidate region. Am J Hum Genet **49**(1): 7–16.

Bendall, S. C., and G. P. Nolan (2012). From single cells to deep phenotypes in cancer. Nat Biotechnol **30**(7): 639–47.

Bick, A. G., J. Flannick, et al. (2012). Burden of rare sarcomere gene variants in the Framingham and Jackson Heart Study cohorts. Am J Hum Genet **91**(3): 513–19.

Bilder, R. M., F. W. Sabb, et al. (2009). Phenomics: the systematic study of phenotypes on a genome-wide scale. Neuroscience **164**(1): 30–42.

Boja, E., T. Hiltke, et al. (2010). Evolution of clinical proteomics and its role in medicine. J Proteome Res **10**(1): 66–84.

Brestoff, J. R., and D. Artis (2013). Commensal bacteria at the interface of host metabolism and the immune system. Nat Immunol **14**(7): 676–84.

Cannon, T. D. (2005). The inheritance of intermediate phenotypes for schizophrenia. Curr Opin Psychiatry **18**(2): 135–40.

Cannon, T. D., T. L. Gasperoni, et al. (2001). Quantitative neural indicators of liability to schizophrenia: implications for molecular genetic studies. Am J Med Genet **105**(1): 16–19.

Chen, R., and M. Snyder (2013). Promise of personalized omics to precision medicine. Wiley Interdiscip Rev Syst Biol Med **5**(1): 73–82.

Churchill, F. B. (1974). William Johannsen and the Genotype Concept. J Hist Biol **7**(1): 5–30.

Collins, F. S. (1992). Positional cloning: let's not call it reverse anymore. Nat Genet **1**(1): 3–6.

Cross-Disorder Group of the Psychiatric Genomics Consortium, C., S. H. Lee, et al. (2013). Genetic relationship between five psychiatric disorders estimated from genome-wide SNPs. Nat Genet **45**(9): 984–94.

Deo, R. C., L. Hunter, et al. (2010). Interpreting metabolomic profiles using unbiased pathway models. PLoS Comput Biol **6**(2): e1000692.

Dolan, J. P., and G. R. Holmes (1984). Some important epochs in medicine. South Med J **77**(8): 1022–26.

Doll, R., and R. Peto (1976). Mortality in relation to smoking: 20 years' observations on male British doctors. Br Med J **2**(6051): 1525–36.

Durand, C., and G. A. Rappold (2013). Height matters-from monogenic disorders to normal variation. Nat Rev Endocrinol **9**(3): 171–77.

Eichler, E. E., J. Flint, et al. (2010). Missing heritability and strategies for finding the underlying causes of complex disease. Nat Rev Genet **11**(6): 446–50.

Falconer, D. S. (1960). Introduction to Quantitative Genetics. London: Oliver and Boyd.

Flannick, J., N. L. Beer, et al. (2013). Assessing the phenotypic effects in the general population of rare variants in genes for a dominant Mendelian form of diabetes. Nat Genet **45**(11): 1380–85.

Freimer, N., and C. Sabatti (2003). The human phenome project. Nat Genet **34**(1): 15–21.

Ganesh, S. K., N. A. Zakai, et al. (2009). Multiple loci influence erythrocyte phenotypes in the CHARGE Consortium. Nat Genet **41**(11): 1191–98.

Garnaas, M. K., C. C. Cutting, et al. (2012). Rargb regulates organ laterality in a zebrafish model of right atrial isomerism. Dev Biol **372**(2): 178–89.

Garver, D. L., J. A. Holcomb, et al. (2000). Heterogeneity of response to antipsychotics from multiple disorders in the schizophrenia spectrum. J Clin Psych **61**(12): 964–72; quiz 973.

Ge, H., A. J. Walhout, et al. (2003). Integrating 'omic' information: a bridge between genomics and systems biology. Trends Genet **19**(10): 551–60.

Gerstein, M. (2012). Genomics: ENCODE leads the way on big data. Nature **489**(7415): 208.

Goh, K. I., M. E. Cusick, et al. (2007). The human disease network. Proc Natl Acad Sci U S A **104**(21): 8685–90.

Goldin, L. R., N. J. Cox, et al. (1984). The detection of major loci by segregation and linkage analysis: a simulation study. Genet Epidemiol **1**(3): 285–96.

Gonzaga-Jauregui, C., J. R. Lupski, et al. (2012). Human genome sequencing in health and disease. Annu Rev Med **63**: 35–61.

Gusella, J. F., N. S. Wexler, et al. (1983). A polymorphic DNA marker genetically linked to Huntington's disease. Nature **306**(5940): 234–38.

Hansen, J., and R. Iyengar (2013). Computation as the mechanistic bridge between precision medicine and systems therapeutics. Clin Pharmacol Ther **93**(1): 117–28.

Hill, A. B. (1965). The environment and disease: association or causation? Proc R Soc Med **58**: 295–300.

Ho, J. E., M. G. Larson, et al. (2013). Metabolite profiles during oral glucose challenge. Diabetes **62**(8): 2689–98.

Ioannidis, J. P. (2005). Why most published research findings are false. PLoS Med **2**(8): e124.

Janssens, A. C., J. P. Ioannidis, et al. (2011). Strengthening the reporting of genetic risk prediction studies: The GRIPS Statement. Ann Intern Med **154**(6): 421–25.

Jeong, H., B. Tombor, et al. (2000). The large-scale organization of metabolic networks. Nature **407**(6804): 651–54.

Jones, D. P., Y. Park, et al. (2012). Nutritional metabolomics: progress in addressing complexity in diet and health. Annu Rev Nutr **32**: 183–202.

Jones, W. H. S. (1868). Hippocrates Collected Works, Cambridge, MA: Harvard University Press.

Kastner, P., J. M. Grondona, et al. (1994). Genetic analysis of RXR alpha developmental function: convergence of RXR and RAR signaling pathways in heart and eye morphogenesis. Cell **78**(6): 987–1003.

Keating, M. T., and M. C. Sanguinetti (2001). Molecular and cellular mechanisms of cardiac arrhythmias. Cell **104**(4): 569–80.

Kemper, K. E., P. M. Visscher, et al. (2012). Genetic architecture of body size in mammals. Genome Biol **13**(4): 244.

Kumar, S., D. Alibhai, et al. (2011). FLIM FRET technology for drug discovery: automated multiwell-plate high-content analysis, multiplexed readouts and application in situ. Chemphyschem **12**(3): 609–26.

Lalouel, J. M., D. C. Rao, et al. (1983). A unified model for complex segregation analysis. Am J Hum Genet **35**(5): 816–26.

Lander, E. S., and D. Botstein (1989). Mapping mendelian factors underlying quantitative traits using RFLP linkage maps. Genetics **121**(1): 185–99.

Lanktree, M. B., Y. Guo, et al. (2011). Meta-analysis of dense genecentric association studies reveals common and uncommon variants associated with height. Am J Hum Genet **88**(1): 6–18.

Lee, T. H. (2008). The future of primary care: the need for reinvention. N Engl J Med **359**(20): 2085–86.

Leshchiner, I., K. Alexa, et al. (2012). Mutation mapping and identification by whole-genome sequencing. Genome Res **22**(8): 1541–48.

Lewis, G. D., L. Farrell, et al. (2010). Metabolic signatures of exercise in human plasma. Sci Transl Med **2**(33): 33ra37.

Lim, J., T. Hao, et al. (2006). A protein-protein interaction network for human inherited ataxias and disorders of Purkinje cell degeneration. Cell **125**(4): 801–14.

Loscalzo, J., I. Kohane, et al. (2007). Human disease classification in the postgenomic era: a complex systems approach to human pathobiology. Mol Syst Biol **3**: 124.

Lynch, M., and B. Walsh (1998). Genetics and Analysis of Quantitative Traits. Sunderland, MA: Sinauer.

MacArthur, D. G., S. Balasubramanian, et al. (2012). A systematic survey of loss-of-function variants in human protein-coding genes. Science **335**(6070): 823–28.

MacRae, C. A., and R. S. Vasan (2011). Next-generation genome-wide association studies: time to focus on phenotype? Circulation. Cardiovasc Genet **4**(4): 334–36.

Mahner, M., and M. Kary (1997). What exactly are genomes, genotypes and phenotypes? And what about phenomes? J Theor Biol **186**(1): 55–63.

Manolio, T. A., F. S. Collins, et al. (2009). Finding the missing heritability of complex diseases. Nature **461**(7265): 747–53.

Masel, J., and M. V. Trotter (2010). Robustness and evolvability. Trends Genet **26**(9): 406–14.

Mayr, E. (1982). The Growth of Biological Thought: Diversity, Evolution and Inheritance. Cambridge, The Belknap Press of Harvard University Press.

Morozova, T. V., D. Goldman, et al. (2012). The genetic basis of alcoholism: multiple phenotypes, many genes, complex networks. Genome Biol **13**(2): 239.

Osler, W. (1892). The Principles and Practice of Medicine. New York: D. Appleton.

Ostrowski, J., and L. S. Wyrwicz (2009). Integrating genomics, proteomics and bioinformatics in translational studies of molecular medicine. Expert Rev Mol Diagn 9(6): 623–30.

Oti, M., and H. G. Brunner (2007). The modular nature of genetic diseases. Clin Genet 71(1): 1–11.

Oti, M., M. A. Huynen, et al. (2009). The biological coherence of human phenome databases. Am J Hum Genet 85(6): 801–8.

Park, E., B. Williams, et al. (2012). RNA editing in the human ENCODE RNA-seq data. Genome Res 22(9): 1626–33.

Peck, D., E. D. Crawford, et al. (2006). A method for high-throughput gene expression signature analysis. Genome Biol 7(7): R61.

Peterson, R. T., and C. A. MacRae (2012). Systematic approaches to toxicology in the zebrafish. Annu Rev Pharmacol Toxicol 52: 433–53.

Poduri, A., G. D. Evrony, et al. (2013). Somatic mutation, genomic variation, and neurological disease. Science 341(6141): 1237758.

Popper, K. R. (1959). The Logic of Scientific Discovery. London: Hutchison.

Pott, P. (1775). Chirurgical Observations Relative to the Cataract, the Polypus of the Nose, the Cancer of the Scrotum, the Different Kinds of Ruptures, and the Mortification of the Toes and Feet. London: Printed by T. J. Carnegy, for L. Hawes, W. Clarke, and R. Collins.

Praneenararat, T., T. Takagi, et al. (2012). Integration of interactive, multi-scale network navigation approach with Cytoscape for functional genomics in the big data era. BMC Genomics 13 Suppl 7: S24.

Raamsdonk, L. M., B. Teusink, et al. (2001). A functional genomics strategy that uses metabolome data to reveal the phenotype of silent mutations. Nat Biotechnol 19(1): 45–50.

Rikke, B. A., and T. E. Johnson (1998). Towards the cloning of genes underlying murine QTLs. Mamm Genome 9(12): 963–68.

Risch, N. J. (2000). Searching for genetic determinants in the new millennium. Nature 405(6788): 847–56.

Robinson, P. N., E. Arteaga-Solis, et al. (2006). The molecular genetics of Marfan syndrome and related disorders. J Med Genet 43(10): 769–87.

Robinson, P. N., and S. Mundlos (2010). The human phenotype ontology. Clin Genet 77(6): 525–34.

Roden, D. M., R. B. Altman, et al. (2006). Pharmacogenomics: challenges and opportunities. Ann Intern Med 145(10): 749–57.

Rual, J. F., J. Ceron, et al. (2004). Toward improving Caenorhabditis elegans phenome mapping with an ORFeome-based RNAi library. Genome Res 14(10B): 2162–68.

Scythes, J. B., and C. M. Jones (2013). Syphilis in the AIDS era: diagnostic dilemma and therapeutic challenge. Acta Microbiol Immunol Hung 60(2): 93–116.

Seidman, J. G., and C. Seidman (2001). The genetic basis for cardiomyopathy: from mutation identification to mechanistic paradigms. Cell 104(4): 557–67.

Sharon, I., and J. F. Banfield (2013). Microbiology: genomes from metagenomics. Science 342(6162): 1057–58.

Shaw, S. Y., D. M. Blodgett, et al. (2011). Disease allele-dependent small-molecule sensitivities in blood cells from monogenic diabetes. Proc Natl Acad Sci U S A 108(2): 492–97.

Shaw, S. Y., E. C. Westly, et al. (2008). Perturbational profiling of nanomaterial biologic activity. Proc Natl Acad Sci U S A 105(21): 7387–92.

Shimizu, W., A. J. Moss, et al. (2009). Genotype-phenotype aspects of type 2 long QT syndrome. J Am Coll Cardiol 54(22): 2052–62.

Singer, E. (2005). Phenome project set to pin down subgroups of autism. Nat Med 11(6): 583.

Snow, J. (1855). On the Mode of Communication of Cholera. London: John Churchill.

Solovieff, N., C. Cotsapas, et al. (2013). Pleiotropy in complex traits: challenges and strategies. Nat Rev Genet 14(7): 483–95.

Sucov, H. M., E. Dyson, et al. (1994). RXR alpha mutant mice establish a genetic basis for vitamin A signaling in heart morphogenesis. Genes Dev 8(9): 1007–18.

Talbot, C. J., A. Nicod, et al. (1999). High-resolution mapping of quantitative trait loci in outbred mice. Nat Genet 21(3): 305–8.

Talbott, J. H. (1961). French's Index of Differential Diagnosis. JAMA 175(3): 259.

Taubes, G. (1995). Epidemiology faces its limits. Science 269(5221): 164–69.

Temporini, C., E. Calleri, et al. (2008). Integrated analytical strategies for the study of phosphorylation and glycosylation in proteins. Mass Spectrom Rev 27(3): 207–36.

Tewari, M., P. J. Hu, et al. (2004). Systematic interactome mapping and genetic perturbation analysis of a C. elegans TGF-beta signaling network. Mol Cell 13(4): 469–82.

Trusheim, M. R., B. Burgess, et al. (2011). Quantifying factors for the success of stratified medicine. Nat Rev Drug Discov 10(11): 817–33.x

Walhout, A. J., J. Reboul, et al. (2002). Integrating interactome, phenome, and transcriptome mapping data for the C. elegans germline. Curr Biol 12(22): 1952–58.

Wang, T. J., M. G. Larson, et al. (2011). Metabolite profiles and the risk of developing diabetes. Nat Med 17(4): 448–53.

Wang, Z., E. Klipfell, et al. (2011). Gut flora metabolism of phosphatidylcholine promotes cardiovascular disease. Nature 472(7341): 57–63.

Watkins, D. A., N. Hendricks, et al. (2009). Clinical features, survival experience, and profile of plakophylin-2 gene mutations in participants of the arrhythmogenic right ventricular cardiomyopathy registry of South Africa. Heart Rhythm 6(11 Suppl): S10–7.

Weckwerth, W., and K. Morgenthal (2005). Metabolomics: from pattern recognition to biological interpretation. Drug Discov Today 10(22): 1551–58.

Williams-Blangero, S., C. D. Criscione, et al. (2012). Host genetics and population structure effects on parasitic disease. Philos Trans R Soc Lond B Biol Sci 367(1590): 887–94.

Wolf, Y. I., G. Karev, et al. (2002). Scale-free networks in biology: new insights into the fundamentals of evolution? Bioessays 24(2): 105–9.

Woolfe, A., M. Goodson, et al. (2005). Highly conserved non-coding sequences are associated with vertebrate development. PLoS Biol 3(1): e7.

6

A New Paradigm for Defining
Human Disease and Therapy

JOSEPH LOSCALZO

Introduction

The reductionist approach to scientific discovery has dominated modern Western thought, and has been successful in the quest to understand observable phenomena. This fundamental principle of scientific investigation has also dominated biomedical research, and has led to the identification of causative mechanisms of and effective therapeutic approaches for many diseases. Yet, as we move into the realm of increasingly complex, chronic diseases, this straightforward approach fails to provide the insight needed to explain disease pathogenesis. In addition, drug discovery, tied as it is to the purely reductionist principle of single drug target identification and validation, has been waning despite great advances in the fields of structural biology and bioinformatics. Owing to these limitations, it is prudent to consider alternative approaches to understanding disease and therapeutics. Network medicine offers such an approach.

Background

Network medicine is a rapidly evolving, new field that strives to apply network science and systems biology principles to disease mechanism and to pharmacotherapeutics (Barabási, Gulbahce, et al. 2011; Silverman and Loscalzo 2013). This field first arose in an effort to address the increasingly obvious shortcomings of conventional disease definition and disease pathogenesis (Loscalzo, Kohane, et al. 2007). Modern definitions of disease have their origins in the late nineteenth century, at which time Osler first applied the principle of clinicopathological correlation to pathogenesis. This approach involved characterizing and categorizing clinical signs and symptoms, then linking those observations to abnormalities observed at autopsy. As a result, what had previously been vaguely contrived descriptions of illness, such as "ague" or "dropsy," could be explained often as being caused by different relatively specific disease processes generally affecting a single organ. This Oslerian approach to disease classification became widespread, and it served as the organizational basis for textbooks of medicine, departments of medicine, and departments of pathology worldwide. Furthermore, this organ-based focus of disease also served as the driving principle underlying basic research into disease pathogenesis at the physiological, biochemical, and molecular levels. Biomedical research into disease was ever in search of the cause (or a limited number of causes) of pathogenic processes as complicated as myocardial infarction, heart failure, or cirrhosis.

This clinical and scientific enterprise in understanding the mechanistic basis of disease was quite successful throughout the previous century, leading to the identification of causes for many complex diseases and to the identification of potential drug targets for those diseases. As a result, the general health of the developed world's population improved with reduced morbidity and mortality, and enhanced longevity.

Yet with this success came the growing realization that there are, to be sure, many shortcomings of this approach to disease characterization. It relies on clinical, rather than preclinical, disease manifestations, often in a single organ system, and often at a point in the course of the disease that nears the end stage. At this stage of any disease process, the drivers of disease expression are not specific to the disease, but represent later-stage mechanisms that underlie all disease—the intermediate (patho)phenotypes of inflammation and immune response, thrombosis or hemorrhage, fibrosis, apoptosis, and cell proliferation. As such, many different diseases may be expressed with common clinical phenotypes—end-stage liver disease in patients who initially were exposed to a hepatotoxin and in patients who were initially infected with hepatitis B virus, or pathological cardiac hypertrophy in patients with mutations in sarcomeric proteins and in patients with a mutant protein kinase, AMP-activated, gamma 2 (PRKAG2) noncatalytic subunit of AMP kinase. Similar reasoning leads to the conclusion that many so-called specific disease therapies actually focus on these common intermediate pathobiological mechanisms rather than on the specific underlying disease determinants, such as the use of antithrombotics in acute myocardial infarction, or the use of anti–tumor necrosis factor therapies for rheumatoid arthritis.

Even classic Mendelian disorders suffer from the shortcomings of reductionism, limiting its usefulness in defining disease presentation. Sickle-cell anemia is one such example. In this disorder, there is homozygosity for a mutation at the sixth position of the hemoglobin beta-chain in which valine substitutes for a glutamic acid, producing hemoglobin S. This form of hemoglobin is susceptible to polymerization under hypoxic conditions, yielding the characteristic change in the shape of the erythrocyte. If Mendelian rules applied, one would expect that all patients with this mutation would have an identical pheno-type. This is not the case. Patients with sickle-cell anemia can present clinically with anemia, hemolytic crisis, acute thrombotic stroke, pulmonary hyperten-sion, acute bone infarction, acute painful crisis, etc. Thus, the lack of correlation between even this straightforward and very well characterized Mendelian ge-netic disorder and its clinical manifestations argues for the need to explore the consequences of disease-causing alleles within the genetic, molecular, and en-vironmental context of a given individual.

Principles of Network Medicine

With the growth of large data sets comprising detailed and comprehensive in-formation about the genome, the transcriptome, the proteome, the metabolome, and the exposome, biomedical research has reached a stage at which a specific disease-causing event can be explored and understood in integrated context. Doing so requires mining these data sets for physical or mechanistic associations among them that comprise the molecular network within which a disease-causing molecular mediator(s) operates to produce a pathophenotype. Network medicine has as its basic operating tenet the identification of disease networks or disease modules within networks responsible for specific pathophenotypes.

To date, -omic datasets have been used to derive simple associations between molecular variants and disease phenotypes. Genome-wide association studies serve as the best example of this straightforward approach and are now viewed as rather limited in the insight they have provided. This conclusion should not be surprising if one considers the importance of the network context within which a variant operates. Simple statistical association studies, if they identify candidate loci or alleles for complex disease traits, typically find that these loci have small effect sizes, raising the concern that such loci are not necessarily important for disease pathogenesis. One can argue, however, that these loci may well have more powerful effects if their function were explored in the network within which they operate. One can, therefore, view genome-wide association studies as providing the "parts list" of potentially important functional variants; however, the assembly diagram is required to appreciate how these variants may affect function or cause dysfunction and disease. Early efforts to explore the net-work context of genes identified by genome-wide association studies for com-plex human diseases have met with some success in identifying genes within the network neighborhood of the gene identified by genome-wide association, and in identifying genes common to different diseases defined by the classic Osle-rian approach (Goh, Cusick, et al. 2007; Barrenas, Chavali, et al. 2009); yet true insight into fundamental disease-causing modules within these networks re-quires a different approach.

Network modeling can be approached either statically or dynamically. Static modeling focuses only on network architecture or topology, generally without regard for the directionality of a link between nodes, the strength of association, or the changes in node expression or activity as a function of network perturbation. Dynamic modeling in the extreme requires knowledge of the formal kinetics and kinetic constants, as well as reaction stoichiometry, for a deterministic approach using systems of nonlinear ordinary differential equations of the form:

$$\frac{d(S)(t)}{dt} = Nv(S,k)$$

where $dS(t)/dt$ refers to the time derivative of the concentration vector for all species in the pathway or network, N is the stoichiometry matrix for all reactions in the pathway or network, and $v(S,k)$ is the flux vector defined by the rate constants (k) governing all reactions in the pathway or network. This approach has had its greatest success in modeling biochemical networks and pathways and, in a more limited way, transcriptional network dynamics. Simulation of network dynamics can provide, for example, an approach for defining stable operating ranges of the network with regard to substrate availability (using ordinary differential equations) or transcription factor activity (using stochastic differential equations given the limited [at least two] number of potential *cis*-binding sites for any given transcription factors).

Static modeling serves as the framework within which disease-determining nodes or modules of nodes are identified and requires only identification of the links between nodes indicative of a physical or functional association. Between these two extremes are approaches that are semiquantitative, yielding information on system dynamics that is not fully deterministic but provides a range of possible solutions owing to limitations in the initial conditions and solution space constraints; these include flux balance analysis and structural kinetic modeling (Figure 6–1). For the purpose of this discussion, we will focus only on static networks.

Networks, Disease Genes/Gene Products, and Disease Modules

Identifying disease modules within networks must begin by first defining the network. The ideal network is one that represents all known interactions between gene products, their metabolite substrates and products, and their post-translationally modified derivatives. Curation of the scientific literature has offered one approach to creating the protein–protein interaction network; however, it is not without its shortcomings, which stem largely from the biases intrinsic to the published literature (Cusick, Yu, et al. 2009). Owing to these

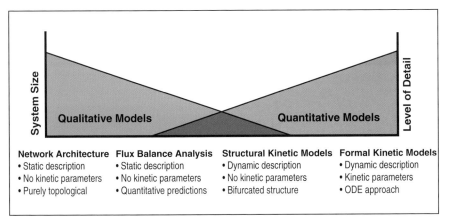

FIGURE 6–1. General approaches to network modeling. Qualitative models and quantitative models are represented, with the comparative level of detail required for each. ODE, ordinary differential equation.

important limitations, unbiased approaches have been adopted that utilize yeast two- and three-hybrid screening with immunoprecipitation and mass spectrometry (Ewing, Chu, et al. 2007; Vidal, Cusick, et al. 2011) to create a comprehensive protein–protein interactome to serve as the basis for identifying novel disease pathways or modules. In our own work, my colleagues and I have attempted to assemble all known physical interactions from a wide variety of sources, which include the following:

(i) protein–protein interactions from three yeast two-hybrid datasets with IntAct (Kerrien, Aranda, et al. 2012) and MINT (Ceol, Chatr Aryamontri, et al. 2010) databases, the sum of which yields 15,315 interactions between 6101 proteins; note that the IntAct and MINT databases provide interactions derived from the curated literature and direct submission;

(ii) literature-curated protein–protein interactions documented by low-throughput experiments, imported from IntAct (Kerrien, Aranda, et al. 2012), MINT (Ceol, Chatr Aryamontri, et al. 2010), BioGrid (Stark, Breitkreutz, et al. 2011), and HPRD (Prasad, Kandasamy, et al. 2009) yielding 10,890 nodes and 74,195 links;

(iii) protein–DNA regulatory interactions from the TRANSFAC database to capture all experimentally demonstrated regulatory interactions, which includes 271 human transcription factors and 564 regulated genes (TRANSFAC 2008.2);

(iv) metabolic enzyme–coupled interactions from the KEGG and BIGG databases; metabolic coupling exists if two enzymes share substrates,

products, or substrate-product couples in these databases, leading to
the addition of 10,642 links between 921 enzymes;

(v) protein complexes from the CORUM database, which is an experimentally verified collection of mammalian protein complexes manually extracted from the literature, yielding 2837 protein complexes
with 2069 proteins connected by 31,276 links (Ruepp, Waegele, et al.
2009); and

(vi) kinase–substrate pairs from the PhosphositePlus, which provides a
network of the best-studied form of post-translational modification,
protein phosphorylation, which yields 327 kinases linked to 1771
substrates (http://www.phosphosite.org).

The resulting network consists of 141,296 interactions (links or edges) between
13,460 gene products. While reasonably comprehensive, it remains incomplete,
incorporating only one form of post-translational modification of the >300
recognized modifications, and excluding epigenetic modifications and interactions with noncoding RNAs. It is also prone to false positives and false nega-
tives and is not without bias given the inclusion of datasets that are derived
from the curated literature. Yet it is the most comprehensive set of interactions
constructed to date and has been used to identify disease modules, as illustrated
below. This interactome displays significant clustering with regions of very dense
interconnectedness, and manifests scale-free topology (see Chapter 2). Owing to
the density of clusters, at most, only a few links separate any node from any
other node. This network structure suggests that perturbations of a single node
can evoke wide-ranging effects through multiple modules, leading to significant consequences for functional (patho)phenotypes.

The identification of the disease module(s) within a network requires first
that one recognize that genes governing chronic, complex diseases are typically nonessential and generally weakly linked within the interactome-derived
network (Figure 6–2). In addition, it requires that one can distinguish among
three types of network modules: topological, or modules that are defined
purely by proximity of nodes to one another; functional, or modules that
comprise nodes with common functional consequences, often acting through
a common pathway; and disease, or modules that reflect altered functional
consequences owing to changes in the behavior of a (mutant) node, the loss of
a links between normally functioning nodes, or the development of new links
between nodes leading to novel, dysfunctional module activities (Figure 6–3).

To construct the disease network (Figure 6–4), one can begin with a collection of
genes or gene products from the curated literature or from unbiased expression

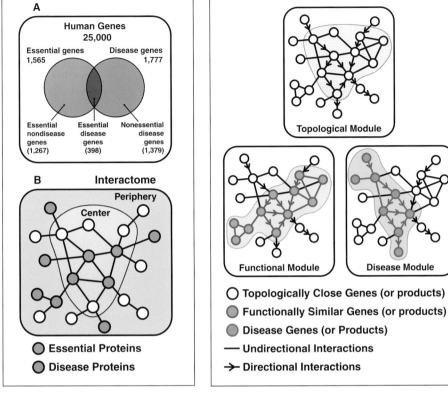

FIGURE 6–2. Essential and disease proteins. A, The relationship between essential (blue) and nonessential (orange) genes (proteins) and disease is illustrated in the Venn diagram. B, Complex, chronic diseases tend to be associated with genes that are nonessential and that are only weakly linked within the interactome. (Reprinted with permission from Barabási, A. L., N. Gulbahce, et al. (2011). Network medicine: a network-based approach to human disease. Nat Rev Genet 12(1): 56–68.)

FIGURE 6–3. Modules within biological networks. Topological modules are subnetworks that are contiguous within the overall network. Functional modules are subnetworks whose links reflect functional consequences, often comprising a definable pathway. Disease modules are subnetworks that may have functional consequences owing to new or altered links between (dys)functional modules. (Reprinted with permission from Barabási, A. L., N. Gulbahce, et al. (2011). Network medicine: a network-based approach to human disease. Nat Rev Genet 12(1): 56–68.)

datasets that appear to distinguish individuals with the disease from those without. This collection of nodes is then mapped onto the consolidated interactome to create the disease network. This approach has been used by us to create the disease network for pulmonary arterial hypertension (Figure 6–5A), and led to the discovery of a novel disease module linking bone morphogenetic protein receptor 2 to interleukin-6 and the rho B/rho kinase pathway via microRNA-21 (Parikh, Jin, et al. 2012) (Figure 6–5C). Doing so required that we use the pool of microRNAs whose expression changes in hypoxia as a filter that provided insight into new linkages among two genes that were orphaned in the original disease network, rhoB

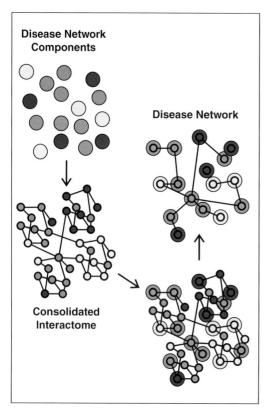

FIGURE 6–4. Disease network derivation. Network components (nodes), derived from the curated literature or from unbiased expression datasets, are mapped onto the consolidated interactome to define the disease network.

and interleukin-6 (Figure 6–5B). In this analysis, we exploited the concept that microRNAs whose expression changes in response to a stress tend to have common mRNA targets and/or common pathway members as targets.

Other approaches to identifying novel disease genes through network analysis are illustrated in Figure 6–6 (Chan and Loscalzo 2012). These approaches include strategies that identify novel disease genes through their direct interaction with known disease genes (linkage-based), by their presence in a disease module (disease module–based), or by their presence in modules or pathways that are in the proximate neighborhood of a known disease module (diffusion-based). By identifying the network location of novel disease genes, the disease network is enriched and potential novel links identified through which disease modules can be characterized more thoroughly.

The Interactome and Relationships between Diseases

The comprehensive interactome can be used not only as a means for identifying novel relationships among disease genes in specific disease modules, but also as a blueprint for identifying the relationships between diseases. This analysis is particularly relevant because many canonically distinct diseases have common mechanisms, co-occur in the same individual, and can be effectively treated with common therapeutic strategies. Proteins common to different diseases tend to localize to similar neighborhoods in the interactome. The higher the degree of localization, the greater the biological similarity of the disease genes, supporting the notion of well-localized disease modules in the interactome. Topology, then, clearly recapitulates functionality within a disease. In addition and importantly, however, is the more generalizable finding that the network-based, interactome-defined location of a disease also determines its pathobiological relationship to other diseases. Topologically overlapping diseases show signifi-

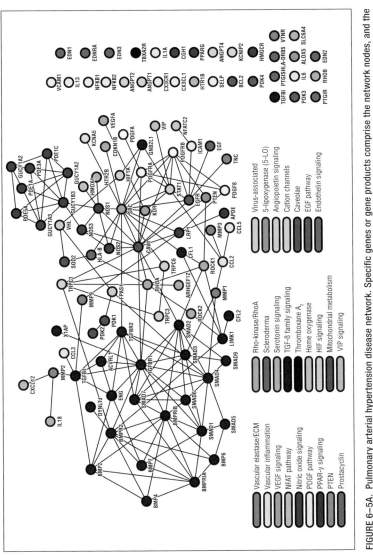

FIGURE 6–5A. Pulmonary arterial hypertension disease network. Specific genes or gene products comprise the network nodes, and the links among them are defined by their position within the consolidated interactome. Functional pathways and known disease pathways are illustrated by color codes, the key for which is contained within the figure. Unconnected (orphaned) nodes on the right of the figure indicate genes or gene products known to be associated with the disease, but without (yet) known links within the disease network. (Reprinted with permission from Parikh, V. N., R. C. Jin, et al. (2012). MicroRNA-21 integrates pathogenic signaling to control pulmonary hypertension: results of a network bioinformatics approach. Circulation **125**(12): 1520–32.)

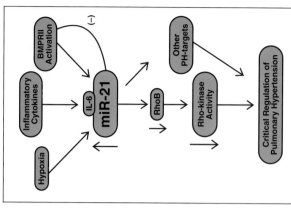

FIGURE 6–5C. A disease module for pulmonary arterial hypertension. Dashed lines indicate sites of incorporation of the previously orphaned proteins (IL6 and RhoB) in the module. (Reprinted with permission from Parikh, V. N., R. C. Jin, et al. (2012). MicroRNA-21 integrates pathogenic signaling to control pulmonary hypertension: results of a network bioinformatics approach. Circulation 125(12): 1520–32.)

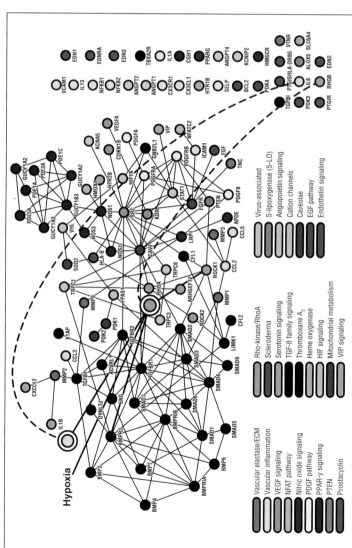

FIGURE 6–5B. Incorporation of two orphaned proteins (IL6 and RhoB) in pulmonary arterial hypertension network through microRNA-based filtering. (Adapted with permission from Parikh, V. N., R. C. Jin, et al. (2012). MicroRNA-21 integrates pathogenic signaling to control pulmonary hypertension: results of a network bioinformatics approach. Circulation 125(12): 1520–32.)

cant gene co-expression, symptoms
similarity, and comorbidity, while
topologically distinct and separated
diseases do not (Menche, Sharma,
et al. 2015). This point is illustrated in
Figure 6–7 for multiple sclerosis, rheumatoid arthritis, and peroxisomal
disorders.

Networks and Therapeutics

Despite increased data sets of potential drug targets and their structural
characterization, drug discovery
has been waning for over a decade
(Loscalzo 2012). In part, this limitation is a consequence of the reductionist approach to discovery, which
seeks a single molecular cause for each
disease that can be targeted with an
Ehrlichian magic bullet. As Figure 6–8
illustrates, however, studying drug targets out of network context is fraught
with challenges, ranging from failing
to appreciate effects that are not as-
sayed in the typical target assay, to the

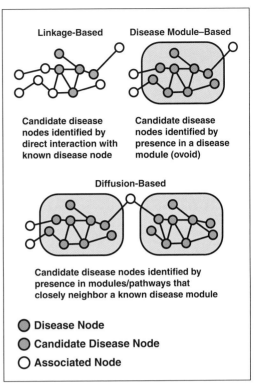

FIGURE 6–6. Discovery of novel disease genes using disease networks. (Reprinted with permission from Chan, S. Y., and J. Loscalzo. (2012). The emerging paradigm of network medicine in the study of human disease. Circ Res 111(3): 359–74.)

potential for unrealized benefits (or toxicities) as a consequence of effects of the
drug against other targets in the network. For these reasons, it is no surprise that
drug discovery strategies that focus on phenotype screening are almost twice as
successful as those that focus on target-based screening, even in the current era
(Swinney and Anthony 2011).

From a network medicine perspective, drugs can be viewed similarly to gene
or gene product variants: they perturb network topology and/or function and, as
such, understanding their actions in network context provides the greatest opportunity for optimal therapeutic restoration of network function (therapeutic
homeostasis) (see Chapter 14). In Figure 6–9, drugs are viewed as network pertur-
bants that can affect the robustness (or ability to withstand perturbations—in
this case by disease agents) of a (cellular) system in response to a disease agent. As
shown in the figure, ideally, a drug affects the pathophenotype landscape to restore homeostasis when diseased or to maintain homeostasis in the face of potential disease stress, preventing its expression. In this paradigm, drugs can also

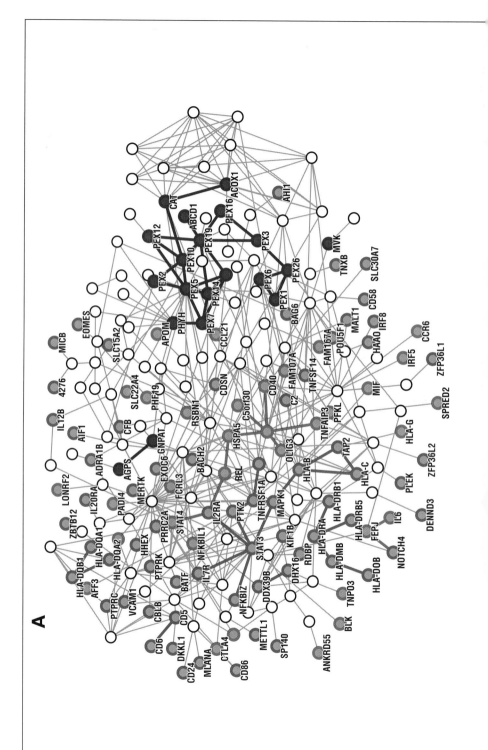

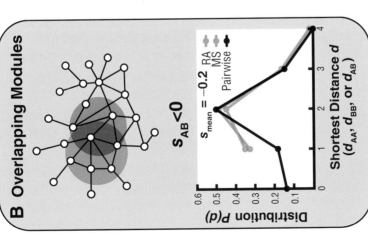

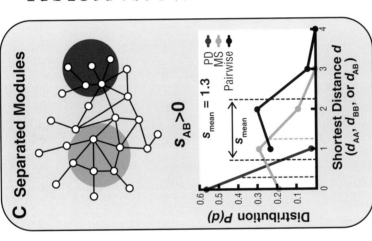

FIGURE 6-7. Network-based interactome-defined relationships between diseases. A, Subnetworks of the full interactome are depicted for multiple sclerosis (blue), peroxisomal disorders (red), and rheumatoid arthritis (orange). B, Quantitation of the overlap of the subnetworks for multiple sclerosis (MS) and rheumatoid arthritis (RA) is illustrated by a Venn diagram (top), where s_{AB} is the network-based separation for a disease pair, A and B, and is defined as $\langle d_{AB} \rangle - (\langle d_{AA} \rangle + \langle d_{BB} \rangle)/2)$, where $\langle d_{AA} \rangle$ and $\langle d_{BB} \rangle$ are the average values for the shortest distances between proteins *within* each disease, A and B, respectively, and $\langle d_{AB} \rangle$ is the average value for the shortest distances between proteins *between* each disease ($s_{AB} < 0$ indicates overlap); and graphically (bottom) by calculating the probability distribution [$P(d)$] as a function of the shortest separation distances. C, Quantitation of the separation of the subnetworks for peroxisomal disorders (PD) and multiple sclerosis (MS) is similarly illustrated by a Venn diagram (top) ($s_{AB} > 0$ indicates no overlap or separation); and graphically (bottom) by calculating the probability distribution [$P(d)$] as a function of the shortest separation distances. (Adapted with permission from AAAS from Menche, J., A. Sharma, et al. (2015). Disease networks: uncovering disease-disease relationships through the incomplete interactome. Science 347(6224): 1257601.)

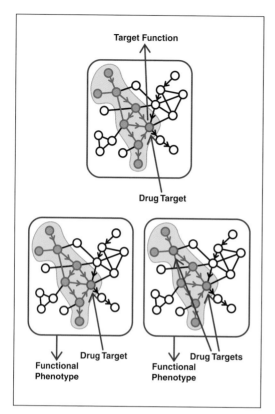

FIGURE 6–8. Drug targets in networks. The top panel demonstrates the conventional approach to drug target identification, in which target function is assessed without regard for its network context. The left panel demonstrates the advantages of phenotype-based, rather than target-based, assessment of drug evaluation. The right panel illustrates a theoretical model within which a drug affects more than one target in a module, the combined effects of which affect phenotype. The disease module is shaded yellow in each panel. (Adapted with permission from Barabási, A. L., N. Gulbahce, et al. (2011). Network medicine: a network-based approach to human disease. Nat Rev Genet **12**(1): 56–68.)

yield system dysfunction and cell death in the worst case (Csermely, Korcsmaros, et al. 2013).

Conclusion

With the advent of modern -omics and the continued expansion of the molecular datasets that are associated with health and disease, biomedicine is undergoing a radical transformation in the diagnostic and therapeutic approach to disease. Rather than simply seeking direct associations between a single effector or pathway that can be analyzed and a specific disease, the field is now presented with the opportunity to explore the integrated molecular underpinnings of disease. To do so requires a very different approach from the reductionist experimentation that has guided the field for more than two centuries. Network medicine is such an approach. It combines elements of systems biology and network science in order to define the complex interactions among molecular determinants of disease phenotypes in an unbiased and integrated manner.

Armed with this integrative map of molecular interactions, network medicine strategies facilitate the unbiased identification of novel disease pathways and modules, and provide support for rational approaches to therapeutics, including rational polypharmacy. As the human interactome becomes increasingly enriched with the growth of more comprehensive datasets, the predictive utility of network medicine will increase significantly, ultimately providing optimal precision in our approach to all human disease.

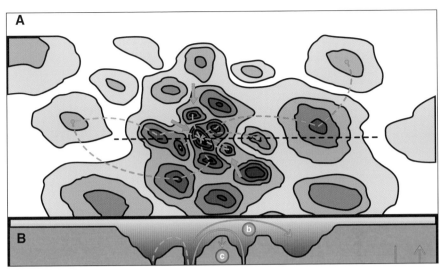

FIGURE 6–9. Drug action and robustness. A, Two-dimensional plot of stability landscape of healthy states, represented by the central and adjacent two minima indicated by orange arrows, and diseased states (all other minima). Thin blue and orange arrows indicate shifts to healthy and disease states, respectively. Dashed arrows refer to less probable state shifts. B, Effect of drug action on robustness. The hills and valleys are representations in the third dimensions of the stability landscape in A along the horizontal black dashed line. Blue symbols refer to drug interactions with disease-prone or affected cells, and orange symbols refer to drug actions on the disease agents (e.g., infective agents, malignant cells). a, counteracting regulatory feedback; b, positive feedback driving the disease agent to another trajectory; c, transient decrease in a specific reaction or pathway restoring a healthy state; d, error-catastrophe, drug action affecting many reactions or pathways, leading to cellular instability and death; e, general increase in (multiple) pathway actions serving as safeguard against disease agent. (Reprinted with permission from Csermely, P., T. Korcsmaros, et al. (2013). Structure and dynamics of molecular networks: a novel paradigm of drug discovery: a comprehensive review. Pharmacol Ther **138**(3): 333–408. © 2013 Elsevier Inc.)

References

Barabási, A. L., N. Gulbahce, et al. (2011). Network medicine: a network-based approach to human disease. Nat Rev Genet **12**(1): 56–68.

Barrenas, F., S. Chavali, et al. (2009). Network properties of complex human disease genes identified through genome-wide association studies. PLoS One **4**(11): e8090.

Ceol, A., A. Chatr Aryamontri, et al. (2010). MINT, the molecular interaction database: 2009 update. Nucleic Acids Res **38**(Database issue): D532–9.

Chan, S. Y., and J. Loscalzo (2012). The emerging paradigm of network medicine in the study of human disease. Circ Res **111**(3): 359–74.

Csermely, P., T. Korcsmaros, et al. (2013). Structure and dynamics of molecular networks: a novel paradigm of drug discovery: a comprehensive review. Pharmacol Ther **138**(3): 333–408.

Cusick, M. E., H. Yu, et al. (2009). Literature-curated protein interaction datasets. Nat Methods **6**(1): 39–46.

Ewing, R. M., P. Chu, et al. (2007). Large-scale mapping of human protein-protein interactions by mass spectrometry. Mol Syst Biol **3**: 89.

Goh, K. I., M. E. Cusick, et al. (2007). The human disease network. Proc Natl Acad Sci U S A **104**(21): 8685–90.

Kerrien, S., B. Aranda, et al. (2012). The IntAct molecular interaction database in 2012. Nucleic Acids Res **40**(Database issue): D841–46.

Loscalzo, J. (2012). Personalized cardiovascular medicine and drug development: time for a new paradigm. Circulation **125**(4): 638–45.

Loscalzo, J., I. Kohane, et al. (2007). Human disease classification in the postgenomic era: a complex systems approach to human pathobiology. Mol Syst Biol **3:** 124.

Menche, J., A. Sharma, et al. (2015). Disease networks: uncovering disease-disease relationships through the incomplete interactome. Science **347**(6224): 1257601.

Parikh, V. N., R. C. Jin, et al. (2012). MicroRNA-21 integrates pathogenic signaling to control pulmonary hypertension: results of a network bioinformatics approach. Circulation **125**(12): 1520–32.

Prasad, T. S., K. Kandasamy, et al. (2009). Human Protein Reference Database and Human Proteinpedia as discovery tools for systems biology. Methods Mol Biol **577:** 67–79.

Ruepp, A., B. Waegele, et al. (2009). CORUM: the comprehensive resource of mammalian protein complexes—2009. Nucleic Acids Res **38**(Database issue): D497–501.

Silverman, E. K., and J. Loscalzo (2013). Developing new drug treatments in the era of network medicine. Clin Pharmacol Ther **93**(1): 26–28.

Stark, C., B. J. Breitkreutz, et al. (2011). The BioGRID Interaction Database: 2011 update. Nucleic Acids Res **39**(Database issue): D698–704.

Swinney, D. C., and J. Anthony (2011). How were new medicines discovered? Nat Rev Drug Discov **10**(7): 507–19.

Vidal, M., M. E. Cusick, et al. (2011). Interactome networks and human disease. Cell **144**(6): 986–98.

7

Complex Disease Genetics and Network Medicine

EDWIN K. SILVERMAN

Introduction

Many leading public health problems, such as asthma, coronary artery disease, and stroke, are complex diseases that are influenced by multiple genetic and environmental factors acting and interacting within a developmental context. If a complex disease is influenced by genetic factors, relatives should be more likely to have the disease than nonrelatives; thus, identifying familial aggregation is an important first step in demonstrating that genetic determinants are likely involved in complex disease pathogenesis (Figure 7–1). For Mendelian disorders, positional cloning studies based on linkage analysis of affected relatives within pedigrees have been quite successful in identifying disease genes; however, this approach has not worked well for complex diseases. Selection of candidate genes based on known biological pathways led to a small number of successes in complex disease genetics (e.g., factor V Leiden in thromboembolic disease), but the number of false-positive reports far outnumbered the validated success stories. Genome-wide association studies (GWAS), enabled by the technological advances that made reliable genotyping of hundreds of thousands of single-nucleotide polymorphisms (SNPs) a feasible study design, have led to many genetic associations that withstand the stringent multiple statistical testing corrections involved in analyzing so many SNPs (Lander 2011). As DNA sequencing costs continue to fall, rare variant studies based on whole-exome or whole-genome DNA sequencing are becoming increasingly important. Whole-genome sequencing identified an uncommon genetic variant in the *EN1* gene significantly associated with bone mineral density (Zheng, Forgetta, et al. 2015); the effect size of this variant was substantially larger than the previously reported GWAS associations for this phenotype. No matter which study design is used, the initial goal of a complex disease gene identification effort is to find the general location of the complex disease determinant or determinants. Subsequent work to identify functional genetic variants could lead to new diagnostic tests, an accurate assessment of the contribution of that genetic locus to disease

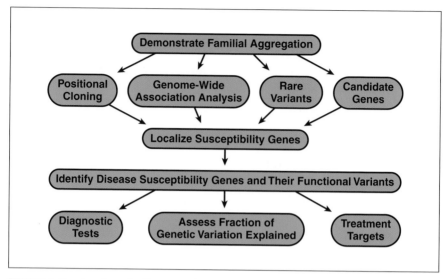

FIGURE 7–1. Overview of complex disease genetics. After demonstrating that a disease clusters in families, approaches to localize the susceptibility genes for a complex disease include positional cloning using linkage analysis, genome-wide association analysis, resequencing or genotyping to assess rare genetic variants, and candidate-gene studies. Further work is required to identify the disease-related gene and its functional genetic variants.

variability, and mechanistic insights that could provide treatment targets. Nelson and colleagues suggested that genetic evidence for a particular drug target's involvement in disease pathogenesis substantially increased the likelihood of that target leading to an FDA-approved drug; while only 2% of all drug targets studied in Phase 1 clinical studies had any genetic support (from the Online Mendelian Inheritance in Man [OMIM] database or GWAS results), 8% of drug targets for approved drugs had some genetic support (Nelson, Tipney, et al., 2015). These results suggest that providing comprehensive assessment of complex disease genetic determinants can assist in the optimal selection of drug targets for new therapies.

Because genes act in a network context, genetic variants can be viewed as perturbations of the cellular molecular interactome network. Vidal and colleagues have interrogated the impact of genetic variants on the interactome using Yeast 2-hybrid assessments (Charloteaux, Zhong, et al. 2011). As shown in Figure 7–2, particular genetic variants could have no effect on interacting gene or protein partners; loss of all interaction edges (i.e., network node removal); loss of some, but not all, interactions of the wild-type allele (an "edgetic" effect); or change in the strength of interactions within the network. As we will discuss, assessment of multiple -omics technologies, such as transcriptomics, proteomics, and metabolomics, can be combined with genetic analysis in a network frame-work to provide insight into complex disease pathogenesis.

Limitations of Complex Disease Studies

The explosion of successful GWAS has provided strong evidence for common genetic determinants of many complex diseases (Manolio, Brooks, et al. 2008). Genetic loci identified by GWAS typically have modest odds ratios and, thus, individual GWAS loci have not been very useful for predicting disease risk. Such loci may still point to important biological pathways (Wang, Baldassano, et al. 2010). However, for most complex diseases, a large percentage of heritability—the fraction of the total phenotypic variation attributed to genetic causes—remains unexplained (Manolio, Collins, et al. 2009). Possible explanations for this missing her-

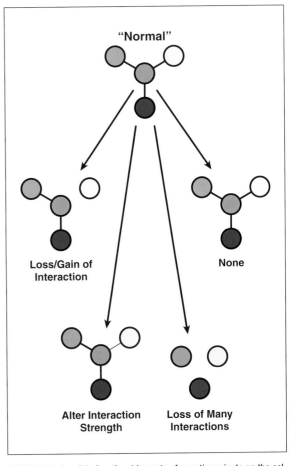

FIGURE 7–2. Possible functional impacts of genetic variants on the cellular molecular interactome network. In this simple hypothetical network of four nodes representing genes or proteins, the perturbations related to genetic variants range in impact from loss of one or more interactions to alteration in interaction strength to no effect.

itability include the potential for large numbers of additional common and rare genetic determinants to be identified (Table 7–1). However, the estimation of complex disease heritability under the assumptions that gene–gene (epistatic) and gene–environment interactions are not present leads to potentially biased estimates of heritability. Zuk and colleagues suggested that epistatic effects could account for much of the missing heritability in complex diseases (Zuk, Hechter, et al. 2012). They argued that the estimation of total narrow sense heritability, which is typically based on assuming additive genetic contributions without interactions, is likely inaccurate. Biological processes that depend on the rate-limiting value of multiple inputs can lead to inaccurate heritability estimates due to the inclusion of this "phantom heritability" in the overall

TABLE 7–1. Potential Contributors to Limited Understanding of Complex Disease Genetics

ETIOLOGY	RATIONALE
Common genetic variants	More common variants are likely to be found in GWAS with larger sample sizes. Functional variants need to be found.
Rare genetic variants	Resequencing studies could identify rare genetic determinants.
Interactions	Gene–gene and gene–environment interactions are likely important.
Inaccurate heritability estimates	Heritability estimates are usually generated under assumptions of no gene–gene or gene–environment interactions.
Phenotypic heterogeneity	Most complex diseases are likely to be syndromes with multiple disease subtypes.

heritability estimate. The phenotypic heterogeneity of complex diseases, which are likely often syndromes composed of multiple, potentially overlapping, disease subtypes, also contributes to our limited understanding of complex disease genetics.

Although genetic association studies of rare and common variants can implicate specific genomic regions in complex diseases, functional validation is needed to confirm which gene within a region of association is actually conferring disease susceptibility and to understand the mechanism by which functional genetic variants affect disease pathogenesis. However, functional variant identification in the post-GWAS era has been relatively slow (Freedman, Monteiro, et al. 2011; Juran and Lazaridis 2011) because: (a) many functional variants are likely regulatory variants of moderate effect (Cooper and Shendure 2011) rather than highly penetrant variants, such as the variants observed in many Mendelian syndromes, which often impose a deleterious effect on protein structure (e.g., major amino acid change) (Gibson 2011); (b) gene transcriptional regulation is complicated by tissue specificity as well as dynamic temporal and spatial controls (Sanyal, Lajoie, et al. 2012); and (c) the impact of genetic variation on gene expression may escape detection with current methods in available tissue samples (Pomerantz, Ahmadiyeh, et al. 2009). The development of new bioinformatic approaches to prioritize potentially functional genetic variants, such as the Bayesian approach using dense genotyping data along a region of interest developed by Fahr and colleagues (Farh, Marson, et al. 2015), will likely assist in the identification of functional genetic variants in complex disease GWAS regions.

In our research on chronic obstructive pulmonary disease (COPD) genetics, my colleagues and I have focused on a locus at chromosome 4q31 that has been significantly associated with lung function in general population samples (Hancock, Eijgelsheim, et al. 2010; Repapi, Sayers, et al. 2010) and with COPD in GWAS (Pillai, Ge, et al. 2009; Wilk, Chen, et al. 2009) as well as in subsequent replication studies (Van Durme, Eijgelsheim, et al. 2010; Young, Whittington, et al. 2010). The region of strongest association is located in a block of genetic variants within an intergenic region which begins ~51 kb away from hedgehog interacting protein (*HHIP*), a sonic hedgehog pathway gene that is crucial for the development of the lungs (Chuang and McMahon 1999; Chuang, Kawcak, et al. 2003; Kawahira, Ma, et al. 2003). Zhou and colleagues performed next-generation sequencing of long-range polymerase chain reaction (PCR) products covering the genomic region upstream from *HHIP* associated with COPD, the intervening DNA sequence, and all of the exons and introns of *HHIP* in 29 patients with severe, early-onset COPD (Zhou, Baron, et al. 2012). A total of 493 SNPs were identified; however, no common nonsynonymous SNPs were found within *HHIP*, suggesting that regulatory elements likely confer COPD susceptibility in this region. We found that *HHIP* gene expression was reduced in COPD as compared with control lung tissue samples. We used chromosome conformation capture (3C) assays, an approach that cross-links DNA to characterize chromatin structure, in both lung epithelial (Beas-2B) and lung fibroblast (MRC5) cell lines to identify a 7-kb region approximately 85 kb upstream from the *HHIP* gene, which showed a long-range interaction with the *HHIP* promoter. Subsequently, we identified enhancer activity in this region, which was narrowed to a 500-bp genomic region. By resequencing, we identified two common SNPs located inside the 500-bp enhancer region (rs6537296 and rs1542725). Electrophoretic mobility shift assays demonstrated that the COPD-associated allele at rs1542725 binds more avidly to the transcription factor Sp3, likely leading to the reduced *HHIP* gene expression levels that we observed in COPD as compared with control lung tissue samples. Further study of complex disease GWAS loci to identify functional genetic variants can confirm which gene is influenced by the functional variant and provide information regarding the biological mechanism for disease susceptibility. Since many genetic determinants of complex diseases appear to influence gene-regulatory networks, approaches like 3C that assess long-range chromatin interactions will likely be essential in defining the relevant genes involved in a particular disease-related network.

Interpretation of GWAS and Sequencing Results using Network Approaches

Vidal and colleagues cited multiple lines of evidence that molecular networks underlie genotype–phenotype relationships in human disease (Vidal, Cusick, et al. 2011), including the prediction of new disease genes from cellular network models (e.g., genes for ataxia syndromes) (Lim, Hao, et al. 2006). Since each individual has multiple private and rare potentially deleterious genetic variants, the identification of a causative genetic variant based on DNA sequencing of a single individual can be quite challenging. Network-based approaches can assist in this process. Erlich and colleagues used disease-network analysis to provide another layer of filtering of genetic variants identified by whole exome sequencing and to implicate *KIF1A* as the causative gene in a small consanguineous pedigree with hereditary spastic paraparesis (HSP) (Erlich, Edvardson, et al. 2011). They compared the characteristics of 15 previously identified HSP genes to the genes located within runs of homozygosity using three different disease-network methods. One of these methods was Endeavor, which includes multiple data types such as protein–protein interactions to rate potential candidate genes. They found that *KIF1A* was consistently ranked as the top candidate gene based on multiple disease-prediction algorithms. O'Roak and colleagues sequenced whole exomes in parent-child trios in which the child was affected by autism to find de novo mutations, then created a protein-protein interaction network of genes with truncating or severe missense mutations using Gene-Mania (O'Roak, Vives, et al. 2012). A high percentage of the mutated genes mapped to a particular interconnected network neighborhood, which may represent a disease network module for autism.

Another approach to the use of network analysis to interpret genetic association results is to perturb the specific gene implicated by genetic association analysis in cell-based or animal model systems and then to assess the impact of this perturbation on the expression of other genes. To identify genes regulated by *HHIP* and potentially related to COPD pathogenesis, my research group performed gene expression microarray analysis in a human bronchial epithelial cell line (Beas-2B) after RNA interference; the Beas-2B cells were stably infected with short hairpin RNAs (shRNAs) targeting the *HHIP* mRNA (Zhou, Qiu, et al. 2013). *HHIP* silencing led to differential expression of 296 genes; enrichment for variants nominally associated with COPD in our GWAS analyses was found. Eighteen of the differentially expressed genes were validated by real-time PCR in Beas-2B cells. Seven of 11 validated genes tested in human COPD and control lung tissues demonstrated significant gene expression differences. Functional annotation indicated enrichment for extracellular matrix and cell-growth genes. Using the Predictive Networks Web application, we found that the extracellular matrix and cell proliferation genes influenced by *HHIP* tended to be interconnected more than expected by chance (Figure 7–3). Subsequent studies in a chronic smoke exposure model demonstrated that the *Hhip* heterozygous gene-targeted mouse ($Hhip^{+/-}$) had increased susceptibility to develop emphysema compared to wild-type mice, with evidence for rewiring of the Klf4 signaling network (Lao, Glass, et al 2015).

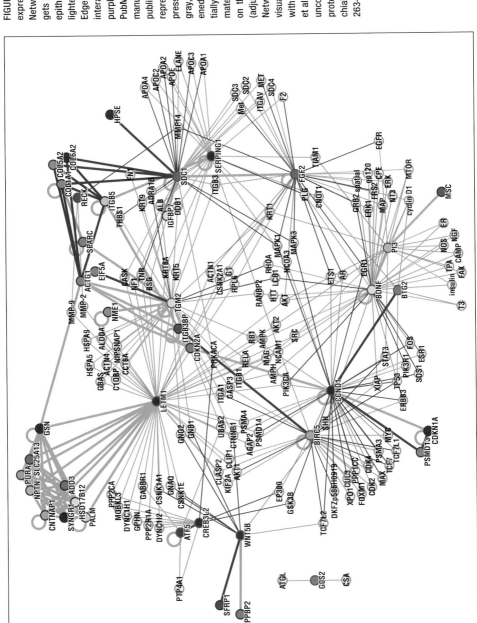

FIGURE 7–3. Network of differentially expressed genes with *HHIP* silencing. Network analysis of validated *HHIP* targets based on gene silencing in a lung epithelial cell line (Beas-2B) (highlighted by pink circles around nodes). Edge colors represent sources of the interaction (gold, Pathway Commons; purple, functional interaction; blue, PubMed or Medline abstract; red, manual curation based on recently published literature) and node colors represent the level of differential expression (purple, highly differential; gray, no expression change). Thickened edges connect pairs of differentially expressed genes. Unbiased, automated literature mining was performed on the differentially expressed genes (adjusted $p < 0.05$) using the Predictive Networks application. Networks were visualized with Cytoscape. (Reprinted with permission from: Zhou, X., W. Qiu, et al. (2013). Gene expression analysis uncovers novel hedgehog interacting protein (HHIP) effects in human bronchial epithelial cells. Genomics **101**(5): 263–72. © 2013 Elsevier Inc.)

Network Analysis of Genetic Data

In order to overcome the low power of GWAS relating a genome-wide SNP panel directly to a complex disease, investigators have attempted to determine whether specific biological pathways are overrepresented among SNPs (within known genes) that do not reach genome-wide significance. Using approaches like Gene Set Enrichment Analysis (Subramanian, Tamayo, et al. 2005), groups of genes with known functions can be assessed for involvement in a disease or other phenotype of interest. These gene-set or pathway-based approaches for genetic analysis were reviewed by Ramanan and colleagues (Ramanan, Kim, et al. 2012); however, these approaches are limited by the relatively small number of genes that have been accurately placed within known biological pathways and the limited information regarding which proteins within a pathway interact. Moreover, these approaches typically do not determine the network structure of gene and protein relationships among pathway members.

Baranzini and colleagues developed a protein interaction, network-based, pathway analysis approach and applied this method to two GWAS of multiple sclerosis (Baranzini, Galwey, et al. 2009). Their approach started by assigning a p value to each gene based on the SNP in that gene with the smallest p value for association. These gene-based p values were integrated with protein–protein interaction network information using the jActive modules component of Cytoscape to identify disease-related modules. The statistical significance of these modules was assessed by comparing them to networks built using randomly distributed p values. They identified 346 significant modules for multiple sclerosis; however, the gene members of some of these modules overlapped substantially. In addition to the known relationships of multiple sclerosis to immunological defects, they identified a neural-based network, which had not been implicated in many previous genetic association studies of multiple sclerosis. Sources of potential bias in genetic networks include gene length and SNP density, because longer genes and genes with a higher density of SNPs genotyped may have SNPs with lower p values based on random chance. In addition, the baseline degree distribution of the gene needs to be considered, since highly connected genes in the interactome may be more likely to be included within disease modules.

Subsequently, Jia and colleagues (Jia, Zheng, et al. 2011) developed dmGWAS, a dense module searching approach utilizing GWAS results and protein–protein interaction networks. As in the Baranzini approach, they picked the single most significant SNP to represent the gene in the network analysis, although alternative approaches including the gene-wise false-discovery rate were also implemented. They used a protein–protein interaction network derived from six public databases; starting with a seed gene from the protein–protein interaction network, they applied a dense module searching approach to maximize the occurrence of disease-associated genes within subnetworks—which they defined as a module. Permutation testing was used to assess the statistical significance of their identified modules. Applying this approach to a breast cancer GWAS from the Nurses' Health Study generated 9212 modules. They focused on the top 1% of modules for further analysis, which included 166 genes in a merged breast cancer subnetwork. As expected, some of these genes were highly associated with breast cancer, while others were weakly associated genes that were linked to strongly associated genes in the network. In later work, Jia and colleagues extended their dmGWAS approach and applied it to schizophrenia (Ramanan, Kim, et al. 2012). They used two schizophrenia GWAS datasets to build and validate their genetic-network modules, and they implemented new approaches to assess the statistical significance of disease modules to overcome the biases related to gene length, SNP density, and baseline degree distribution. They found a disease module composed of 205 genes for schizophrenia; 76 of those genes showed nominal evidence for association in a third schizophrenia GWAS. Subsequently, dmGWAS has been updated to include edge-weighting based on differential gene co-expression levels along with the node-weighting by GWAS evidence (Wang, Yu, et al. 2015).

A variety of other computational methods have been developed to analyze GWAS results within a network context, including Network Interface Miner for Multigenic Interactions (NIMMI) (Akula, Baranova, et al. 2011), Disease Association Protein-Protein Link Evaluator (DAPPLE) (Rossin, Lage, et al. 2011), and NetworkMiner (Garcia-Alonso, Alonso, et al. 2012). These genetic-network approaches assume that genetic association studies and protein–protein interaction networks offer complementary information regarding a complex disease. These methods have provided strong evidence that protein products of genes associated with a complex disease are likely to have a physical interaction. However, the optimal genetic network approach for assigning a statistical significance level to each gene, or, better yet, using all of the SNPs within each gene for network analysis, has not yet been determined. Nonetheless, these efforts to analyze all of the GWAS data, not just the top SNPs from the GWAS, within a network framework have great potential.

Studies of Gene–Gene Interactions

Epistasis refers to the interaction between different genes. *Epistasis* was originally defined in biological terms, to denote an interfering effect of one genetic variant on the phenotypic impact of another variant (Cordell 2002). However, testing for epistasis has typically been performed statistically; deviation from independent effects of genetic loci on a phenotype is assessed. This statistical deviation can be compared to either additive or multiplicative effects, and the scale of measurement can influence the detection of an interaction. Testing for statistical evidence of epistasis may not capture a relevant biological interaction, such as binding between two proteins.

Given the likely great importance of gene–gene interactions in complex diseases, it has been surprisingly difficult to demonstrate epistasis in human complex-disease research. However, an interesting demonstration of epistasis was provided by Hinkley and colleagues with the protease and reverse transcriptase enzymes of HIV (Hinkley, Martins, et al. 2011). They defined epistasis as the impact of one genetic variant depending on the presence or absence of variants located elsewhere in the HIV genome—even if they were located within the same gene. They assessed the replicative capacity of clinical HIV isolates exposed to antiviral drugs, and they sequenced amplification products of protease and reverse-transcriptase genes to identify nonsynonymous SNPs. They compared the effects of models for replicative capacity that included only main effects with models that also included pairwise epistatic interactions. Their model including epistatic effects had 18.3% better predictive power than the model without epistatic effects. They found that intragenic interaction effects were generally greater than intergenic effects in HIV, and the strongest interactions were between nearby variants within the same protein structural domain.

In a model-organism investigation, Huang and colleagues studied genetic determinants of three quantitative traits (starvation resistance, startle response, and chill coma recovery time) in Drosophila (Huang, Richards, et al. 2012). They performed genome-wide association analysis in both a set of inbred Drosophila lines and a laboratory-derived outbred population created by crossing a subset of those inbred lines. Multiple GWAS signals were identified for each trait in both populations, but, surprisingly, the overlap in genetic signals between the two populations was minimal. By performing pairwise interaction tests using significant SNPs from their GWAS, they found that epistatic effects were widespread. Of interest, when they mapped the SNPs involved in significant epistasis to genes, they found that many overlapping genes were found in both of their study populations. Moreover, these interacting genes represented highly connected networks of similar function, including signaling and metabolic pathways. They point out that epistatic effects can contribute to the additive genetic variance as well as the interaction genetic variance, especially when minor allele frequencies are low.

In one of the few positive findings of epistasis in human disease, Emily and colleagues performed gene–gene interaction tests for seven complex diseases that had undergone GWAS analysis in the Wellcome Trust Case-Control Consortium (Emily, Mailund, et al., 2009). They prioritized SNPs based on the protein–protein interaction network and assessed markers only in genes expected to interact biologically. After adjustment for multiple statistical testing, they found four significant pairwise interactions, one each for Crohn's disease, hypertension, rheumatoid arthritis, and bipolar disorder.

One of the limitations of efforts to identify epistasis in human complex diseases has been the statistical approach of searching for a nonadditive contribution of pairwise SNP effects, typically by testing for significant cross-product interaction terms between allele counts for these SNPs in regression models. These approaches require pairwise tests of millions of SNPs, and the multiple statistical testing penalty has likely been a limiting factor in epistasis detection. To minimize this multiple testing penalty, some investigators have proposed focusing only on SNPs that have a significant main effect for epistasis analysis (Musani, Shriner, et al. 2007). A more promising alternative approach is to model statistical epistasis within a network context (Hu, Sinnott-Armstrong, et al. 2011). Hu, Moore and colleagues developed a method to use information theory measures to assess the main and interaction effects between SNPs within a statistical epistasis network. They applied this method to a candidate SNP panel of 1422 SNPs genotyped in patients with bladder cancer as compared with control subjects. Network properties that they assessed included the numbers of edges and nodes, the number of genes in the largest connected component (Figure 7–4), and the degree distribution of the nodes. They assessed the statistical significance of their interaction network by permutation of disease status and found evidence for increased numbers of edges and nodes, as well as a large connected component, within the bladder cancer network. They also found that their epistasis network had scale-free properties. However, even with these more elegant network-based statistical approaches, the assessment of statistical epistasis may not capture the biological epistasis (e.g., physical interaction between proteins), which is likely of greater relevance for disease pathogenesis. Subsequently, Hu, Moore, and colleagues developed ViSEN, a software package to visualize both two-way and three-way statistical epistasis networks; network analysis using small candidate SNP panels can also be performed using this software (Hu, Chen, et al. 2013).

Integration of Genetic Variants with Single -Omics Approaches

Since there is such a long biological path between a genetic risk variant and development of a complex disease, it is not surprising that genetic association

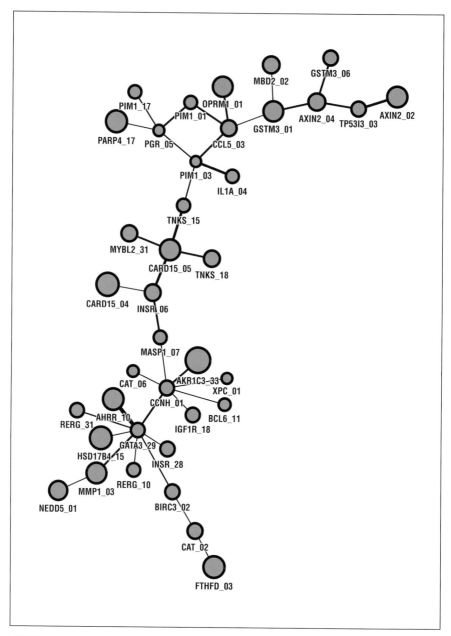

FIGURE 7–4. Epistasis network in bladder cancer. Hu and colleagues created an epistasis network based on a panel of SNPs genotyped in bladder cancer cases and controls. The largest connected component of their epistasis network, shown here, includes 39 SNPs, which are represented by nodes in this network. The size of the nodes corresponds to the strength of the main effect and the width of the edge connecting two nodes corresponds to the strength of the interaction between those SNPs. (Reprinted from Hu, T., N.A. Sinnott-Armstrong, et al., (2011). Characterizing genetic interactions in human disease association studies using statistical epistasis networks. BMC Bioinformatics 2011; 12: 364. (CC BY 2.0))

studies relating genotypes to complex diseases have low statistical power. These first-generation genetic studies (Silverman and Loscalzo 2012) (Figure 7–5) have typically required large samples to identify genetic determinants of modest effect size. Genetic studies have also been performed using many of the -omics data types that are described elsewhere in this book, including quantitative levels of messenger RNA (mRNA), proteins, and metabolites. The genetic architecture of these "intermediate phenotypes" or "endophenotypes," which are biologically more proximal to the genetic variant, can be used to gain insight into the biological networks relevant for complex diseases. My colleagues and I have referred to these genetic analyses of -omics data types as second-generation genetic studies. Although these approaches have been quite successful in identifying statistically and biologically significant genetic determinants of these intermediate phenotypes, using these associations to identify genetic determinants of disease remains challenging.

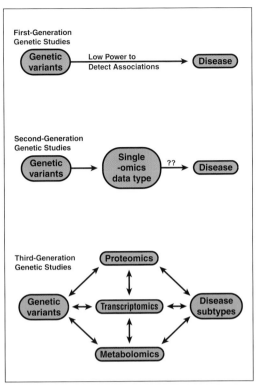

FIGURE 7–5. Evolution of complex-disease genetic studies. Most genetic-association studies attempt to relate genetic variants directly to disease, but these first-generation genetic studies have low power. Second-generation genetic studies attempt to identify genetic determinants of an -omics data type (e.g., gene expression levels) and then relate those genetic variants to disease. Ultimately, third-generation genetic studies that integrate genetic variants with multiple -omics data types in a network framework will be required. (Reprinted with permission from: Silverman, E. K., and J. Loscalzo. (2012). Network medicine approaches to the genetics of complex diseases. Discov Med **14**(75): 143–52. © 2012 Discovery Medicine.)

Transcriptomics and Genetics

Genetic determinants of gene expression levels, known as expression quantitative trait loci, or eQTLs, can be located near the coding gene (*cis* effects) or at a great distance on the same chromosome or on different chromosomes from the coding gene (*trans* effects). Stranger and colleagues performed integrative genomics analysis in a total of 270 HapMap phase II lymphoblastoid cell lines, with genome-wide gene expression microarray analysis (representing 13,643 genes) and more than 2 million SNPs in European, Asian, and African HapMap subjects (Stranger, Nica, et al. 2007). Despite the small sample size within each HapMap population, 1348 genes had a *cis*-eQTL and 180 genes had a *trans*-

eQTL in at least one of the racial groups. Several factors likely contributed to the smaller number of *trans*-eQTLs observed, including the inclusion of only a subset of SNPs for *trans*-eQTL analysis and the reduced power to detect *trans*-acting effects. However, it was noteworthy that the identified *trans*-eQTLs were often found to act also as *cis*-eQTLs. Multiple investigators have shown that eQTLs are enriched for complex-disease susceptibility loci. For example, Fehrmann and colleagues performed an integrative genomics study using gene expression microarray analysis of peripheral-blood samples with genome-wide SNP genotyping data in 1,469 individuals and found substantial enrichment for reported trait-associated GWAS SNPs among eQTLs (Fehrmann, Jansen, et al. 2011). Among all common SNPs, 17% were *cis*-eQTLs and 0.2% were *trans*-eQTLs; however, among trait-associated SNPs, 40% were *cis*-eQTLs and 6% were *trans*-eQTLs. Surprisingly, 48% of the *trans*-eQTL SNPs that they identified were located within the HLA region. Integrative genomics studies can provide functional insights into complex disease genetic associations; *cis*-eQTLs associated with disease can implicate a specific gene in disease pathogenesis and suggest that disease susceptibility is influenced by regulation of that gene, while *trans*-eQTLs can provide insight into the network of interacting genes and proteins involved in a complex disease (Figure 7–6). Hemani and colleagues identified many epistatic effects between eQTLs on gene expression levels (Hemani, Shakhbazov, et al. 2014)—in contrast to the paucity of epistatic effects noted above for disease phenotypes—potentially due to the large effect sizes of many eQTLs on gene expression levels. However, alternative explanations for these observed eQTL interactions include linkage disequilibrium with a functional SNP not included in the panel of analyzed variants (Wood, Tuke, et al., 2014).

Chen and colleagues used genotypic and gene expression microarray data from a murine cross between the C57BL6/J and C3H/HeJ strains to identify eQTLs (Chen, Zhu, et al. 2008). They built liver and adipose co-expression networks from these mice and found enrichment for eQTLs within a region on mouse chromosome 1 that had been previously implicated in metabolic traits, including body weight and cholesterol levels. They identified a macrophage-enriched metabolic network that influenced many metabolic phenotypes, and they validated the novel metabolic impact of several genes in this network using transgenic or knockout mice. Their results suggested that network analysis could implicate key genes in disease-related phenotypes that would not have been identified using traditional genetic methods.

Small and colleagues studied metabolic syndrome in humans, which encompasses a variably represented group of conditions, including obesity, insulin resistance, hypertension, type 2 diabetes mellitus, and hyperlipidemia (Small, Hedman, et al. 2011). Although genetic determinants for individual components

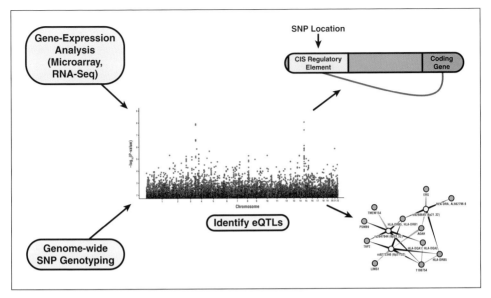

FIGURE 7–6. Genetic network insights from expression quantitative trait loci. Gene expression results from microarray analysis or RNA-seq can be tested for association with a genome-wide SNP panel to identify expression quantitative trait loci (eQTLs). SNPs that affect *cis*-acting regulatory elements, such as transcription factor binding sites, can implicate a specific gene in a phenotype of interest. SNPs may have *cis*- and/or *trans*-eQTL effects, and a network of interacting genes can be identified based on eQTL relationships. A network constructed from eQTL SNPs in type 1 diabetes mellitus is shown at the bottom right. Black arrows indicate *cis*-eQTL effects; gold arrows indicate *trans*-eQTL effects; and grey edges indicate co-expression in peripheral blood. (Reprinted with permission from: Fehrmann, R.S.N., R.C. Jansen, et al. (2011). Trans-eQTLs Reveal That Independent Genetic Variants Associated with a Complex Phenotype Converge on Intermediate Genes, with a Major Role for the HLA. PLoS Genetics 7: 31002197. (CC BY 3.0))

of the metabolic syndrome have been reported, key overall regulators of the metabolic syndrome had not been identified. They studied *KLF14*, a transcription factor that had a known *cis*-eQTL in adipose tissue. They performed *trans*-eQTL analysis using this *cis*-eQTL SNP in gene expression microarray data from adipose tissue. They identified 10 genes that showed *trans*-eQTL effects from this *KLF14* SNP; many of these affected genes were associated with metabolic syndrome traits. Thus, this *trans*-eQTL analysis identified part of the metabolic syndrome network, which was regulated by *KLF14*.

Statistical genetic assessment of the relationships between gene expression and genetic variants within a network framework was proposed by Chu and Raby and their colleagues (Chu, Weiss, et al. 2009). They used a Gaussian graphical network modeling approach based on partial correlation coefficients between gene expression levels, which included genetic association testing conditional on the gene expression graphical network. They later extended this approach to compare gene–gene connectivity patterns across disease states (Chu, Lazarus, et al. 2011). The application of statistical methods to test network relationships between genetic variants and gene expression levels will be helpful in rigorously delineating genetic networks.

Proteomics and Genetics

Proteomics has been linked to genetics by using protein levels as phenotypes for genetic analysis in an effort to identify protein quantitative trait loci (pQTLs). For example, Naitza and colleagues used serum levels of several protein biomarkers related to inflammation (interleukin-6 [IL-6], monocyte chemoattractant protein 1 [MCP-1], and high sensitivity C-reactive protein [CRP]) as phenotypes in a two-stage GWAS including a total of 6,148 Sardinians (Naitza, Porcu, et al. 2012). As expected, some of the significant associations with protein levels were located within the corresponding coding gene (e.g., a SNP in *CRP* was significantly associated with CRP levels). Other associations recapitulated known biological relationships, such as the association of a SNP near the MCP-1 receptor gene (*CCR2*) with MCP-1 levels. However, some significant associations revealed novel biological relationships; for instance, a rare SNP (minor allele frequency 0.003) near the inducible T-cell costimulator ligand (*ICOSLG*) and autoimmune regulator (*AIRE*) genes had a large effect size and was significantly associated with CRP levels.

To identify genetic variants influencing circulating protein biomarkers and novel genetic determinants of COPD, my research group performed GWAS for two pneumoproteins, club cell secretory protein (CC16) and surfactant protein D (SP-D), and five systemic inflammatory markers (CRP, fibrinogen, IL-6, IL-8, and tumor necrosis factor α) in 1,951 patients with COPD from the ECLIPSE study (Kim, Cho, et al. 2012). Genome-wide significant susceptibility loci affecting biomarker levels were found only for the two pneumoproteins. As shown in Figure 7–7, two discrete loci affecting CC16, one region near the CC16 coding gene (*SCGB1A1*) on chromosome 11 and another ~25 Mb away from *SCGB1A1*, were identified, whereas multiple SNPs on chromosomes 6 and 16, in addition to SNPs near *SFTPD* (the coding gene for SP-D), had genome-wide significant associations with SP-D levels. Several SNPs highly associated with CC16 or SP-D levels were nominally associated with COPD in a collaborative GWAS ($p = 0.001$ to 0.049), although these COPD associations were not replicated in two additional cohorts. We concluded that distant genetic loci as well as biomarker-coding genes affect circulating levels of COPD-related pneumoproteins. A subset of these protein quantitative trait loci may influence COPD susceptibility.

Most of the reported pQTL studies have focused on a small number of proteins of interest. More recently, genetic-association analysis of a more comprehensive set of proteomics data was reported by Wu and colleagues (Wu, Candille, et al.

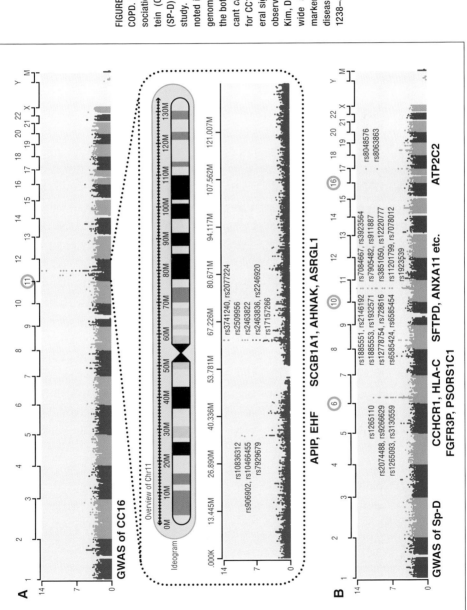

FIGURE 7–7. Protein quantitative trait loci in COPD. Manhattan plots for genome-wide association analysis of Club cell secretory protein (CC16) (A) and surfactant protein D (SP-D) (B) bloodstream levels in the ECLIPSE study. Genome-wide significant SNPs are noted in gold, and the nearest genes to the genome-wide significant regions are listed at the bottom of the plots. In addition to significant *cis* associations near the coding genes for CC16 (*SCGB1A1*) and SP-D (*SFTPD*), several significant *trans* associations were also observed. (Reprinted with permission from Kim, D. K., M. H. Cho, et al. (2012). Genome-wide association analysis of blood biomarkers in chronic obstructive pulmonary disease. Am J Respir Crit Care Med **186:** 1238–47.)

2013). They performed isobaric tandem mass tag-based mass spectrometry to analyze the proteins within 95 HapMap lymphoblastoid cell lines from European, Yoruba, and Asian subjects, and they measured 5,953 protein levels. These protein levels were tested for genetic association with potential *cis*-acting genetic variants located within 20 kb of the gene. Multiple pQTLs were identified. Some pQTLs were identified in only one of the HapMap populations (e.g., European or Yoruba), while others were found in all populations. Of interest, there was substantial but incomplete overlap between eQTL and pQTL signals. Although the small sample size analyzed makes it difficult to exclude the possibility that a SNP that appears to influence protein levels but not mRNA levels in their study will not influence both mRNA and protein levels in a larger sample, it appears likely that at least some genetic factors influence mRNA and protein levels differentially. Thus, the networks of genetic determinants of mRNA and protein levels are likely overlapping but not identical.

In a study of 590 COPDGene and 750 SPIROMICS subjects, Sun and colleagues assessed pQTLs for 88 blood proteins (Sun, Kechris, et al. 2016). Many pQTLs were identified that replicated in both study populations; some pQTLs explained a large percentage of variation in protein level. Of interest, including both a pQTL SNP (in the *AGER* gene) and the sRAGE protein biomarker level together provided substantially stronger associations to emphysema than either the SNP or protein biomarker level alone.

Mendelian randomization is a statistical approach that uses instrumental variable analysis to assess whether a biomarker is causally related to disease risk (Lawlor, Harbord, et al. 2008). Using this approach, Voight and colleagues demonstrated that genetic determinants of LDL cholesterol were related to myocardial infarction, while genetic determinants of HDL cholesterol were not—suggesting that only LDL cholesterol is likely to be causally related to myocardial infarction risk (Voight, Peloso, et al. 2012). Mendelian randomization approaches can assist in determining whether a significant genetic determinant of a protein level is also related to disease risk, thus addressing one of the key challenges of second-generation genetic studies. However, there are multiple assumptions inherent to Mendelian randomization approaches that can lead to substantial biases in the results (VanderWeele, Tchetgen Tchetgen, et al. 2014), and these assumptions should be carefully evaluated to determine whether the application of Mendelian randomization is appropriate in a particular study.

Metabolomics and Genetics

Metabolomic studies can provide complementary information to transcriptomics and proteomics, but because affordable, high-throughput metabolomic assay systems have been developed only recently, efforts to identify genetic determinants of large panels of metabolites have been more limited. Suhre and colleagues performed GWAS of more than 250 metabolites from fasting serum in 2820 individuals in two study populations (Suhre, Shin, et al. 2011). They used liquid and gas chromatography with tandem mass spectrometry to measure metabolites. They analyzed genome-wide SNP genotyping data and all individual metabolites and ratios of metabolites in a screening stage with log-transformed metabolite values. They subsequently performed meta-analysis of both study populations and found 37 loci that were significant genome-wide after Bonferroni correction for multiple statistical testing. In many of these loci, the observed effect size per allele was surprisingly high (> 10%). At 30 loci, the associated SNP mapped to a protein previously known to be biochemically related to the metabolite. At 15 of their genome-wide significant loci, a SNP was associated with a disease-related or drug-response phenotype. For example, a *NAT8* SNP was associated with *N*-acetylornithine levels in their study, a locus that was previously associated with renal function. They measured *N*-acetylornithine levels and found that they were correlated with renal function in their study populations, suggesting a potential role for this metabolite in chronic renal insufficiency. Of interest, six of their 37 genome-wide significant associations to metabolites have previously been related to adverse drug effects; further study of these metabolites and their genetic determinants could provide insight into the mechanisms for drug toxicity.

Conclusion

In this chapter, we have reviewed the main approaches that have been used to analyze genetic variants related to complex diseases within a network context (Figure 7–8). Network information can be used to interpret SNP associations with complex diseases, thus placing new genetic findings, which may have never previously been considered to be involved in disease pathogenesis, into biological context. By incorporating information about the strength of association for the full panel of SNPs tested in a GWAS, disease-related networks can be built that may help to overcome the limited power of first-generation genetic association studies relating genetic variants directly to a complex disease. Epistasis networks hold great promise to identify the gene–gene interactions that seem likely to be involved in complex disease pathogenesis but that have been quite difficult to identify. Functional validation of GWAS associations is essential to confirm the gene that influences disease susceptibility and also to provide information regarding the biological mechanism by which those genetic variants influence disease pathogenesis.

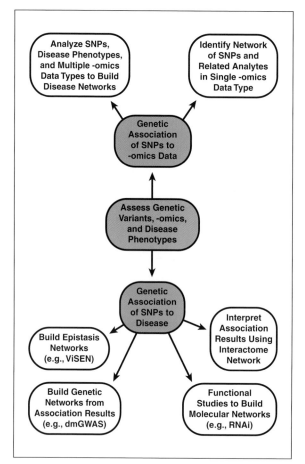

FIGURE 7–8. Approaches to analyze genetic variation and complex diseases in networks. Approaches related to the two major classes of genetic network analysis methods are shown, which begin with either genetic association analysis of disease or of -omics data types. New methodology will be required for truly integrated analyses of genetic variants with multiple -omics data and disease-related phenotypes.

Diseases are typically expressed by creating changes throughout the cellular machinery that can be captured using various -omics technologies. Using different -omics data types has the potential to provide mechanistic insights regarding how the impact of genetic variants is biologically transduced to cause disease. Comprehensive analysis of multiple -omics data types with genetic variants and disease-relevant phenotypes in third generation genetic studies (Figure 7-5) will likely require new network analysis methodologies, and has great potential to revolutionize the diagnosis and treatment of complex diseases.

Califano and colleagues pointed out some of the key challenges facing researchers who are trying to perform these types of systems genetics research studies (Califano, Butte, et al. 2012). Our knowledge of the molecular networks influenced by disease-related genetic variants is typically fragmentary. Moreover, these molecular networks are cell-type specific and dynamic; there is no single cellular molecular interactome, but rather an infinite array of possible interactomes throughout the body and throughout growth, development, and aging. Reconstruction of context-specific gene regulatory networks may be necessary to understand genetic predisposition to complex diseases.

Despite these challenges, assessment of multiple -omics data types within humans is becoming increasingly feasible. Chen and colleagues performed multiple -omics analysis in blood samples from a single individual repeatedly over more than 1 year of observation. In addition to performing whole-genome DNA sequencing, they obtained repeated assessments of transcriptomics (using

RNA-seq), proteomics (including autoantibody profiles), and metabolomics, thus creating an integrative personal -omics profile (iPOP) (Chen, Mias, et al. 2012). From this longitudinal assessment, which included sampling during two viral infections and the development of type 2 diabetes mellitus, they found marked dynamic changes over time in many of the -omics assessments. Integrated analyses of these -omics data types revealed that some disease pathways were detected with only one -omics data type (e.g., the insulin secretion pathway was only seen using proteomics). Future complex disease studies will need to consider the value of longitudinal multiple -omics assessments in uncovering the etiologies of those diseases.

Most complex diseases are syndromes that are likely collections of multiple disorders that share a common set of physiological and/or pathological characteristics. One of the key goals of network medicine is to create more meaningful classification systems for complex diseases based on etiology. An early effort to apply network science principles to disease classification used information about disease genes from the OMIM database (Goh, Cusick, et al. 2007). Two networks were created—one with nodes as diseases with edges placed between nodes if the same gene was implicated in both diseases (Human Disease Network) and one with nodes as genes and edges included if the same disease was implicated for both genes (Disease Gene Network). The Human Disease Network indicated that diseases are not isolated entities; 68% of diseases were connected to at least one other disease. Several of the genes, including *TP53* and *PAX6,* were connected to multiple diseases. More recently, Arnedo and colleagues developed an approach to integrate genetic networks of interacting SNPs with unsupervised assessments of phenotypic heterogeneity, and they reported eight potential subtypes of schizophrenia (Arnedo, Svrakic, et al. 2015). Key ongoing challenges in applying such genetic networks include addressing the impact of linkage disequilibrium between SNPs as well as population stratification on network structure and subtype identification. Although the utility of genes with the smaller effect sizes found in complex disease GWAS for disease classification is less certain than for Mendelian syndromes, the integrated analysis of disease-associated SNPs with multiple -omics data types could lead to useful reclassification of complex diseases.

Finally, network analyses of genetic determinants may have important implications for complex disease treatment (Silverman and Loscalzo 2013). Pharmacogenetics may assist in identifying individuals likely to benefit from specific pharmacological treatment and in avoiding treatment of individuals at high risk for adverse events. For example, genetic association analysis identified a functional variant in *GLCCI1* that was associated with reduced therapeutic response to inhaled corticosteroids in patients with asthma (Tantisira, Lasky-Su, et al. 2011). By identifying the biological networks related to a complex disease, network medicine approaches may provide multiple targets for therapy, which may require treatment with a sequential and dynamic approach to rewire disease-related networks and restore health.

References

Akula, N., A. Baranova, et al. (2011). A network-based approach to prioritize results from genome-wide association studies. PLoS ONE **6**(9): e24220.

Arnedo, J., D. M. Svrakic, et al. (2015). Uncovering the hidden risk architecture of the schizophrenias: confirmation in three independent genome-wide association studies. Am J Psychiatry **172**(2): 139–53.

Baranzini, S. E., N. W. Galwey, et al. (2009). Pathway and network-based analysis of genome-wide association studies in multiple sclerosis. Human Molec Genet **18**(11): 2078–90.

Califano, A., A. J. Butte, et al. (2012). Leveraging models of cell regulation and GWAS data in integrative network-based association studies. Nat Genet **44**(8): 841–47.

Charloteaux, B., Q. Zhong, et al. (2011). Protein-protein interactions and networks: forward and reverse edgetics. Methods Mol Biol **759**: 197–213.

Chen, R., G. I. Mias, et al. (2012). Personal omics profiling reveals dynamic molecular and medical phenotypes. Cell **148**(6): 1293–307.

Chen, Y., J. Zhu, et al. (2008). Variations in DNA elucidate molecular networks that cause disease. Nature **452**(7186): 429–35.

Chu, J. H., R. Lazarus, et al. (2011). Quantifying differential gene connectivity between disease states for objective identification of disease-relevant genes. BMC Syst Biol **5**: 89.

Chu, J. H., S. T. Weiss, et al. (2009). A graphical model approach for inferring large-scale networks integrating gene expression and genetic polymorphism. BMC Syst Biol **3**: 55.

Chuang, P. T., T. Kawcak, et al. (2003). Feedback control of mammalian Hedgehog signaling by the Hedgehog-binding protein, Hip1, modulates Fgf signaling during branching morphogenesis of the lung. Genes Dev **17**(3): 342–47.

Chuang, P. T., and A. P. McMahon (1999). Vertebrate Hedgehog signalling modulated by induction of a Hedgehog-binding protein. Nature **397**(6720): 617–21.

Cooper, G. M., and J. Shendure (2011). Needles in stacks of needles: finding disease-causal variants in a wealth of genomic data. Nat Rev Genet **12**(9): 628–40.

Cordell, H. J. (2002). Epistasis: what it means, what it doesn't mean, and statistical methods to detect it in humans. Human Molec Genet **11**(20): 2463–68.

Emily M., T. Mailund, et al. (2009). Using biological networks to search for interacting loci in genome-wide association studies. Eur J Human Genet **17**(10):1231–40.

Erlich, Y., S. Edvardson, et al. (2011). Exome sequencing and disease-network analysis of a single family implicate a mutation in KIF1A in hereditary spastic paraparesis. Genome Res **21**(5): 658–64.

Farh, K. K., A. Marson,, et al. (2015). Genetic and epigenetic fine mapping of causal autoimmune disease variants. Nature **518**(7539): 337–43.

Fehrmann, R. S., R. C. Jansen, et al. (2011). Trans-eQTLs reveal that independent genetic variants associated with a complex phenotype converge on intermediate genes, with a major role for the HLA. PLoS Genet **7**(8): e1002197.

Freedman, M. L., A. N. Monteiro, et al. (2011). Principles for the post-GWAS functional characterization of cancer risk loci. Nature Genet **43**(6): 513–18.

Garcia-Alonso, L., R. Alonso et al. (2012). Discovering the hidden sub-network component in a ranked list of genes or proteins derived from genomic experiments. Nucleic Acids Res **40**(20): e158.

Gibson, G. (2011). Rare and common variants: twenty arguments. Nat Rev Genet **13**(2): 135–45.

Goh, K. I., M. E. Cusick, et al. (2007). The human disease network. Proc Natl Acad Sci U S A **104**(21): 8685–90.

Hancock, D. B., M. Eijgelsheim, et al. (2010). Meta-analyses of genome-wide association studies identify multiple loci associated with pulmonary function. Nat Genet **42**(1): 45–52.

Hemani, G., K. Shakhbazov, et al. (2014). Detection and replication of epistasis influencing transcription in humans. Nature **508**(7495): 249–53.

Hinkley, T., J. Martins, et al. (2011). A systems analysis of mutational effects in HIV-1 protease and reverse transcriptase. Nat Genet **43**(5): 487–89.

Hu, T., Y. Chen, et al. (2013). ViSEN: methodology and software for visualization of statistical epistasis networks. Genet Epidemiol **37**(3): 283–85.

Hu, T., N. A. Sinnott-Armstrong, et al. (2011). Characterizing genetic interactions in human disease association studies using statistical epistasis networks. BMC Bioinform **12**: 364.

Huang, W., S. Richards, et al. (2012). Epistasis dominates the genetic architecture of Drosophila quantitative traits. Proc Natl Acad Sci U.S.A. **109**(39): 15553–59.

Jia, P., S. Zheng, et al. (2011). dmGWAS: dense module searching for genome-wide association studies in protein-protein interaction networks. Bioinformatics **27**(1): 95–102.

Juran, B. D., and K. N. Lazaridis (2011). Genomics in the post-GWAS era. Semin Liver Dis **31**(2): 215–22.

Kawahira, H., N. H. Ma, et al. (2003). Combined activities of hedgehog signaling inhibitors regulate pancreas development. Development **130**(20): 4871–79.

Kim, D. K., M. H. Cho, et al. (2012). Genome-wide association analysis of blood biomarkers in chronic obstructive pulmonary disease. Am J Respir Crit Care Med **186**(12): 1238–47.

Lander, E. S. (2011). Initial impact of the sequencing of the human genome. Nature **470**(7333): 187–97.

Lao T., K. Glass, et al. (2015). Haploinsufficiency of Hedgehog interacting protein causes increased emphysema induced by cigarette smoke through network rewiring. Genome Med 7(1):12.

Lawlor, D. A., R. M. Harbord, et al. (2008). Mendelian randomization: using genes as instruments for making causal inferences in epidemiology. Stat Med **27**(8): 1133–63.

Lim, J., T. Hao, et al. (2006). A protein-protein interaction network for human inherited ataxias and disorders of Purkinje cell degeneration. Cell **125**(4): 801–14.

Manolio, T. A., L. D. Brooks, et al. (2008). A HapMap harvest of insights into the genetics of common disease. J Clin Invest **118**(5): 1590–605.

Manolio, T. A., F. S. Collins, et al. (2009). Finding the missing heritability of complex diseases. Nature **461**(7265): 747–53.

Musani, S. K., D. Shriner, et al. (2007). Detection of gene x gene interactions in genome-wide association studies of human population data. Hum Hered **63**(2): 67–84.

Naitza, S., E. Porcu, et al. (2012). A genome-wide association scan on the levels of markers of inflammation in Sardinians reveals associations that underpin its complex regulation. PLoS Genet **8**(1): e1002480.

Nelson MR, H. Tipney, et al. (2015). The support of human genetic evidence for approved drug indications. Nat Genet **47**(8):856–60.

O'Roak, B. J., L. Vives, et al. (2012). Sporadic autism exomes reveal a highly interconnected protein network of de novo mutations. Nature **485**(7397): 246–50.

Pillai, S. G., D. Ge, et al. (2009). A genome-wide association study in chronic obstructive pulmonary disease (COPD): identification of two major susceptibility loci. PLoS Genet **5**(3): e1000421.

Pomerantz, M. M., N. Ahmadiyeh, et al. (2009). The 8q24 cancer risk variant rs6983267 shows long-range interaction with MYC in colorectal cancer. Nat Genet **41**(8): 882–84.

Ramanan, V. K., S. Kim, et al. (2012). Genome-wide pathway analysis of memory impairment in the Alzheimer's Disease Neuroimaging Initiative (ADNI) cohort implicates gene candidates, canonical pathways, and networks. Brain Imag Behav **6**(4): 634–48.

Repapi, E., I. Sayers, et al. (2010). Genome-wide association study identifies five loci associated with lung function. Nat Genet **42**(1): 36–44.

Rossin, E. J., K. Lage, et al. (2011). Proteins encoded in genomic regions associated with immune-mediated disease physically interact and suggest underlying biology. PLoS Genet 7(1): e1001273.

Sanyal, A., B. R. Lajoie, et al. (2012). The long-range interaction landscape of gene promoters. Nature 489(7414): 109–13.

Silverman, E. K., and J. Loscalzo (2012). Network medicine approaches to the genetics of complex diseases. Discov Med 14(75): 143–52.

Silverman, E. K., and J. Loscalzo (2013). Developing new drug treatments in the era of network medicine. Clin Pharmacol Therap 93(1): 26–28.

Small, K. S., A. K. Hedman, et al. (2011). Identification of an imprinted master trans regulator at the KLF14 locus related to multiple metabolic phenotypes. Nat Genet 43(6): 561–64.

Stranger, B. E., A. C. Nica, et al. (2007). Population genomics of human gene expression. Nat Genet 39(10): 1217–24.

Subramanian, A., P. Tamayo, et al. (2005). Gene set enrichment analysis: a knowledge-based approach for interpreting genome-wide expression profiles. Proc Natl Acad Sci U.S.A. 102(43): 15545–50.

Suhre, K., S. Y. Shin, et al. (2011). Human metabolic individuality in biomedical and pharmaceutical research. Nature 477(7362): 54–60.

Sun, W., K. Kechris, et al. (2016). Common genetic polymorphisms influence blood biomarkers in COPD. PLoS Genetics (In Press).

Tantisira, K. G., J. Lasky-Su, et al. (2011). Genomewide association between GLCCI1 and response to glucocorticoid therapy in asthma. N Engl J Med 365(13): 1173–83.

Van Durme, Y. M., M. Eijgelsheim, et al. (2010). Hedgehog-interacting protein is a COPD susceptibility gene: the Rotterdam Study. Eur Respir J 36(1): 89–95.

VanderWeele, T. J., E. J. Tchetgen Tchetgen, et al. (2014). Methodological challenges in Mendelian randomization. Epidemiology 25(3): 427–35.

Vidal, M., M. E. Cusick, et al. (2011). Interactome networks and human disease. Cell 144(6): 986–98.

Voight, B. F., G. M. Peloso, et al. (2012). Plasma HDL cholesterol and risk of myocardial infarction: a mendelian randomisation study. Lancet 380(9841): 572–80.

Wang, K., R. Baldassano, et al. (2010). Comparative genetic analysis of inflammatory bowel disease and type 1 diabetes implicates multiple loci with opposite effects. Hum Mol Genet 19(10): 2059–67.

Wang, Q., H. Yu, Z. Zhao, and P. Jia (2015). EW_dmGWAS: edge-weighted dense module-search for genome-wide association studies and gene expression profiles. Bioinformatics 31(15): 2591–94.

Wood, A.R., M.A. Tuke, et al. (2014). Another explanation for apparent epistasis. Nature 514: E3–E5.

Wilk, J. B., T. H. Chen, et al. (2009). A genome-wide association study of pulmonary function measures in the Framingham Heart Study. PLoS Genet 5(3): e1000429.

Wu, L., S. I. Candille, et al. (2013). Variation and genetic control of protein abundance in humans. Nature 499(7456): 79–82.

Young, R. P., C. F. Whittington, et al. (2010). Chromosome 4q31 locus in COPD is also associated with lung cancer. Eur Respir J 36(6): 1375–82.

Zheng, H. F., V. Forgetta, et al. (2015). Whole-genome sequencing identifies EN1 as a determinant of bone density and fracture. Nature 526(7571): 112–17.

Zhou, X., R. M. Baron, et al. (2012). Identification of a chronic obstructive pulmonary disease genetic determinant that regulates HHIP. Hum Molec Genet 21(6): 1325–35.

Zhou, X., W. Qiu, et al. (2013). Gene expression analysis uncovers novel hedgehog interacting protein (HHIP) effects in human bronchial epithelial cells. Genomics 101(5): 263–72.

Zuk, O., E. Hechter, et al. (2012). The mystery of missing heritability: Genetic interactions create phantom heritability. Proc Natl Acad Sci U S A 109(4): 1193–98.

8

Transcriptomics and Network Medicine

JOHN QUACKENBUSH AND KIMBERLY GLASS

Introduction

The first reference human genome was announced complete in June 2000, and scientific papers describing two versions—public and private—appeared early in 2001. Although there were some basic differences in what was presented—and despite the fact that "finishing" the draft genome sequence would require a number of years of additional work—sequencing the human genome provided us with a tremendous resource for advancing medicine and biomedical research in the twenty-first century. There was immense excitement about the potential for new discoveries and approaches to patient care; however, progress has been slower than anticipated. Early hopes that identifying alterations in the DNA sequence (genetic variants) would lead us quickly to the root cause of human disease or that simply looking at patterns of gene expression could inform us about the functional underpinnings of the phenotypes we observe were quickly dashed. These are now recognized as overly simplistic assumptions about the link between the genome and phenotype, and they represent a major impediment to more substantial progress.

Encoded within the human genome are approximately 20,000 protein-coding genes, something on the order of fivefold more isoforms, more than 1000 microRNAs, and multiple noncoding epigenomic states, all of which can affect the functioning of the cell. The challenge is to use the data that we can collect about these components effectively to make informative connections between the genes encoded in the genome and the (healthy and disease) phenotypes we observe.

Much of the progress we have made in understanding disease phenotypes has come from analyzing gene transcriptional data—making static measurements of the abundance of RNA levels for different cellular states and using these data to develop network models representing the dynamical processes driving biological systems. One might argue that transcriptomic data do not fully capture either the complexity of gene regulation or the dynamics of cellular processes. However, given experimental constraints, gene expression data represent the best resource available today for modeling regulatory networks and for building predictive models of cellular response in a wide range of situations.

Although inference of cellular networks is one of the areas in which we have made the most significant advances in creating models that may be useful in a network medicine context, it remains both a challenge and an area of active research (Chuang, Hofree, et al. 2010; Marbach, Costello, et al. 2012). This work has made it increasingly clear that we need integrated datasets that capture the various components that contribute to the gene regulatory process. Fortunately, new DNA-sequencing technologies are allowing the generation of increasingly large and complex datasets comprising multiple -omic assays from individual samples, including genome-sequence data, transcriptomic data, and genome-wide data on patterns of epigenetic modification.

In this chapter we begin by exploring transcriptomic data and then review a representative subset of the many methods that have been developed for network inference and modeling using transcriptional data. We also explore emerging methods that can be extended to integrate multiple types of genomic and other data with transcriptional information. Finally, we discuss how these network models are being used to characterize diseases, their possible medical applications, and their emerging potential to suggest alternative treatment strategies.

Measuring the Transcriptome

The transcriptome is defined as the collection of all RNA molecules in the cell, including messenger RNA (mRNA). The abundance levels of these molecules, commonly referred to as "gene expression," are widely used as the primary input values for algorithms that seek to model transcriptional networks.

Gene expression microarrays were developed in the 1990s as an efficient, high-throughput way to measure gene expression levels. Microarrays quantify the amount of mRNA that is captured, or bound, to a set of complementary sequences (probes) that are themselves attached to a solid substrate (Figure 8–1). In principle, the observed level of RNA hybridization to a particular probe represents the amount of mRNA produced from the corresponding gene. In practice, the measured levels can be influenced by a variety of factors, including the sequence of the probes, where they are located within their target genes, how well the corresponding mRNA binds to the chosen complementary sequence, and even where the probes are physically located on the array, among

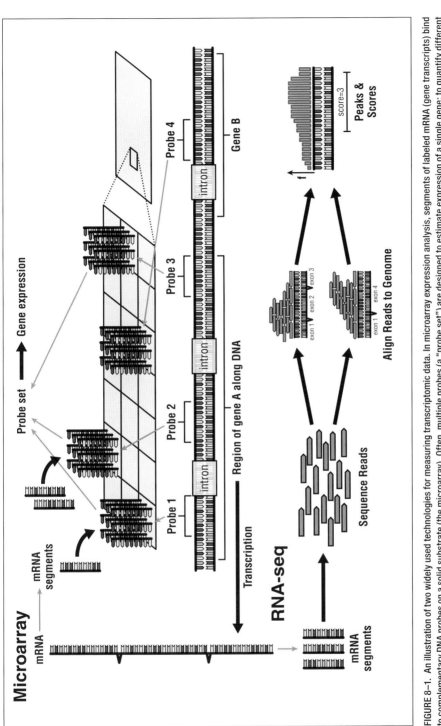

FIGURE 8–1. An illustration of two widely used technologies for measuring transcriptomic data. In microarray expression analysis, segments of labeled mRNA (gene transcripts) bind to complementary DNA probes on a solid substrate (the microarray). Often, multiple probes (a "probe set") are designed to estimate expression of a single gene; to quantify different gene isoforms, different probes can be combined to reflect the isoform's unique exonic structure. In RNA-seq, mRNA fragments are sequenced and mapped back to a catalog of representative gene sequences (or the genome) to estimate gene or isoform expression levels, typically presented as read counts per transcript.

other factors. Fortunately, these and other potential artifacts have been well studied, and, as array technologies have evolved, so have the methods for normalizing the data and extracting robust gene expression measures (Irizarry, Hobbs, et al. 2003; Leek, Scharpf, et al. 2010).

As new sequencing technologies have become more robust and cost-efficient, the sequencing of RNA (or RNA-seq) has begun to replace microarrays as a means of assessing gene-transcript levels. RNA-seq starts by determining the base sequence of individual RNA molecules and then maps those sequences to a reference genome to determine the abundance of individual gene transcripts (Figure 8–1). As opposed to the continuous values measured using microarrays, RNA-seq data represent counts of the RNA sequence reads that map to a given gene. One advantage of this technology is that it can, in principle, measure the expression levels of all genes (not just those represented by a set of arrayed probes). However, a variety of factors can affect the quality and fidelity of RNA-seq measurements, including the gene sequence, biases in sequencing library construction, the total number of sequenced reads (which affects the depth of coverage in mapping reads to the genome), and even the method used to map sequence reads to the genes.

While there are advantages and disadvantages to both microarrays and RNA-seq, and the analysis of data from each requires careful preprocessing to eliminate artifacts in order to estimate gene expression levels accurately, both have been widely used in transcriptomic network modeling. Importantly, there is a wealth of such data archived in public databases including the Gene Expression Omnibus at the National Center for Biotechnology Information (NCBI) and the European Bioinformatics Institute's (EBI) Array Express.

Transcriptomics as a Measure of Network Output

Part of the challenge of linking genomic information with observed phenotypes is the complexity of biological processes. For gene regulatory networks, transcription is the output of an underlying process wherein the concentration of mRNA in a cell or population of cells is mediated by the context-specific behavior of a variety of controlling factors (Figure 8–2). For a particular gene, transcriptional activation begins with the collective binding of various transcription factors (TFs), a class of regulatory proteins, to special control regions of the DNA (Figure 8–3); these are most often located immediately upstream of (before) the target gene, in its promoter, but they can also be located distally (far away) in what are called "enhancers." Once bound to the promoter/enhancer, TFs work together to recruit RNA polymerase (RNAP), which can then "transcribe" the gene, producing a pre-mRNA that is further processed to become a mature mRNA capable of being "translated" into the corresponding protein. Still other factors, including microRNAs, influence mRNA stability, and ultimately affect the level of the protein that is translated from a particular gene. While one might want to measure the proteins that result from this process, RNA levels are far more easily measurable in a comprehensive assay and, thus, are often treated as surrogates for the corresponding protein levels.

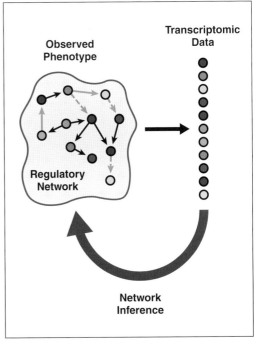

FIGURE 8–2. Gene expression is considered an output of an underlying (and often unknown) gene regulatory network. Network inference algorithms seek to reconstruct the regulatory processes that are associated with a particular phenotype or disease outcome using this information.

It is worth noting that some proteins are TFs and have the potential to further regulate other genes, including, occasionally, themselves. One consequence of this process is that the quantity of specific TFs found in the cell is affected through the same mechanisms as the genes these TFs regulate. It is clear that gene regulation cannot be thought of as a single interaction, or even a single pathway, but rather as a complex set of interacting genes and gene products. One way to conceptualize these regulatory interactions is as a network wherein individual components of the system, namely the genes and TFs, are "nodes" connected to each other by directed "links" or "edges." In principle, it is this network and the interactions between its components that we would like to understand, since this is what underlies the way in which organisms respond to environmental and other cues and may determine how functional biological systems are altered as disease develops. Deducing these networks and understanding their properties has become one of the most exciting and challenging areas of research in computational and systems biology.

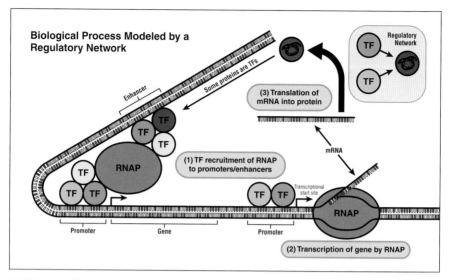

FIGURE 8–3. An illustration of the basic gene regulatory process and how that process is modeled by edges in a gene regulatory network. First, sets of transcription factors bind to either promoters, located in the immediate vicinity of the transcription start site of a gene, or enhancers, which have many of the same properties as promoters but are more distantly located from genes in the genome. Regulation by enhancers may occur, as the DNA can form loops that bring enhancers close to the genes they regulate. Bound transcription factors recruit RNA-polymerase (RNAP), which transcribes the gene sequence to messenger RNA (mRNA). These mRNAs are processed, exported from the nucleus, and translated into protein at the ribosomes located in the cell's cytoplasm. Some genes code for transcription factors, leading genes to regulate other genes. It is this link, between transcription factors and the genes/proteins they target, that is most often modeled in a gene regulatory network of the transcriptional process.

Correlation/Mutual Information-Based Approaches
for Reconstructing Gene Regulatory Networks
from Gene Expression Data

The analysis of microarray data in the early 1990s quickly revealed sets of genes that exhibited strikingly similar patterns of expression across large numbers of samples. Much of the initial work in correlation-based expression analysis used clustering techniques (Weinstein, Myers, et al. 1997; Eisen, Spellman, et al. 1998; Michaels, Carr, et al. 1998) to group genes and samples together so as to identify sets of genes with common profiles that characterized particular sample groups (Perou, Jeffrey, et al. 1999; Perou, Sorlie, et al. 2000). The grouped samples were often examined to find some clinically or phenotypically relevant endpoint, and the grouped genes were examined to identify common biological themes or known pathways that were significantly overrepresented relative to an expected background distribution (Hosack, Dennis, et al. 2003; Subramanian, Tamayo, et al. 2005; Jiang and Gentleman 2007). A common assumption in this analysis is that genes whose expression was highly correlated across samples were under common regulatory control and hence "coregulated."

As a result, methods were developed for inference of co-expression networks (Sabatti, Rohlin, et al. 2002; Shi, Derow, et al. 2010). These often begin by computing a similarity score, such as a Pearson correlation coefficient, between each pair of genes (Figure 8–4) by comparing their expression across samples. One then specifies a threshold value for the minimum value at which one would consider genes to be "correlated" (or coregulated). If we set every element in the matrix to either zero (below the threshold) or one (at or above the threshold), the result is an adjacency matrix (see Chapter 1) in which the rows and columns represent genes and the matrix entries represent the presence or absence of an edge connecting them.

Since these correlation-based similarity matrixes are sym-

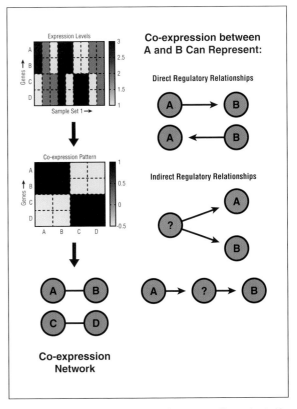

FIGURE 8–4. Gene co-expression networks are generally constructed by transforming gene expression data into a gene-by-gene matrix representing the pairwise similarity in the expression profiles of all genes in the system; thresholding transforms this into an adjacency matrix representing an undirected network. Edges in such networks may represent direct regulatory relationships (between a transcription factor and a downstream target gene whose expression levels are mediated by that transcription factor), correlations between genes that are themselves regulated by the same transcription factors, a series of transcription factors and their individual targets that are correlated, or coincidental correlations between gene expression levels.

metric across the diagonal, networks generated using these measures are generally undirected. They also include information relating every pair of genes, instead of just relationships between TFs and target genes; thus, regulatory relationships are confounded with coregulatory correlations. To produce a putative regulatory network from this matrix, edges between two genes, neither of which is a TF, can be pruned. For the remaining edges, additional specificity can be assigned using TF binding site (TFBS) motifs to eliminate unlikely relationships, and directionality can be assigned by assuming that edges point from TFs to non-TFs (or to correlated genes with appropriate TFBSs).

It soon became obvious that networks created in this way did not accurately represent the underlying regulatory processes. Highly correlated pairs of genes, which were the most common associations in the networks, were likely to be commonly targeted by an upstream TF rather than to regulate each other (see Figure 8–4). Furthermore, co-expression networks estimated from the Pearson correlation did not retain many of the properties that were already beginning to be associated with biological networks, such as a scale-free degree distribution.

WGCNA (weighted gene co-expression network analysis) was developed to address this latter issue. In WGCNA, the computed co-expression values between pairs of genes are modified by using a power adjacency function and taking the absolute value of the correlation to a power (β): $a_{ij} = |cor(x_i,x_j)|^\beta$. Since correlation values are bounded at a maximum of one, the least correlated gene pairs will have their weight converge to zero for increasing values of β, while perfect correlation will be unaffected. Note that setting $\beta = 1$ results in a co-expression network equivalent to using the absolute value of the Pearson correlation without any further modification. By comparing weighted co-expression networks using the topological overlap dissimilarity and clustering the resulting matrix, Horvath and colleagues have identified abnormal spindle homolog, microencephaly-associated (*ASPM*), as a molecular target for glioblastoma (Horvath, Zhang, et al. 2006), identified conserved modules of genes between human and chimpanzee brains (Oldham, Horvath, et al. 2006), and characterized the functional organization of genes in different brain regions (Oldham, Konopka, et al. 2008); they continue to apply their approach in a variety of systems. It is important to note that WGCNA is specifically tuned for finding sets of co-expressed genes with greater accuracy rather than modeling the regulatory network connecting those genes.

While linear correlation is a useful measure of relatedness, some scientists recognized that biological interactions may be nonlinear and that these would be missed by simple linear measures such as Pearson correlation (Figure 8–5). Alternative methods were developed that use measures of correlation such as mutual information to capture such complex relationships and to use them to infer networks (Butte and Kohane 1999; Margolin, Nemenman, et al. 2006; Meyer, Kontos, et al. 2007; Reshef, Reshef, et al. 2011). Although these measures are able to capture more complex information, they generally require large datasets to approximate the correct underlying probability distribution and accurately estimate relationships.

One of the first algorithms to use mutual information to reconstruct a gene regulatory network was ARACNe (Algorithm for the Reconstruction of Accu-

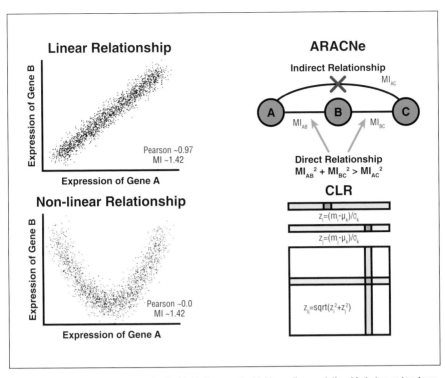

FIGURE 8–5. On the left is an example of a highly linear and a highly nonlinear relationship between two hypothetical gene expression profiles. In practice, each point in these plots represents the result of an experiment measuring gene expression levels. Linear measures, such as the Pearson correlation, can easily capture the relationship between A and B in the top plot, but for nonlinear relationships, such as the one shown in the bottom plot, a measure such as mutual information (MI) is more informative. Two methods that use mutual information as a starting point to infer gene regulatory networks are Algorithm for the Reconstruction of Accurate Cellular Networks (ARACNe) and Context Likelihood of Relatedness (CLR).

rate Cellular Networks; Margolin, Nemenman, et al. 2006). In addition to modeling more complex interactions, ARACNe recognizes that a high mutual information value between two genes may be the result of indirect as well as direct relationships. In other words, if gene A regulates (and thereby has an expression profile that correlates with that of) gene B, and if the same is true of genes B and C, then we might expect that the expression profiles of gene A and gene C are also correlated, even though this is completely mediated by gene B (Figure 8–5). ARACNe seeks to address this issue by evaluating all such "triads" of nodes in a network, and removes the edge in this triad for which there is the least evidence of direct regulation. Califano and colleagues applied ARACNe to analyze gene expression from human B cells, and found v-myc avian myelocytomatosis viral oncogene homolog (*MYC*) to be a hub in the network (Margolin, Nemenman, et al. 2006). They were subsequently able to verify a large percentage of the predicted *MYC* interactions as well as the importance of the MYC protein in their system. Unfortunately, ARACNe's ability to reconstruct useful networks in other contexts has been limited. One reason for this limitation may be a consequence of the algorithm removing all triads in the network, a structure that is important in feedback and feed-forward loops (Milo, Shen-Orr, et al. 2002; Alon 2007).

In 2007, Faith and colleagues developed another approach based on mutual information called CLR (Context Likelihood of Relatedness; Faith, Hayete, et al. 2007). Rather than pruning specific edges by comparing triads, CLR instead prunes edges based on local structure in the mutual information by normalizing the mutual information matrix by recasting it into z-score units. More specifically, for each gene k, CLR recasts the distribution of mutual information into z-scores: $z_i = (m_i - \mu_k)/\sigma_k$, where μ_k/σ_k are the mean/standard deviation of the mutual information gene k has with all other genes, and m_i is the mutual information gene k has with gene i. To maintain symmetry, z-scores for pairs of genes are combined such that: $z_{ij} = sqrt(z_j^2 + z_i^2)$. One interesting feature of this z-score calculation is that, in order to ensure that strongly negative z_i and z_j values do not result in a strongly positive z_{ij}, edges that are derived from negative z_i and z_j values are removed from the final weighted adjacency matrix.

In their paper, Faith and colleagues demonstrated that CLR outperformed ARACNe in a benchmark *Escherichia coli* gene expression dataset. However, like many correlation-based approaches (Marbach, Costello, et al. 2012), CLR has had only limited success in accurately reconstructing networks in larger, more complex organisms and systems. Despite their limitations, both CLR and ARACNe have been applied to the reconstruction of networks in many varied systems and remain well cited in the field of transcriptomics.

While intuitive, simple, and appealing, correlation-based approaches do not address the question of what drives regulatory processes in cells. Co-expression networks may well capture direct regulatory relationships, but these cannot be distinguished from indirect associations based on similarity of expression patterns. The result is often a series of many-to-many associations between genes with correlated expression in which the strongest associations are not necessarily those that are most relevant to understanding regulatory processes. Nevertheless, many studies have found that clusters of highly correlated genes are enriched for particular biological processes (based on a representational analysis (Hawse, Hejtmancik, et al. 2003; Subramanian, Tamayo, et al. 2005; Irizarry, Wang, et al. 2009) using gene ontology terms or pathway databases) that are relevant for understanding at least part of a disease process.

Statistical-Modeling Approaches for Estimating Regulatory Relationships from Transcriptomics Data

Statistical methods have also been adapted for use in the reconstruction of gene regulatory network models. One of the main motivations for using these is that the score predicted for each edge in the network has a probabilistic interpretation with weights and errors. Also, unlike correlation-based approaches, these models typically predict directed relationships, which is more consistent with the biological processes involved in gene regulation.

Statistical approaches for modeling gene regulatory networks generally fall into two main classes. The first frames network inference as a series of regression problems wherein the expression level of each target gene is predicted by a combination of the expression levels across a set of potential upstream regulators. The second casts the problem of finding regulators as a classification problem in which new targets of a TF are predicted by comparing each potential target gene's expression profile to the profiles of known "true" and "false" targets.

Similar to correlation-based approaches to regulatory network reconstruction, regression-based approaches assume that the expression level of a gene is a function of the expression levels of its upstream regulators (De Smet and Marchal 2010). To use transcriptomics data to predict a gene regulatory network, regression approaches generally define a linear equation describing the expression level of gene i as a function of the expression levels of its upstream regulators: $E_j = \Sigma_{wt} E_t + \varepsilon$, where $t \in T$ (the set of regulators) and ε is noise in the system. By considering a series of equations of this form, one for each given experimental condition, one can solve for the coefficients w_t, thereby determining the set of regulators whose expression is most indicative of the expression of the downstream target gene across the experiments. Note that in order to solve this system of equations, the number of measured conditions must be greater than the number of TF regulators, otherwise the problem is underdetermined.

Because each gene is likely only regulated by a small number of TFs, regression approaches often consider this a sparse problem, wherein they limit solution of the linear model to consider the influence of only a small number of potential regulators (Haury, Mordelet, et al. 2012). Standard methods such as LASSO (least absolute shrinkage and selection operator) and least angle regression (LARS) are used to prevent overfitting when the number of given experimental conditions is much greater than the number of regulators being fit.

Regression approaches generally employ a resampling scheme, such as bootstrapping, to determine a score for each regulatory interaction that assesses the probability that the coefficients in the regression equation w_t are nonzero. This score in turn gives a probabilistic interpretation for the edges in the resulting network model. It is worth noting that regression approaches are often sensitive to the choice of resampling method. These methods often have several tuning parameters related to the number of regulators included in the sparse regression, how to sample from the underlying data, and the number of sampling runs. Further, when predicting both in silico and real-world biological networks, the accuracy of regression-based approaches is highly variable, with no particular regression method for fitting these equations consistently achieving higher predictive accuracy (compared to known regulatory interactions) when applied to different types of transcriptomics data or in different species (Marbach, Costello, et al. 2012).

In contrast to regression-based approaches that try to predict the regulators of each gene, classification approaches look at the problem from the opposite direction and try to predict the targets of each TF by conceptualizing regulatory network reconstruction as a feature-selection model (Ernst, Beg, et al. 2008; Mordelet and Vert 2008). To do this, these methods require some prior knowledge about known true and false targets of each TF. Each gene is then examined and assigned as either a target or a nontarget of a particular TF based on whether the gene's expression levels across a given set of conditions is more similar to those in the predefined set of true or false targets.

Classification methods rely heavily on the "prior" information used to build regulatory network predictions. With chromatin immunoprecipitation (ChIP-chip), ChIP-seq, and other sources of data, information on the true interactions is becoming increasingly available. However, it is less obvious how to best define the required set of false interactions. Further, as explicated below, despite the large increase in genomic information over the past decade, only a subset of all known TF regulators have high-quality, condition-specific, validated regulatory interactions.

One limitation of both regression-based and classification-based approaches is that after predicting each gene's regulators, or each TF's targets, it is necessary to perform a postprocessing step to stitch together these sets of predictions into a global network. Consequently, although regression and classification methods perform well in identifying the specific TF–target interactions, assimilating all genes and TF classifications into a single model is often problematic and the resulting global network model is not significantly better than a model based on combining the results of other approaches with the starting set of prior predictions.

Bayesian Networks: A Data-Driven Approach to Network Mapping

Bayesian networks represent an alternative approach to network modeling that requires edges to be directed. Formally, a Bayesian network is a directed acyclic graph (DAG) whose vertices are random variables $X_1, \ldots, X_n$ that are probabilistic, can be discrete or continuous, and describe variation across conditions. In this context, each variable has a conditional distribution given its parents $P(X_i|Parents(X_i))$ and is independent of its nondescendants given its parents. Consequently, Bayesian networks allow only dependencies between a node and its parents, and conditional independence statements encoded by the network structure define the conditional probability distributions.

An example of a Bayesian network is shown in Figure 8–6. In this example, the outcome of whether it is cold inside, for example in an office space or conference room, is dependent on two other factors, whether it is cold outside (for example, during the winter months) and whether the air conditioning is on. In truth, these other two factors are not themselves independent, as the weather may influence whether the air conditioning is on. In the context of gene regulatory networks, the nodes in a Bayesian network are various genes represented in the system. The edges, which are directed, represent "causal" (in truth and importantly, inferential) interactions between the elements in the system.

In the context of transcriptomics data, with each gene we can associate a measured gene expression level, and the conditional probability distributions that define a Bayesian network are the factors that influence

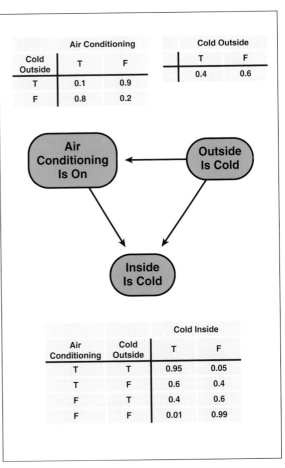

FIGURE 8–6. An example of a simple Bayesian network with three nodes and their interdependencies noted in contingency tables.

Air Conditioning

Cold Outside	T	F
T	0.1	0.9
F	0.8	0.2

Cold Outside

T	F
0.4	0.6

Cold Inside

Air Conditioning	Cold Outside	T	F
T	T	0.95	0.05
T	F	0.6	0.4
F	T	0.4	0.6
F	F	0.01	0.99

gene expression. Part of the attraction of these models is that the edges do not necessarily represent direct interactions but can represent the influence of a number of undetected genes, proteins, or metabolites that, in many ways, allow us to overcome the imperfect knowledge of the relationships that exist in the systems we study and incompleteness in the experimental data.

Bayesian networks were first applied to gene expression studies in the analysis of the yeast cell cycle (Friedman, Linial, et al. 2000), using a dataset that consisted of expression experiments collected over a carefully planned time-course (Spellman, Sherlock, et al. 1998). Friedman and colleagues were able to deduce a predictive model of the cell cycle machinery in yeast from these data, a result that generated a great deal of excitement within the research community. However, application of Bayesian network analysis to more "realistic" datasets (such as tumor vs. normal, treated vs. control) failed to provide similarly useful insights and, as a result, is rarely used in analysis of expression profiling data. The most significant reason for this is the computational complexity of learning the structure of the networks, a problem that has been shown to be nondeterministic polynomial time (NP)–hard (Chickering 1996), implying that an exact computational solution is not possible. Consequently, although Bayesian networks are still considered very powerful models, their applicability to estimating networks that contain more than a handful of genes is severely limited.

To overcome these limitations, one alternative is to "seed" the search for network structure based on integration of prior knowledge, an idea that has support from the computer science literature. For example, Wolpert and Macready (1997) noted that the use of domain-specific knowledge can provide a useful bias that leads to near-optimal solutions in exploring the state space of a particular problem. In the context of Bayesian network analysis of microarray data, a useful bias can be introduced through the use of preliminary network topologies as soft constraints to seed the search for a network graph (Castelo and Siebes 1998; Hartemink, Gifford, et al. 2002; Imoto, Higuchi, et al. 2003), an approach that has been applied in a variety of related problems (Le Phillip, Bahl, et al. 2004; Bastos and Guimarães 2005; Gevaert, Van Vooren, et al. 2007; Husmeier and Werhli 2007; Werhli and Husmeier 2007). Although a network seed biases the search for the best topology, it does not limit the search so that new potential interactions between genes can be identified. An extensive analysis of the use of seeds in learning Bayesian networks (Djebbari and Quackenbush 2008) demonstrated that by using static snapshots of gene expression in various leukemia datasets, one can learn realistic Bayesian networks that capture many of the subtle interrelationships in these systems and, in doing so, produce realistic models of the networks and pathways controlling disease development and progression.

Despite these advances, Bayesian networks have significant limitations that have prevented their widespread adoption. Although Bayesian networks allow high resolution of correlation structure in large datasets, they are fundamentally acyclic graphs and therefore cannot include feedback loops that are important for many biological processes, including the cell-cycle processes that Friedman and colleagues first studied. There have been a number of extensions of the Bayesian network framework to include cyclic structures, including factor graph approaches (Gat-Viks, Tanay, et al. 2006) and dynamic Bayesian networks (DBNs) that model a series of networks in which nodes at time $t+1$ have parents only at time t, resulting in a network that is both acyclic and tractable (Husmeier 2003; Kim, Imoto, et al. 2003; Yu, Smith, et al. 2004; Zou and Conzen 2005). These networks are sometimes augmented by hidden nodes (Perrin, Ralaivola, et al. 2003) which can describe TF activity (Nachman and Regev 2009) or other effects that might perturb expression (Beal, Falciani, et al. 2005).

Additional Emerging Sources of Gene Regulatory Information

It has become increasingly clear that inferring regulatory networks from gene expression data alone results in, at best, an incomplete model. Consequently, regulatory network reconstruction algorithms have been developed that include, as inputs, regulatory edges predicted *a priori* from external data sources (Conlon, Liu, et al. 2003; Margolin, Nemenman, et al. 2006; Chang, Payton, et al. 2008). One common source of network prior information is derived from scanning the genome for TFBSs in the neighborhood of genes (typically defined within the promoter or another specific sequence window around a gene's annotated transcription start site). These TFBS sequences are generally short (5 to 15 base pairs in length) and are often represented as "motifs" (observed nucleic acid base frequency distributions at each location in the TFBS region). Unfortunately, only a small fraction of identified TFs (as little as 1 in 10) have well-defined and highly accurate TFBS motifs. Nevertheless, combining TFBS motif data with protein–DNA binding information from ChIP-chip/ChIP-seq experiments or epigenetic information regarding chromatin structure has been applied to seed network models (Beyer, Workman, et al. 2006; Pique-Regi, Degner, et al. 2011), especially in predicting networks for higher organisms such as mice and humans (Gerstein, Kundaje, et al. 2012).

It is also becoming increasingly recognized that enhancers are crucial for gene regulation in higher eukaryotes. However, methods for incorporating distal regulatory elements like enhancers into network models are still being developed. Current approaches generally start by defining a set of enhancers for a particular cell type and then mapping those enhancers to the genes they control (often assumed to be the gene nearest to the enhancer). This nearest-neighbor approach is known not to be completely accurate, as enhancers can regulate genes that are much more distal in linear genome sequence units by being in physical proximity through DNA looping and changes in chromatin structure. Some approaches try to map enhancers to all genes within a given region to account for the fact that enhancers can sometimes regulate multiple genes. Other methods include gene expression information when doing enhancer mapping in an attempt to incorporate even more distal enhancers that may be regulating a target gene; these complex methods are much more computationally intensive and do not lead to a significant improvement in functional predictions based on validation experiments. Nevertheless, the use of enhancers and other epigenetic modifiers of gene expression in network inference is likely to grow as projects such as the Encyclopedia of DNA Elements (ENCODE) continue large-scale efforts to map and catalog functional elements across the genome.

Determining Regulatory Networks by Integrating Transcriptomic Data with Other Sources of Regulatory Information

As noted previously, many network inference methods using only expression data cannot distinguish between direct and indirect regulatory events (de la Fuente, Bing, et al. 2004; Marbach, Prill, et al. 2010), while models that integrate multiple data types can more accurately predict regulatory mechanisms as compared with methods that use any individual data type alone (Hecker, Lambeck, et al. 2009).

PANDA (Passing Attributes between Networks for Data Assimilation; Figure 8–7) (Glass, Huttenhower, et al. 2013) is a promising new method that borrows an idea called message passing (or affinity propagation) from communication theory (Frey and Dueck 2007) to integrate diverse sources of genomic data and to model the flow of information in complex regulatory networks. Message passing assumes communication between transmitters and receivers and requires that both are active for information to flow. In the context of PANDA's regulatory network models, TFs are the transmitters and the receivers are their downstream target genes. PANDA recognizes that although a TF is "responsible" for regulating a target gene, the gene must also be "available" to be regulated. By constructing a prior regulatory network consisting of potential routes for communication (by mapping TF motifs to a reference genome) and integrating other sources of regulatory information (such as protein–protein interaction and gene expression data), one can estimate two mathematical functions for each potential

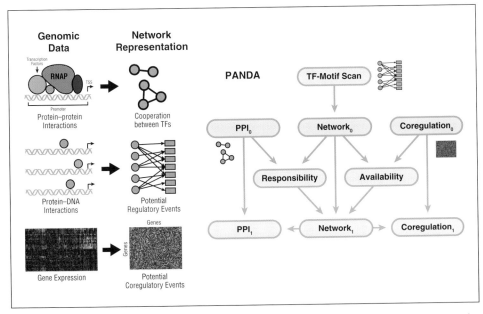

FIGURE 8–7. An illustration of the Passing Attributes between Networks for Data Assimilation (PANDA) message-passing method for data integration and gene regulatory network inference. PANDA starts with input protein-protein interaction (PPI_0) data, coregulation data (C_0, based on gene expression), and initial estimates of the network (W_0) based on transcription factor mapping to the genome. It then iteratively updates each of these (as suggested on the right) until the method converges on a final model that optimizes information flow through the network.

interaction (the responsibility and the availability) and deduce condition-specific network structures. In this model, the quintessential elements are not the genes, but the edges that represent active channels of gene regulation.

One key feature of PANDA is its emphasis on agreement between data elements in a network neighborhood. For example, a regulatory relationship between a TF and a downstream target gene is not inferred solely from co-expression information. Instead, a gene's availability to be regulated by a TF is determined based on whether or not that gene is co-expressed with other known targets of the TF. As such, PANDA can better distinguish between multiple TFs that may regulate a particular gene. PANDA also allows a robust estimation of the effects of combinatorial regulation and can identify TFs that, although not differentially expressed themselves, alter the behavior of their downstream regulatory targets differently depending on the overall cellular state. This allows for a soft coupling between TFs and genes, as PANDA simultaneously evaluates both upstream regulatory events, modeled by protein-interaction information, and downstream regulatory effects, modeled in gene coregulatory information. The result is that relationships between TFs and target genes, which are often imperfectly correlated in expression data, can still be recovered, since PANDA explicitly models the fact that each gene is potentially regulated by multiple TFs while each TF often affects the transcriptional output of many different genes.

Because PANDA considers multiple types of relationships between both regulators and their targets, the method can incorporate multiple independent data sources. For example, microRNAs can be included in much the same way as TFs and epigenetic modifications can be used to modify prior values of the responsibility and availability. Finally, PANDA is often used to first reconstruct condition-dependent regulatory network models, which are then subsequently compared. In this context, it has been shown to identify condition-specific regulatory modules that are often informative as to the functional processes that produce phenotypic differences. This ability to identify relevant alterations in regulatory network structure has crucial implications for developing targeted therapies for disease and illustrates how transcriptomic networks continue to play an important role in future network medicine applications.

Conclusion

Although a wealth of gene expression data has been generated over the past decade, most biological inference has been based on statistical tests at the level of individual genes (with high rates of spurious associations) followed by functional meta-analysis using gene set enrichment techniques. Network analysis provides a more nuanced exploration of the underlying regulatory mechanisms associated with the differential activity of gene regulatory programs. By associating differences in regulatory patterns with differences in gene expression, we can define subsets of genes that are activated or repressed by their regulators. Then, by identifying and exploring relationships between a set of key transcriptional regulators, we can identify putative mechanisms by which they might be coordinately working to activate, or repress, the expression of their target genes. These network methods can also help identify potential areas of therapeutic intervention—not only global hubs in the network, but also local drivers of subnetworks unique to individual phenotypes.

The structures in cellular networks are not static, but rather they are perturbed by disease. Therefore, once transcriptomic networks are reconstructed, it is almost equally crucial to be able to compare them. Changes such as the appearance or disappearance of edges or groups of edges can help define differences between disease phenotypes. One interesting feature that emerges from comparing inferred regulatory networks is that the TFs or their targets may not significantly alter their expression levels between phenotypes, but the most likely regulatory associations may change. In other words, the expression of a gene can be mediated by different upstream TFs. In the context of disease, identifying these differences has the potential to lead to new therapies that would not have been discovered outside of the network medicine paradigm.

Clearly, the field of gene regulatory network inference is in its early days and fails to capture the full complexity of the cellular processes that mediate the link between genotype and phenotype. However, the growing body of comprehensive, multi-omic data integrated with extensive clinical and phenotypic data promises to enable the development of new methods and approaches that may ultimately improve the ways in which we understand and treat disease.

References

Alon, U. (2007). Network motifs: theory and experimental approaches. Nat Rev Genet **8**(6): 450–61.

Bastos, G., and K. Guimarães (2005). Analyzing the Effect of Prior Knowledge in Genetic Regulatory Network Inference. Pattern Recognition and Machine Intelligence. Berlin/Heidelberg, Springer: 611–16.

Beal, M. J., F. Falciani, et al. (2005). A Bayesian approach to reconstructing genetic regulatory networks with hidden factors. Bioinformatics **21**(3): 349–56.

Beyer, A., C. Workman, et al. (2006). Integrated assessment and prediction of transcription factor binding. PLoS Comput Biol **2**(6): e70.

Butte, A. J., and I. S. Kohane (1999). Unsupervised knowledge discovery in medical databases using relevance networks. Proc AMIA Symp: 711–15.

Castelo, R., and A. Siebes (2000). Priors on network structures: Biasing the search for Bayesian networks. Int J Approx Reason **24**(1): 39–57.

Chang, L. W., J. E. Payton, et al. (2008). Computational identification of the normal and perturbed genetic networks involved in myeloid differentiation and acute promyelocytic leukemia. Genome Biol **9**(2): R38.

Chickering, D. M. (1996). Learning Bayesian networks is NP-Complete. In: V. D. Fisher and H. Lenz, eds., Learning from Data: Artificial Intelligence and Statistics. New York: Springer, pp. 121–30.

Chuang, H. Y., M. Hofree, et al. (2010). A decade of systems biology. Annu Rev Cell Dev Biol **26**: 721–44.

Conlon, E. M., X. S. Liu, et al. (2003). Integrating regulatory motif discovery and genome-wide expression analysis. Proc Natl Acad Sci U S A **100**(6): 3339–44.

de la Fuente, A., N. Bing, et al. (2004). Discovery of meaningful associations in genomic data using partial correlation coefficients. Bioinformatics **20**(18): 3565–74.

De Smet, R., and K. Marchal (2010). Advantages and limitations of current network inference methods. Nat Rev Microbiol **8**(10): 717–29.

Djebbari, A., and J. Quackenbush (2008). Seeded Bayesian Networks: constructing genetic networks from microarray data. BMC Syst Biol **2**: 57.

Eisen, M. B., P. T. Spellman, et al. (1998). Cluster analysis and display of genome-wide expression patterns. Proc Natl Acad Sci U S A **95**(25): 14863–68.

Ernst, J., Q. K. Beg, et al. (2008). A semi-supervised method for predicting transcription factor-gene interactions in Escherichia coli. PLoS Comput Biol **4**(3): e1000044.

Faith, J. J., B. Hayete, et al. (2007). Large-scale mapping and validation of Escherichia coli transcriptional regulation from a compendium of expression profiles. PLoS Biol **5**(1): e8.

Frey, B. J., and D. Dueck (2007). Clustering by passing messages between data points. Science **315**(5814): 972–76.

Friedman, N., M. Linial, et al. (2000). Using Bayesian networks to analyze expression data. J Comput Biol **7**(3–4): 601–20.

Gat-Viks, I., A. Tanay, et al. (2006). A probabilistic methodology for integrating knowledge and experiments on biological networks. J Comput Biol **13**(2): 165–81.

Gerstein, M. B., A. Kundaje, et al. (2012). Architecture of the human regulatory network derived from ENCODE data. Nature **489**(7414): 91–100.

Gevaert, O., S. Van Vooren, et al. (2007). A framework for elucidating regulatory networks based on prior information and expression data. Ann N Y Acad Sci **1115:** 240–48.

Glass, K., C. Huttenhower, et al. (2013). Passing messages between biological networks to refine predicted interactions. PloS One **8**(5): e64832.

Hartemink, A. J., D. K. Gifford, et al. (2002). Combining location and expression data for principled discovery of genetic regulatory network models. Pac Symp Biocomput: 437–49.

Haury, A. C., F. Mordelet, et al. (2012). TIGRESS: Trustful Inference of Gene REgulation using Stability Selection. BMC Syst Biol **6**: 145.

Hawse, J. R., J. F. Hejtmancik, et al. (2003). Identification and functional clustering of global gene expression differences between human age-related cataract and clear lenses. Mol Vis **9**: 515–37.

Hecker, M., S. Lambeck, et al. (2009). Gene regulatory network inference: data integration in dynamic models-a review. Biosystems **96**(1): 86–103.

Horvath, S., B. Zhang, et al. (2006). Analysis of oncogenic signaling networks in glioblastoma identifies ASPM as a molecular target. Proc Natl Acad Sci U S A **103**(46): 17402–7.

Hosack, D. A., G. Dennis, Jr., et al. (2003). Identifying biological themes within lists of genes with EASE. Genome Biol **4**(10): R70.

Husmeier, D. (2003). Sensitivity and specificity of inferring genetic regulatory interactions from microarray experiments with dynamic Bayesian networks. Bioinformatics **19**(17): 2271–82.

Husmeier, D., and A. V. Werhli (2007). Bayesian integration of biological prior knowledge into the reconstruction of gene regulatory networks with Bayesian networks. Comput Syst Bioinformatics Conf **6**: 85–95.

Imoto, S., T. Higuchi, et al. (2003). Combining microarrays and biological knowledge for estimating gene networks via Bayesian networks. Proc IEEE Comput Soc Bioinform Conf **2**: 104–13.

Irizarry, R. A., B. Hobbs, et al. (2003). Exploration, normalization, and summaries of high density oligonucleotide array probe level data. Biostatistics **4**(2): 249–64.

Irizarry, R. A., C. Wang, et al. (2009). Gene set enrichment analysis made simple. Stat Methods Med Res **18**(6): 565–75.

Jiang, Z., and R. Gentleman (2007). Extensions to gene set enrichment. Bioinformatics **23**(3): 306–13.

Kim, S. Y., S. Imoto, et al. (2003). Inferring gene networks from time series microarray data using dynamic Bayesian networks. Brief Bioinform **4**(3): 228–35.

Le Phillip, P., A. Bahl, et al. (2004). Using prior knowledge to improve genetic network reconstruction from microarray data. In Silico Biol **4**(3): 335–3.

Leek, J. T., R. B. Scharpf, et al. (2010). Tackling the widespread and critical impact of batch effects in high-throughput data. Nat Rev Genet **11**(10): 733–39.

Marbach, D., J. C. Costello, et al. (2012). Wisdom of crowds for robust gene network inference. Nat Methods **9**(8): 796–804.

Marbach, D., R. J. Prill, et al. (2010). Revealing strengths and weaknesses of methods for gene network inference. Proc Natl Acad Sci U S A **107**(14): 6286–91.

Margolin, A. A., I. Nemenman, et al. (2006). ARACNE: an algorithm for the reconstruction of gene regulatory networks in a mammalian cellular context. BMC Bioinformatics **7 Suppl 1:** S7.

Meyer, P. E., K. Kontos, et al. (2007). Information-theoretic inference of large transcriptional regulatory networks. EURASIP J Bioinform Syst Biol: 79879.

Michaels, G. S., D. B. Carr, et al. (1998). Cluster analysis and data visualization of large-scale gene expression data. Pac Symp Biocomput: 42–53.

Milo, R., S. Shen-Orr, et al. (2002). Network motifs: simple building blocks of complex networks. Science **298**(5594): 824–27.

Mordelet, F., and J. P. Vert (2008). SIRENE: supervised inference of regulatory networks. Bioinformatics **24**(16): i76–82.

Nachman, I., and A. Regev (2009). BRNI: Modular analysis of transcriptional regulatory programs. BMC Bioinformatics **10**: 155.

Oldham, M. C., S. Horvath, et al. (2006). Conservation and evolution of gene coexpression networks in human and chimpanzee brains. Proc Natl Acad Sci U S A **103**(47): 17973–78.

Oldham, M. C., G. Konopka, et al. (2008). Functional organization of the transcriptome in human brain. Nat Neurosci **11**(11): 1271–82.

Perou, C. M., S. S. Jeffrey, et al. (1999). Distinctive gene expression patterns in human mammary epithelial cells and breast cancers. Proc Natl Acad Sci U S A **96**(16): 9212–17.

Perou, C. M., T. Sorlie, et al. (2000). Molecular portraits of human breast tumours. Nature **406**(6797): 747–52.

Perrin, B. E., L. Ralaivola, et al. (2003). Gene networks inference using dynamic Bayesian networks. Bioinformatics **19 Suppl 2:** ii138–148.

Pique-Regi, R., J. F. Degner, et al. (2011). Accurate inference of transcription factor binding from DNA sequence and chromatin accessibility data. Genome Res **21**(3): 447–55.

Reshef, D. N., Y. A. Reshef, et al. (2011). Detecting novel associations in large data sets. Science **334**(6062): 1518–24.

Sabatti, C., L. Rohlin, et al. (2002). Co-expression pattern from DNA microarray experiments as a tool for operon prediction. Nucleic Acids Res **30**(13): 2886–93.

Shi, Z., C. K. Derow, et al. (2010). Co-expression module analysis reveals biological processes, genomic gain, and regulatory mechanisms associated with breast cancer progression. BMC Syst Biol **4**: 74.

Spellman, P. T., G. Sherlock, et al. (1998). Comprehensive identification of cell cycle-regulated genes of the yeast Saccharomyces cerevisiae by microarray hybridization. Mol Biol Cell **9**(12): 3273–97.

Subramanian, A., P. Tamayo, et al. (2005). Gene set enrichment analysis: a knowledge-based approach for interpreting genome-wide expression profiles. Proc Natl Acad Sci U S A **102**(43): 15545–50.

Weinstein, J. N., T. G. Myers, et al. (1997). An information-intensive approach to the molecular pharmacology of cancer. Science **275**(5298): 343–49.

Werhli, A. V., and D. Husmeier (2007). Reconstructing gene regulatory networks with bayesian networks by combining expression data with multiple sources of prior knowledge. Stat Appl Genet Mol Biol **6**: Article15.

Wolpert, D. H., and W. G. Macready (1997). No free lunch theorems for optimization. IEEE Transactions on Evolutionary Computation **1**(1): 67–82.

Yu, J., V. A. Smith, et al. (2004). Advances to Bayesian network inference for generating causal networks from observational biological data. Bioinformatics **20**(18): 3594–603.

Zou, M., and S. D. Conzen (2005). A new dynamic Bayesian network (DBN) approach for identifying gene regulatory networks from time course microarray data. Bioinformatics **21**(1): 71–79.

9

Post-translational Modifications of the Proteome: The Example of Tau in the Neuron and the Brain

Guy Lippens, Jeremy Gunawardena, Isabelle Landrieu,
Caroline Smet-Nocca, Sudhakaran Prabakaran,
Benjamin Parent, Arnaud Leroy, and Isabelle Huvent

Introduction

In this chapter, we will outline the role that post-translational modifications (PTMs) can play in information processing at the cellular level and at the protein level. These modifications can not only lead to enhanced or decreased activity of a biomolecule, but can also generate novel interaction sites or destroy previously existing ones and thereby change the biomolecule's position in the network of interactions that characterizes the cell. They can determine, in a direct or indirect manner, the stability of the protein and hence its cellular concentration. In contrast to protein modifications resulting from genomic alterations, the information content of PTMs is inherently dynamic, with a demodifying enzyme class identified for each class of modifying enzymes. The action of these enzymes in the cell is not random, but is tightly regulated through the use of scaffolding proteins that control the spatial proximity of the many enzymes involved in generating a functional outcome of the signal. Understanding this order and how its possible perturbations can lead to disease is a central research effort pursued for various pathologies.

An overview of all PTMs linked to disease would require a full encyclopedia that would need updating on an almost daily basis. The importance of novel PTMs is indeed a recurring theme in the present biomedical literature. Novel methodology, especially based on innovative mass spectrometry techniques aimed at getting an unbiased view of all proteome changes that accompany selected diseases, is being developed at a fast pace. In this chapter, we do not aim to present such an enumeration. Rather, trying to "See a World in a Grain of Sand" (Blake 1803), we want to focus on the PTMs of the neuronal Tau protein and their relationship to Alzheimer disease. Recent results have only started to show the complexity of the possible PTM patterns in different stages of the disease and how its PTMs couple to other related processes in the neuronal cell. We hope through this example to underline the conceptual importance of PTMs as a time- and space-dependent distribution of modifications over individual molecules, the technological challenges associated with the study of PTMs in physiological and pathological conditions, and the true challenge of learning how to interpret these modifications in terms of cellular outcome.

Information Processing through Allostery and Post-translational Modifications

Life is all about information processing. At length scales varying over 9 orders of magnitude, from the full organism to the individual (macro)molecule over the intermediate scales of organs and cells, we integrate signals from the exterior world and process them to yield a specific action. The physical nature of information processing at the molecular level takes on many forms. Allostery and PTMs are major mechanisms in which a protein can modify its form and function as a consequence of a given signal, engage in novel interactions with other biomolecules, and, thereby, pass the information to different compartments of the cell. Here we define *allostery* as a conformational change stabilized or induced by ligand binding, leading to altered function of the resulting complex at a site different from the allosteric ligand binding site. Better or worse binding to a third partner is one such possible function, but many other functions can result.

A classical example of proteins that undergo allosteric changes upon ligand binding is the large class of nuclear receptors that act as transcription factors with a ligand-binding domain. Binding of a small ligand to the ligand-binding domain modulates, directly or indirectly, target gene transcription (Billas and Moras 2013). A second important example in which ligand binding at one site modifies the structure at a different site, but for which information has to be transmitted from outside to inside the cell, is that involving the large family of G-protein–coupled receptors (GPCRs). With its 800 members in the human genome, these receptors are essential for signal transduction over the plasma membrane (Rosenbaum et al. 2009). The signal here is a chemical entity, in the form of a ligand molecule that will bind in a stoichiometric manner to the extracellular domain of the receptor, inducing a conformational switch across the plasma membrane that leads to differential interaction with cytosolic signaling proteins such as G proteins, GPCR kinases, or arrestins (Katritch et al. 2012). When the ligand diffuses from the receptor, statistical fluctuations in the macromolecule will bring it back to its default conformation, indicating that the lifetime of the complex is an important factor for the information transfer.

Once outside information enters the cell but before it can mediate down-stream effects such as altered gene expression, the signal must enter the appropriate compartment, such as the nucleus. This step in the information transfer process is typically where PTMs come into play, because they allow both for amplification of the signal and for its physical stabilization during the diffusion time of the macromolecule from the cytoplasm to the nucleus (Prabakaran et al. 2012). Seeking an equivalent in computer science, the transistor provides the same function as regulated amplification. Phosphorylation appears to be the main (although not the only) PTM for the transfer of information toward the nucleus and is effected by one of the roughly 500 kinases encoded by the human genome (Manning et al. 2002). Recently, many other PTMs have been described, some of which we will discuss in the framework of Tau biology below.

When combining both mechanisms of allostery and PTM, the resulting complexity is tremendous, especially as we have to consider not a single macromolecular species, but thousands of different ones. Nevertheless, detailed structural studies of many signaling molecules in different states of activation have led to a deep understanding of the importance of both allostery and PTM at the level of the protein as an individual component of the circuitry. The complex interplay between genomic alterations and the resulting changes in PTM distribution is of direct importance to disease, but it equally emphasizes the technological challenges that will have to be overcome to merge the information into a coherent picture. When we consider that unraveling the human genome was a major endeavour only 10 years ago and now genomic sequencing of individual patients is about to enter the clinic, it is not easy to predict at what pace proteomics technology will (have to) develop to become a clinically useful tool in the near future. However, understanding how the individual components can comprise a network of information transfer, how context can decide that seemingly similar complex networks lead to differential cellular outcomes, and how this complexity is related to pathobiology is and will be a major aim of modern medicine. To what level of detail we will need to understand the individual components and/or the modules to make meaningful predictions about cellular outcome is still unclear, but we argue that both a quantitative view of the PTMs and introduction of a spatial and temporal picture of the different determinants and mediators will probably be required to understand signal transduction in terms of cellular, organ, and patient outcomes. In this chapter, we will focus on a single protein, Tau, as an example of the molecular and functional complexities of PTMs. We will use Tau as a specific lens through which to view the process and consequences of covalent modification of proteins in terms of cellular (neuronal) and organ (brain) function and dysfunction.

Alzheimer Disease: A Toxic Interplay of Amyloid-β and Tau?

Alzheimer disease (AD) is a progressive neurodegenerative disorder. Starting at the clinical level with impairment of memory and learning, it ultimately leads to a severe form of dementia and complete loss of independence. Age is the primary risk factor for the disease, and as such, the disease will truly threaten our aging societies. Dementia in people over the age of 60 in the Western world currently exceeds 5%, about two-thirds of which are due to AD (Reitz et al. 2011). The age-specific prevalence of AD moreover, nearly doubles every 5 years after age 65, leading to a prevalence of greater than 25% in those over the age of 90 (Qiu et al. 2009).

At the histopathological level, the disease is characterized by the presence of two types of abnormal protein deposits: amyloid plaques and neurofibrillary tangles. Amyloid plaques are extracellular deposits consisting primarily of amyloid-β (Aβ) peptides generated by successive proteolytic cleavage of the Alzheimer precursor protein (APP) (De Strooper et al. 2010). Neurofibrillary tangles are intraneuronal aggregates of hyperphosphorylated Tau (Flament-Durand and Brion 1985; Grundke-Iqbal et al. 1986; Kosik et al. 1986). The latter protein, Tau, was discovered as a "tubulin associated unit" (Weingarten et al. 1975) and is a family of six proteins generated by alternative splicing from a single gene on chromosome 17 (Figure 9–1) (Lee et al. 1988).

The amyloid cascade hypothesis states that the accumulation of amyloid β (Aβ), a peptide derived from the amyloid precursor protein (APP), would initiate AD and start the pathogenesis (Selkoe 1991) and has structured research in the disease over the past 20 years, with the ultimate goal being efficient disease-modifying treatments. Both the identification of the protein machinery leading to the production of the Aβ peptide and the identification of mutations in the proteolytic machinery or APP substrate that cause an early-onset form of the disease are undeniably a strong argument in favour of the cascade theory (Hardy 2009). However, the toxicity of Aβ alone is not sufficient to explain the clinically observed neuronal loss, for which reason Tau is believed to be a crucial partner for relaying this toxicity. Many mechanisms have been proposed, but they all seem to require PTMs, and notably phosphorylation of Tau.

After age, the second most important risk factor for AD is genetic in nature, and it concerns the polymorphism of apolipoprotein E (Corder et al. 1993). Homozygous carriers of the apolipoprotein E (ApoE) 4 allele are at a 10-fold greater risk for late-onset AD as compared with the more common ApoE3 carriers, and even a single copy of ApoE4 increases the risk threefold. A recent study used differential co-expression analysis of whole-transcriptome datasets derived from

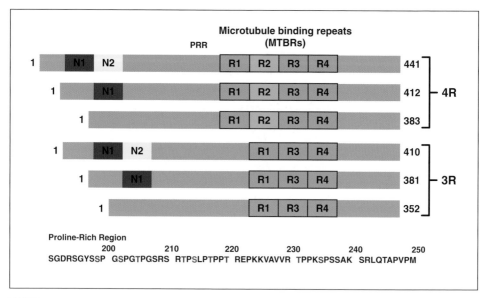

FIGURE 9–1. Alternative splicing of the tau gene can lead to six different isoforms that differ by the presence or absence of two N-terminal inserts and the presence of three or four microtubule binding repeats (MTBRs). The proline-rich region comes upstream of the first repeat and contains eight potential sites for proline-directed kinases and the Ser214 site that can be phosphorylated by protein kinase A.

ApoE4 or ApoE3 carriers with and without the disease and interpreted the resulting cluster of differentiating genes in terms of Aβ production and transport (Rhinn et al. 2013). Nevertheless, the differential regulation of proteins, such as the Fyn kinase or protein tyrosine kinase PTKB2, can equally directly influence the phosphorylation pattern of Tau (see below) and, hence, regulate its cellular function. This finding underlines the need to consider results from unbiased studies in the framework of both Aβ and Tau. Another attempt to obtain an unbiased view of the distinct molecular features of AD combined several comparative proteomics studies of healthy and diseased brains (Korolainen et al. 2010). Although subject to large technical and even conceptual problems—the tissues mainly come from patients in the final stage of the disease, and, hence, do not necessarily inform on the causal factors—the resulting dataset of 109 differentially expressed proteins could be cast in a network around Aβ or Tau. The resulting network, here depicted as a subnetwork for Tau (Figure 9–2), contains no less than 26 proteins or protein subunits involved in the phosphorylation process (kinases or phosphatases), but also contains enzymes, such as the O-linked N-acetylglucosamine (GlcNAc) transferase or the prolyl cis–trans isomerase Pin1, which play an important role in the other possible PTMs of Tau.

An important bottleneck in the development of a disease-modifying treatment for AD is the extremely slow evolution of the disease—which might range

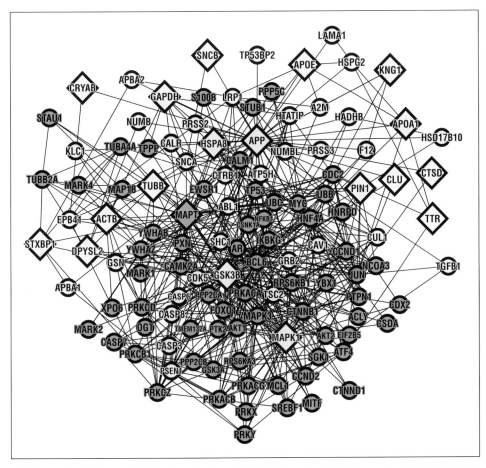

FIGURE 9–2. Protein changes in the brain and cerebrospinal fluid between healthy elderly people and those with AD are connected in a network of protein/protein interactions. The original network focused on three candidates (APP, tau, and Gsk3β) as AD-related nodes. The tau subnetwork depicted here (gray and orange, with tau [or microtubule-associated protein tau {MAPT}] as a blue diamond) contains many enzymes involved in its PTMs. Diamonds represent proteins detected in differential proteomics studies (gray for tau interactors, yellow for APP or Gsk3β) and circles their interaction partners. (Reprinted with permission from Korolainen, M. A., T. A. Nyman, et al. (2010). An update on clinical proteomics in Alzheimer's research. J Neurochem **112**(6): 1386–414. © 2010 The Authors.)

from 10 to 20 years—and the absence of clear biomarkers in the earliest stage of the disease that would indicate that a person is at risk. At present, next to early cognitive tests, the best biomarker seems the quantity of Aβ peptide and Tau in the cerebrospinal fluid (CSF). Although more invasive than a blood test, CSF also can be collected at several time points. CSF dosage of the Ab and Tau biomarkers hence should allow monitoring of disease progression in the presence of potential drug candidates. Whereas the concentration of Aβ typically decreases as the disease progresses from the early mild cognitive impairment stage to its more severe forms, concentrations of Tau and phospho-Tau typically

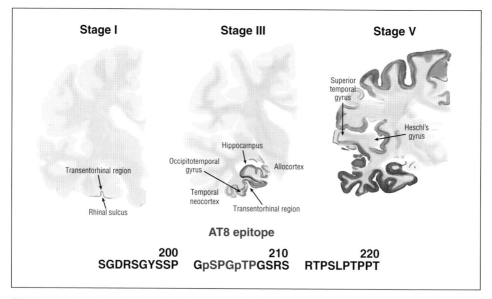

FIGURE 9–3. The AT8 antibody recognizes the pS202/pT205 epitope on tau, and its staining of different brain regions is used to classify postmortem in a histopathological manner the disease progression. (Reprinted with permission from Braak H., I. Alafuzo. (2006). Staging of Alzheimer disease-associated neurofibrillary pathology using paraffin sections and immunocytochemistry. Acta Neuropathol 112: 389–404. Figure 3 (a. c. f.). © Springer-Verlag 2006.)

increase (Blennow 2005). As we will see later in this chapter, phospho-Tau levels are detected and quantified by a phospho-Tau–specific antibody and, as such, is currently also the postmortem visualization of the disease stage. Initially based on the technically demanding Gallyas silver staining assay (Braak and Braak 1991), Braak and Alafuzo proposed in 2006 an immunohistochemical method to detect disease progression based on the AT8 antibody (Figure 9–3). This latter antibody recognizes the pS202/pT205 epitope on Tau, and will be discussed in detail when we address the currently available tools to probe the PTM status of Tau.

Recent work has suggested that Tau has multiple functions (Morris and Maeda 2011), with possibly distinct functions at different places in the neuron, and that it should be seen in terms of an integrated system whereby Tau and its interaction partners are anchored spatially together (Hashiguchi and Hashiguchi 2013) or even considered as parts of one single molecular machine composed of a finite number of biomolecules (Juhàsz et al. 2011). We want to focus on our current understanding of how Tau fits in the organized system that is the axon or the dendritic spine, how its position in these organized networks is regulated by PTMs, and how these same PTMs can contribute to the integration of Tau into the neurofibrillary tangles that characterize AD.

Tau in the Axon: Microtubule Stability and Axonal Transport

Tau, the tubulin-associated unit, was initially discovered as a protein that stabilizes tubulin assembly into microtubules (Weingarten et al. 1975) and as such is a key regulator of neuronal morphogenesis (Drubin et al., 1985) and neurite polarity (Caceres and Kosik, 1990). Through assembling and stabilizing the microtubules in the axons, Tau is a key player in the axonal transport that connects the neuron cell body with the synapses. Splicing is developmentally regulated, with a dominant role for the shortest variant (hTau352–0N3R, see Figure 9–1) early in development, whereas in adult life, all six isoforms are present (Kosik et al. 1989; Goedert et al. 1989). At the molecular level, the splicing of exon 10, which yields the second microtubule binding repeat (MTBR), was found to be regulated by the dual specificity Dyrk1a kinase through phosphorylation of the splicing factor SRp55 (Yin et al., 2012). Because the shortest isoform does not stabilize microtubules to the same extent as the 4R isoforms, the changing expression pattern was initially linked to brain maturation (Goode and Feinstein, 1994), although more recent work dissecting brain region-specific expression patterns did not find a similar correlation (Bullmann et al. 2009).

Tau can regulate axonal transport not only through the stabilization of microtubules, but also by directly interfering with the cytoplasmic motor proteins, kinesin and dynein. Kinesin movements can not only be reduced by the presence of Tau, but Tau can also promote the detachment of the motor protein from the microtubule (MT) surface (Dixit et al. 2008). The different isoforms interfere in a differential manner with kinesin-driven axonal transport, with the 3R isoforms interfering more substantially with multiple motor-driven transport processes than the 4R isoforms (Vershinin et al. 2007). Beyond the isoforms, the spatial distribution of Tau finely regulates the transport process, and the observed proximal-to-distal gradient of Tau as observed in a healthy neuron (Kempf and Clement 1996) can explain selective cargo release in the distal regions of the axon. Combining this finding with the observation that Tau messenger RNA is equally transported by the KIF3A motor protein over the MT to the region where novel Tau will be produced in situ (Aronov et al. 2001) leads to a potential feedback loop.

Not only is the isoform distribution of Tau developmentally regulated, but also is its phosphorylation pattern, which brings us to the heart of the present topic. Phosphorylation of Tau was initially detected through the increased gel mobility of the protein after its dephosphorylation by alkaline phosphatase. The more pronounced change upon phosphatase treatment for the fetal protein when compared to the adult forms indicated that phosphorylation is more pronounced in early life stages (Goedert et al. 1993). Together with the widespread notion that phosphorylation decreases binding to microtubules, the enhanced phosphorylation together with the dominant production of the 3R form both would lead to a more dynamic microtubule network during development (Mattsson et al. 2010).

The same differential mobility in sodium dodecyl sulfate–polyacrylamide gel electrophoresis (SDS PAGE) after alkaline phosphatase treatment was equally observed for Tau in the paired helical filaments (PHFs) found in AD brain tissue (Lee et al. 1991), suggesting that Tau can become more extensively modified at both ends of the lifespan. Mass spectrometry allowed detection of some phosphorylation sites (Hasegawa et al. 1992) and confirmed the intriguing overlap between the phosphorylation patterns of Tau in fetal and AD neurons. Further evidence for neuronal cell cycle reentry came in the mid-1990s, when several phospho-epitopes characteristic of dividing cells were discovered in an AD brain, but not in age-matched normal brain (Vincent et al. 1997). However, all this evidence does not go beyond the factual description of potential common phosphorylation sites. The exact stoichiometry and, even more, the distribution of distinct phosphorylation events over the Tau protein population remains a true analytical challenge, to which we will devote a separate discussion below.

Phosphorylation can regulate the interference of Tau with the kinesin-driven transport of cargo in several ways. The microtubule affinity–regulating kinase (MARK) phosphorylates Tau at the Ser262 residue in the first repeat, thereby reducing the affinity of Tau toward the MT surface (Drewes et al. 1997) and potentially removing the physical barrier that is a Tau molecule anchored to the microtubule. Whether other phosphorylation patterns in the nearby proline-rich region that do not necessarily affect the affinity of Tau for the microtubule surface (Amniai et al. 2009) also interfere with this process is currently not known. Phosphorylation of Tau at its Tyr18 residue, notably catalyzed by the Fyn kinase, does not affect the binding of Tau to the MT surface, but does reduce the impact of Tau on kinesin-driven transport (LaPointe et al. 2009). Whether this altered regulation of MT transport through Tyr18 phosphorylation contributes to erroneous cell cycle reentry and, hence, neurodegeneration remains to be proven. The N-terminal Tyr18 phosphorylation of Tau as catalyzed by the Fyn kinase is, however, impaired by other phosphorylation events. The anchoring of Fyn through a physical interaction of its SH2 domain to the canonical $P_{233}XXP_{236}$ recognition motif in the Tau proline-rich region (PRR) disappears when Tau is phosphorylated by glycogen synthase kinase 3β (Gsk3β) on the neighboring Thr231 (Kanaan et al. 2012). As this same motif is equally recognized by the protein phosphatase 2A (Sontag et al. 2012), it is clear that the resulting pattern of phosphorylation will be the outcome of many interacting partners that cluster around Tau (Hashiguchi and Hashiguchi 2013).

Tau in the Dendritic Spine: Mediating Amyloid β Oligomer Toxicity

Whereas an axonal sorting of Tau was thought to accompany neuronal differentiation (Bullmann et al. 2009), more recent findings have shown that a fraction of Tau is also located at the dendritic spines (Ittner et al. 2010). The presence of Fyn at this location is conditioned by this pool of Tau in the synaptic density, as it anchors Fyn through the physical interaction of the Fyn sarcoma homology 3 (SH3) domain with the aforementioned Tau $P_{233}XXP_{236}$ motif. Aβ oligomers, the first toxic species in the amyloid cascade hypothesis (Hardy 2009), would relay their toxicity through this dendritic pool of Tau and Fyn. Only recently, however, possible molecular mechanisms that link Aβ oligomers to Tau have begun to emerge and seem to suggest that Aβ can exert its toxicity via multiple receptors. Soluble oligomers of Aβ interact with the prion PrP^c protein (Laurén et al. 2009), and this complex activates not only the Fyn kinase but also the cyclic AMP–regulated protein kinase A and calcium-calmodulin kinase II that then generate a specific phosphorylation pattern on Tau (Seward et al. 2013). The resulting cell-cycle reentry recapitulates the aforementioned parallel between fetal and diseased Tau phosphorylation patterns.

Other mechanisms of Aβ toxicity have also been described, with other receptors and downstream effects (Benilova and De Strooper 2013), but most seem relayed at a given moment by Tau and its phosphorylation status. The intervening kinases and resulting Tau phosphorylation pattern thereby vary according to the model used, but they also seem to depend crucially on the timing after the Aβ challenge. Twenty years ago, Takashima and colleagues (1993) cultured primary rat hippocampal neurons for 5 days before subjecting them to a solution of Aβ peptide and found that the pronounced neuronal death observed after 24 hours could be reduced by an antisense oligonucleotide against Gsk3β. The toxic Aβ species was recently identified as Aβ dimers, whereby the AD cortex–derived dimeric species was toxic at subnanomolar concentrations, 100-fold less than synthetic oligomers (Jin et al. 2011). Nevertheless, Gsk3β inhibitors did not prevent the Aβ-promoted cell-cycle reentry, suggesting that this kinase comes later in the toxic cascade (Seward et al. 2013). In agreement with this inference, the specific phospho-patterns of Tau induced by Aβ oligomers after three hours in the dendritic spines correspond to an increased kinase activity for MARK and cyclin-dependent kinase (CDK) 5, but not Gsk3β (Zempel et al. 2010); they could be localized to the dendritic Tau pool, but would not necessarily concern axonal Tau species that migrate to the somatodendritic compartment of the neuron. Rather, they would be newly synthesized at the dendritic location, implying, again, a perturbation of transport over the microtubules as a potential problem. Because the MARK kinase activity notably lags one hour behind microtubule destabilization, the dissociation of MARK-phosphorylated Tau from the MT surface cannot be at the origin of the MT disruption. The authors rather focused on an active process whereby spastin recruited after polyglutamylation of tubulin would actively disrupt the microtubules (Zempel et al. 2013).

Quantitative mass spectrometry has most recently been applied to epidermal growth factor (EGF)–induced signaling networks and has revealed their temporal regulation by the SH2 containing protein Shc1 scaffold protein (Zheng et al. 2013). A similar approach applied to the postsynaptic density of neurons challenged by Aβ dimers or oligomers will be essential for understanding how the toxicity is relayed and for elucidating the temporal and spatial role of the enzyme network of distinct Tau kinases and phosphatases.

Tau in the Alzheimer Disease–Characterizing Filaments: Role for Phosphorylation

The realization that Tau is the main component of the neurofibrillary tangles that characterize neurons in the brains of patients with AD evidently established a link between microtubule stability and AD. Still, at first a central role of Tau in the disease was challenged, as no genetic linkage had been found, and no clinical mutation in the Tau gene had been identified for patients diagnosed with bona fide AD. Mutations in the Tau gene have been identified in other forms of dementia, notably hereditary frontotemporal dementia and parkinsonism linked to chromosome 17 (FTDP-17). Whereas in certain of these diseases, the balance between the 3R and 4R isoforms is perturbed through differential mRNA stability and concomitant splicing in the second MTBR (Varani et al. 1999), other mutations such as the P301L mutant do not significantly change the balance between the isoforms, but produce a more aggregation-prone protein. Some of the related tauopathies also occur in the absence of amyloid plaque burden, suggesting that Tau in itself can also develop a neurotoxic species.

In the neurons of patients with AD, the Tau protein is invariably found in an abnormally hyperphosphorylated state. Although commonly used, both notions do not carry a precise definition. "Abnormal" phosphorylation points to sites on Tau that carry a phosphate moiety only in diseased neurons, whereas *hyperphosphorylation* suggests sites for which the stoichiometry of phosphate incorporation changes (and mostly increases) with disease. Both notions are related to the general description of Tau as a phospho-protein carrying 2 to 3 moles of phosphate per mole in "normal" neurons, but with 8 to 9 moles of phosphorylated

Ser/Thr sites per mole in diseased neurons. A more precise definition in terms of distributions of phospho-patterns has been difficult to obtain, mainly owing to technical limitations.

Initially, the definite diagnosis of AD and the stage of advancement of the disease were assessed on thick paraffin-embedded brain slices using Gallyas silver staining, which detects the amyloid tangles and their progression in different brain areas. This procedure has evolved into the technically easier immunocytochemical detection with the AT8 antibody, which recognizes an epitope around pSer202/pThr205 in Tau (Braak et al. 2006). This same AT8 antibody also stains Tau isolated from neuronal axons found in the human fetal spinal cord; after birth and in normal life, however, the same phospho-epitope disappears. This observation suggests some parallel between the disease and a normal developmental stage (Goedert et al. 1993). More than 20 years ago, these authors wrote that phosphorylation at this site "presumably serves some presently unknown control function, possibly related to microtubule binding." Akin to what was postulated for transforming growth factor β (TGFβ) signalling (Massagué 2000), the neuronal cell somehow determines the outcome of this PTM. At present, however, we still do not know why these sites again become phosphorylated in AD neurons and whether or how this precise pattern functionally affects neuronal function.

The mechanistic scenario of the effect of Tau phosphorylation seemed simple at first. Indeed, both in vitro and in vivo, it was found that certain phosphorylation patterns decreased the affinity of Tau for the microtubule surface. The hypothesis that the ensuing detachment would lead to a soluble form of Tau poised to aggregate seemed logical; however, when this hypothesis was tested for the protein kinase A (PKA)–promoted phosphorylation event at Ser214 or for the MARK-promoted phosphorylation event at Ser262, reality proved more complex. Indeed, these phosphorylation patterns did not stimulate the aggregation of Tau in an in vitro test, but actually prevented it (Schneider et al. 1999). Moreover, for other patterns, including those recognized by the AT8 and AT180 antibodies, the affinity toward the MT surface did not vary noticeably, despite the fact that the potential of Tau to promote MT assembly was severely impaired when three or more sites in the PRR were phosphorylated (Amniai et al. 2009). Yet after incubating recombinant Tau with a rat brain extract for a long period of time, a hyperphosphorylated form of Tau (defined by a stoichiometry of 12 to 15 phosphates incorporated per Tau molecule) was described that in itself could form paired helical and straight filaments (Alonso et al. 2001). This finding suggests that phosphorylation could be the driving force for the aggregation of Tau. As the nucleation of fibers with AD PHFs but otherwise recombinant unphosphorylated Tau equally leads to novel fibers of the same morphology as the initial seeds (Morozova et al. 2013), hyperphosphorylation might be necessary for nucleation but not fiber elongation.

As in the proposed histone code (Strahl and Allis 2000), the Tau field is faced with a combinatorial pattern of possible modifications that we currently cannot interpret. Distinct reading modules for the different phosphorylation patterns and for the different histone modifications are not yet clearly identified. Bulk electrostatics with the negatively charged microtubule interface seems an important factor and, hence, might be modified by the amount of phosphate incorporation rather than by a precise pattern (Serber and Ferrell 2007). In the absence of mechanistic insights in the Tau-tubulin interaction, however, a deeper understanding of how phosphorylation translates to altered function remains challenging.

Other Post-translational Modifications of Tau

Extensive cross-talk between different PTMs has been described previously, with a notable emphasis on the link between phosphorylation and ubiquitination (Hunter 2007). Reduced proteasomal degradation of Tau might be associated with AD (Keck et al. 2003). Further evidence that a failure of the ubiquitin–proteasome system could play an early role in initiating the formation of degradation-resistant PHF tangles came from mass spectrometric characterization of AD-brain–derived SDS-soluble Tau, where in addition to phosphorylation at distinct sites, poly-ubiquitination was identified at Lys254, Lys311, and Lys353, all of which lie within the microtubule-binding region of Tau (Cripps et al. 2006). More recently (Tai et al., 2012), the simultaneous presence of phosphorylated and ubiquitinated Tau oligomers at the synaptic densities derived from AD brains suggested that a defective ubiquitin–proteasome system also plays a role in the synaptic aspects of the disease. The early observation that ubiquitinated Tau is a component of PHFs (Mori et al. 1987) finally confirmed that phosphorylation and ubiquitination of Tau occur at the different stages of the disease.

One example of negative regulation between different PTMs is the addition of β-N-acetylglucosamine to Ser/Thr residues, a reversible PTM controlled by two unique enzymes: the O-GlcNAc transferase (OGT) and β-N-acetylglucosaminidase (OGA). Many proteins are modified by this PTM, raising the question of how these single enzymes attain specificity. OGT-interacting proteins have been identified as regulatory partners that target OGT to a specific substrate (Iyer et al. 2003a, b; Cheung et al. 2008), in agreement with the common structural architecture between OGT and the protein phosphatase 2A (PP2A), which equally contains specific regulatory subunits for recognition of the different substrates (Smet-Nocca et al. 2011). Similarly, although

O-GlcNAcylation of Tau was described 20 years ago (Arnold et al., 1996), its precise sites were identified only recently. As they were shown to coincide with potential phoshorylation sites (Wang et al. 2010; Smet-Nocca et al. 2011), O-GlcNAcylation and phosphorylation clearly represent an example of negative cross-talk between two PTMs. This notion suggests that the defective glucose metabolism associated with AD might tip the balance between both PTMs in favor of phosphorylation, thereby contributing to the hyperphosphorylation of pathological Tau. Tau O-GlcNAcylation affects not only the extent of phosphorylation, but also directly decreases its aggregation capacity, thereby interfering with the pathological neurodegeneration in a phospho-independent manner (Yuzwa et al. 2012). An inhibitor of the O-GlcNAcase in a mouse model led to enhanced O-GclNAcylation, and was concomitant with reduced pathological Tau-induced neurodegeneration (Yuzwa et al. 2012). Nevertheless, the relationship between the two PTMs seems more complex than these simple relationships initially suggested, as decreased O-GlcNAc incorporation in an ogt⁻ *Caenorhabditis elegans* FTDP-17 worm model actually improved the tauopathy (Wang et al. 2012).

Acetylation is another PTM recently shown to be as ubiquitous as phosphorylation (Choudhary et al. 2009). It was found in many instances to interfere negatively with ubiquitination of the same lysines (Xu et al. 2010). Tau acetylation also follows this trend, and acetylation has been identified as a factor that hinders its degradation and thereby positively contributes to the tauopathy (Min et al. 2010). Since that original report, more direct roles for Tau acetylation have been determined, notably by affecting its function as a microtubule stabilizer and by enhancing its aggregation potential (Cohen et al. 2011). Tau acetylation is found at every pathological stage of AD and correlates specifically with insoluble Tau aggregates. Although the sequence of PTM events is far from being fully understood, it has been shown that pathological acetylation and hyperphosphorylation follow a similar distribution and regional severity in AD and other tauopathies (Irwin et al. 2012). Most recently, an antibody recognizing the acetylated Lys274 of Tau failed to recognize Tau in brains from patients with argyrophilic grain disease, suggesting that the complex PTM pattern of Tau can directly influence the clinical form of the tauopathy (Grinberg et al. 2013).

All of these PTMs of Tau (including those that we have not described, such as nitration [Horiguchi et al. 2003], methylation [Thomas et al. 2012], proteolytic cleavage, and others [Martin et al. 2011] are covalent in nature. One last modification, however, concerns its conformation rather than its chemical composition. The *cis–trans* conformation of the prolines following a phosphorylated Ser or Thr residue has, indeed, been proposed as a second level of regulation beyond the actual phosphorylation itself (Zhou et al. 1999). Pin1, a prolyl *cis–trans* isomerase of the parvulin family, can catalyze the interconversion between both conformations, and would, therefore, control the extent and timing of this second level of signaling. Other prolyl *cis–trans* isomerase such as FKBP52 (Chambraud et al. 2010) or cyclophilin A (Rhein et al. 2009) have also been linked to Tau pathology, suggesting the potential importance of a catalyzed conformational modification. Unlike all other PTMs, the prolyl conformation leaves no trace detectable modification by mass spectrometry. Nuclear magnetic resonance (NMR) spectroscopy of isolated Tau peptides (Smet et al. 2004) and, recently, a *cis*-conformation–specific antibody (Nakamura et al. 2012) represent the only tools we have to detect this unconventional modification.

Detection of Tau Post-translation Modification Patterns: A Toolbox for in Vitro and in Vivo Studies

Searching PubMed for *Tau phosphorylation* yields nearly 4000 references; narrowing the search to *Tau phosphorylation sites* still yields nearly 700 references. Detecting the phosphorylation status of the 80 possible phosphorylatable residues in a protein such as Tau as isolated from a brain section, indeed, has been and remains a formidable technical challenge. Defining at a second level possible patterns that consist of two or more simultaneous (or exclusive) phosphorylation events has become feasible only recently with novel sophisticated mass spectrometry (MS) approaches that combine measurements on the intact proteins (top-down MS) and on its trypsin-digested peptides (bottom-up MS) with known reference standards (Witze and Old 2007; Siuti and Kelleher, 2007; Gillette & Carr, 2013). Nevertheless, the need to obtain a site-specific and quantitative description of the population of proteins that characterize a given cell phenotype is increasingly recognized. We have called the specific pattern of modifications on all modifiable residues in a protein its "mod-form" (Prabakaran et al. 2012), whereas the term *proteoform* includes, beyond the PTM pattern, the possible alternative splice forms of a protein (Smith and Kelleher, 2013). The underlying reason is that the distribution of different PTMs, generated by the multiple enzymes involved, carries the information in the complex system that is the cell. Our "digital world feeling" has indeed led us to reductionist, linear statements such as "under this condition, protein X becomes phosphorylated at site Y." This leads to a simple schematic drawing, but does not consider that different copies of protein X may or may not carry the phosphate moiety at this position. We tend to write (and think) digitally, but our language might not be in line with our own physical reality that is profoundly analog. We moreover have a tendency to believe that there is only one mod-form, usually the maximally phosphorylated one, when, in reality, there is a distribution of potential mod-forms, each of which may have an analog frequency in the molecular population—hence the "mod-form distribution." When we consider that a protein such as Tau contains 80 potential phosphorylation sites, it is clear that all these combinatorial phospho-patterns cannot co-exist, but it is equally difficult to imagine that all molecules at a given moment will be in exactly the same state. Is one single erroneously phosphorylated molecule in a given neuron enough to trigger aggregation? Is there a threshold population above which the process becomes irreversible? Does Aβ-oligomer–triggered excitotoxicity present a switch that turns on a program for Tau? *Trigger,* and *switch* are, again, engineering terms that might not recognize the fuzziness of the real situation and are probably less sharply defined in the biological context of a neuron than an electrical engineer might conceive (Pauwels 2013).

What tools are available to evaluate the distribution of PTM patterns on a protein such as Tau? In vitro, kinase specificity for the different sites has been established by the (laborious) approach of radioactive ATP incorporation followed by digestion and peptide identification (Illenberger et al. 1996). Combinations of two kinases have been studied and were shown to lead to novel patterns whereby one kinase incorporates a phosphate at a given position, rendering a neighboring site a suitable substrate for the second kinase (Zheng-Fischhöfer et al. 1998). An example is the CDK5-promoted phosphorylation of the Ser235 residue that turns the Thr231 site into a substrate for Gsk3β (Landrieu et al. 2010). This observation, however, does not take into account the structured nature of the cell. Indeed, whereas this priming mechanism can easily be observed in vitro, the same event in a neuron requires that both kinases encounter in a time-ordered manner the same Tau molecule. As CDK5 is localized in the nucleus to keep the neurons in a postmitotic state, an erroneous reentering of the cell cycle possibly triggered by the Aβ peptide with concomitant cytoplasmic release of CDK5 (Zhang et al. 2008) might be a mechanism that generates a similar phosphorylation pattern of Tau in the fetal and diseased states.

Recently, we showed that NMR spectroscopy could, in a single experiment, yield similar information, allowing us to map the phospho-pattern generated by different kinases or combinations of them (Figure 9–4). We found, for example, that the Ser404 site can be independently modified by Gsk3β, whereas other sites in the PRR cannot be modified by this kinase without previous phosphorylation (by PKA or CDK5, for example) (Leroy et al. 2010). A surprising result was the discovery of an equivalent of priming for the PP2A phosphatase, whereby phosphorylation at the Thr231 site influences the dephosphorylation rate at the distinct pS202/pT205 motif (Landrieu et al. 2011). The method requires the incorporation of a stable isotope (e.g., ^{15}N) in the protein and is, as such, applicable

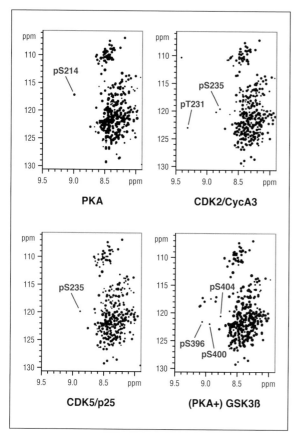

FIGURE 9–4. NMR spectroscopy allows monitoring of the Tau phosphorylation patterns generated by different kinases in a quantitative and time-dependent manner. Panels show the [¹H], [¹⁵N] two-dimensional spectrums of [¹⁵N]-labeled Tau, after phosphorylation by different recombinant kinases. Selected phospho-sites are labeled. The last panel shows the result of a successive incubation with first PKA and then Gsk3β. (Reprinted with permission from Leroy, A., I. Landrieu, et al. (2010). Spectroscopic studies of GSK3β phosphorylation of the neuronal tau protein and its interaction with the N-terminal domain of apolipoprotein E. J Biol Chem **285**(43): 33435–44. © The American Society for Biochemistry and Molecular Biology.)

only when recombinant protein is available. However, the labeled protein can be combined with an extract of cells or even rat brain and, thereby, can allow for the detection of a complex phosphorylation pattern. Similar spectral perturbations have been mapped for other PTMs (Theillet et al. 2012), for which reason we foresee that NMR might gain further prominence in the characterization of complex PTM patterns.

Because of their relatively easy use and high sensitivity, antibodies are not only the historical alternatives to biophysical methods but also remain the tool of choice for most studies. Combined with modern imaging techniques, they allow for a site-specific evaluation of the epitope against which they were raised. Nevertheless, a number of fundamental issues hinder their use for obtaining a view of the distribution of possible PTMs. First, they are rarely characterized in a quantitative manner, and a positive response is impossible to translate into a stoichiometry, even at a single site. This absence of quantitative response was initially recognized and even led to question the link between PHF–Tau and hyperphosphorylated Tau (Wischik et al. 1995). Second, epitope mapping through the use of synthetic peptides is reductive and can miss potential secondary sites. When more than a single PTM is involved, the amount of different peptides required to confirm the epitope grows exponentially. Porzig et al. (2007) mapped the epitope of the AT8 antibody to the pS202/pT205 motif, although the initial report had concluded that the phosphorylation of Ser199 and/or Ser202 was required (Biernat et al. 1992).

Third, establishing a correlation between different epitopes would require the purification with an initial antibody, followed by blotting with a second one, but, again, runs into the problem of difficult quantification of the response. Finally, antibodies can give only a (partial) answer about the status of the site they were raised, and can, therefore, completely miss a given PTM site. Phosphorylation of the T153 residue was readily detected in our NMR spectrum of CDK phosphorylated Tau (Amniai et al. 2009), but went largely unnoticed as most antibodies concentrate on epitopes in the PRR or extreme C-terminal of Tau.

Approaches that make use of advanced mass spectrometry methods, and combine top-down mass spectrometry and synthetic peptide-calibrated bottom-up methods have allowed the characterization of a complete phospho-proteome (Manning et al. 2002; Prabakaran et al. 2012; Salek and Acuto 2012). However, we know of no studies that have resolved positional isomers by multistage MS on proteins of similar size and complexity as Tau. The first attempts to apply quantitative methods to Tau have appeared in the literature only very recently, but they still mostly concern the quantification of a limited number of phospho-sites (Zhang et al. 2013).

Tau Integrates Information at the Level of the Neuron and the Brain

Focusing on the PTMs of a single protein such as Tau might seem very reductive in the framework of "network medicine" as a nascent discipline that attempts to model the (dys)function of the cell as a network of interacting biochemical entities. However, when we consider that Tau is capable of integrating the information content of the tubulin network, the many kinases and phosphatases that cluster around it, glucose homeostasis, etc., into a given pattern of PTMs, its central role as a hub protein translates this information functionally. Tau also does this through its effect on transport, its anchoring of other components such as the Fyn kinase, etc., and leads to its playing a central network role in the functioning of the neuron both in the axonal and synaptic compartments. Although at this time, we cannot read the different PTM patterns in sufficient detail to interpret their functional consequences, the available knowledge can be used to extend the network to other functional aspects of the neuron. A first example of this point was the quantitative comparison at the proteomic level of a triple transgenic AD mouse model harboring the Tau P301L mutation next to two mutations in the APP and presenilin genes to its counterpart with only the two Aβ-related mutations. This study pointed to mitochondrial defects, with notably a Tau-dependent deregulation of complex I of the oxidative phosphorylation system (Rhein et al.

2009). Second, using the levels of Tau and Tau phosphorylated at the Thr181 position as surrogate markers for disease, a recent genome-wide association study first confirmed the correlation between disease and the genomic variations in the ApoE gene but concluded that DNA variants in the ApoE gene region influence Tau pathology independently of Aβ or even AD disease status (Cruchaga et al. 2013). The same study furthermore found other genetic factors associated with the levels of Tau/pTau, notably genes in the Triggering Receptor Expressed on Myeloid cells (TREM) cluster, but the observation that the levels of Tau expression did not vary at all with any of the identified genetic factors led the authors to the hypothesis that the genes identified modify Tau protein levels through PTM rather than gene expression (Cruchaga et al. 2013).

Gsk3β is considered to be a central information processor of the cell and integrates information through its phosphorylation status, altered protein–protein interactions, or subcellular localization in many pathways (Jope and Johnson 2004). Identified early on as the Tau protein kinase I that generates several epitopes of paired helical filaments (Ishiguro et al. 1993), it is one of the kinases that appears always to be associated with diverse pathological aspects of Alzheimer disease. Regulation of its activity through altered Ser9 (de)phosphorylation by the PP2A/B phosphatase can indirectly lead to a different pattern of Tau phosphorylation (Louis et al. 2002). We expect that Tau as a substrate for Gsk3β and its many other modifying enzymes plays a similar central role, and, as such, actively coordinates the information flow.

The intriguing similarity between Tau's phosphorylation patterns in the fetal and diseased state suggests an analogy with the free-energy landscapes that characterize the protein-folding problem (Figure 9–5), which may be helpful as a summary of the dynamics of the underlying complex Tau network. In the fetal state, before differentiation, we consider the neuron to be in a first potential well. In a way similar to the multiple physical interaction terms that determine the folding of a protein, many factors define the stability of this state, which we can integrate in a readout via the Tau protein, both at the level of its isoform balance (with a prominent 3R isoform population) and its phosphorylation distribution, which contains a sizable fraction of Tau molecules phosphorylated at the Ser202/Thr205 residues. After differentiation, this state becomes less stable, and the neuron in a healthy brain evolves into a second state, characterized by the presence of all isoforms of Tau and by an altered phosphorylation pattern. However, the erroneous cell-cycle reentry that is associated with the earliest forms of the disease would bring the neuron back into the first potential well, as is shown by the specific readout of the Tau phosphorylation pattern. Although shown here as a two-dimensional problem, the neuronal state is evidently determined by many degrees of freedom. The genes currently discovered by different genome-wide association studies can influence both the depth and spread of the potential wells or the barrier that separates them, thereby increasing or decreasing the probability that a neuron evolves from one well into another.

The spatial and temporal progression of the disease over distinct brain areas (see Figure 9–3) was initially thought to originate in the entorhinal cortex, and then spread in a cell-autonomous manner toward neighboring neuronal regions; however, more recent evidence suggests a prion-like propagation, whereby the misfolded Tau would escape from a given neuron, and be internalized by a second target neuron. The initial seeds of Tau pathology would start early in life in some selected neurons of the locus ceruleus, and spread from these neurons via their long projecting axons toward the entorhinal cortex (Braak and Del Tredici 2011). Owing to the long distance between both regions, initial spreading would happen through the synapses of the

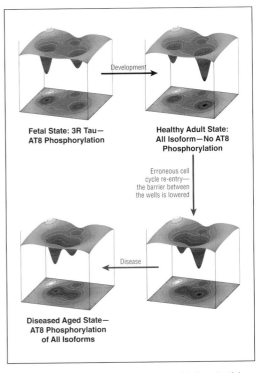

Fetal State: 3R Tau—
AT8 Phosphorylation

Healthy Adult State:
All Isoform—No AT8
Phosphorylation

Erroneous cell
cycle re-entry—
the barrier between
the wells is lowered

Development

Disease

Diseased Aged State—
AT8 Phosphorylation
of All Isoforms

FIGURE 9–5. Analogy of the neuronal state with the potential energy surface of protein folding. The proteo-form of Tau thereby serves as a readout, with dominant population of the 3R isoforms and phosphorylation at the AT8 epitope in the fetal state (top left), that shifts to a 3R/4R balanced population without AT8 phosphorylation after differentiation (top right). AD at the level of an individual neuron starts as an erroneous cell-cycle reentry, possibly triggered by Aβ oligomers (bottom right), and can evolve into a state that is read out by the AT8 phosphorylation pattern (bottom left).

neurons in which the pathology began. Whether the precise objects that leave a neuronal cell and enter another are species of Tau with or without a specific PTM pattern, pretangle Tau, or full-grown fibers is not clear at this moment. We have previously shown that the Gsk3β catalyzed ordered phosphorylation pattern at the extreme C-terminus of Tau (pS404/pS400/pS396) creates an ApoE interaction surface (Leroy et al. 2010). Because spreading of Tau depends on its interaction with the heparan sulfate proteoglycans (HSPGs) at the surface of the receptor neurons (Holmes et al. 2013) and that cell attachment of viruses such as HCV via the HSPGs is mediated by ApoE, (Jiang et al., 2012) a possible role for ApoE in the spreading merits further investigation. Because acetylated Tau was detected in all tauopathies except for the argyrophilic grain disease, an atypical tauopathy characterized by a more reduced spreading in the brain whereby 30%

of the patients do not develop any clinical symptoms (Ferrer et al. 2008), it was suggested that acetylation might be a necessary PTM for the spreading of the tauopathy over the brain.

Conclusion

We have illustrated how Tau through its PTMs can integrate information at the level of the individual neuron. The dynamic character of this pattern, both in space and time, contributes to physiological functioning of the cell. The transition toward a diseased neuron can equally be detected by a change in its PTM pattern. An accurate and quantitative reading of the PTM mod-form of Tau at all levels of the neuron and the brain will be required to understand whether this is a cause or a consequence of AD.

Acknowledgments

We thank our many colleagues who contributed to this work through insightful discussion, notably L. Buée (University of Lille2, France), B. Chambraud (Inserm, France), A. Van de Voorde and E. Van Mechelen (Innogenetics, Belgium). The research leading to these results was supported by the Centre National de la Recherche Scientifique (CNRS, France), the Agence Nationale de la Recherche (ANR-05-Blanc-6320–01, program MALZ-TAF), the LABEX (laboratory of excellence program investment for the future), DISTALZ grant (Development of Innovative Strategies for a Transdisciplinary Approach to Alzheimer disease), and the CNRS Large Scale Facility NMR THC Fr3050.

References

Alonso, A., T. Zaidi, et al. (2001). Hyperphosphorylation induces self-assembly of tau into tangles of paired helical filaments/straight filaments. Proc Natl Acad Sci U S A **98**(12): 6923–28.

Amniai, L., P. Barbier, et al. (2009). Alzheimer disease specific phosphoepitopes of Tau interfere with assembly of tubulin but not binding to microtubules. FASEB J **23**(4): 1146–52.

Arnold, C.S., G.V. Johnson, et al. (1996) The microtubule-associated protein tau is extensively modified with O-linked N-acetylglucosamine. J Biol Chem **271**(46):28741–44.

Aronov, S., G. Aranda, et al. (2001). Axonal tau mRNA localization coincides with tau protein in living neuronal cells and depends on axonal targeting signal. J Neurosci **21**(17): 6577–87.

Benilova, I., and B. De Strooper (2013) Promiscuous Alzheimer's amyloid: yet another partner. Science **341**(6152): 1354–55.

Biernat, J., E. M. Mandelkow, et al. (1992). The switch of tau protein to an Alzheimer- like state includes the phosphorylation of two serine-proline motifs upstream of the microtubule binding region. EMBO J **11**: 1593–97.

Billas, I., and D. Moras. (2013) Allosteric controls of nuclear receptor function in the regulation of transcription. J Mol Biol **425**(13): 2317–29.

Blake, W. (1803) The avguires of innocence. In Poets of the English language, Viking Press, 1950. http://www.poetryfoundation.org/poems-and-poets/poems/detail/43650.

Blennow, K. (2005). CSF biomarkers for Alzheimer's disease: use in early diagnosis and evaluation of drug treatment. Expert Rev Mol Diagn **5**(5): 661–72.

Braak, H., F. Braak.(1991). Neuropathological staging of Alzheimer-related changes. Acta Neuropathol **82**: 239–59.

Braak, H., and I. Alafuzo (2006). Staging of Alzheimer disease-associated neurofibrillary pathology using paraffin sections and immunocytochemistry. Acta Neuropathol **112**: 389–404.

Braak, H., and K. Del Tredici (2011), The pathological process underlying Alzheimer's disease in individuals under thirty. Acta Neuropathol **121**(2): 171–81.

Bullmann, T., M. Holzer, et al. (2009). Pattern of tau isoforms expression during development in vivo. Int J Dev Neurosci **27**: 591–97.

Caceres, A., and K. S. Kosik (1990). Inhibition of neurite polarity by tau antisense oligonucleotides in primary cerebellar neurons. Nature **343**: 461–63.

Chambraud. B., E. Sardin, et al. (2010). A role for FKBP52 in Tau protein function. Proc Natl Acad Sci U S A **107**(6): 2658–63.

Cheung, W. D., K. Sakabe, et al. (2008). O-linked beta-N acetylglucosaminyltransferase substrate specificity is regulated by myosin phosphatase targeting and other interacting proteins. J Biol Chem **283** (49): 33935–41.

Choudhary, C., C. Kumar, et al. (2009). Lysine acetylation targets protein complexes and co-regulates major cellular functions. Science **325**: 834–40.

Cohen, T. J., J. L. Guo, et al. (2011). The acetylation of tau inhibits its function and promotes pathological tau aggregation. Nature Commun **2**: 252.

Corder, E. H., A. M., et al. (1993). Gene dose of apolipoprotein E type 4 allele and the risk of Alzheimer's disease in late onset families. Science **261**(5123): 921–3.

Cripps, D., S. N. Thomas. S. N., et al. (2006). Alzheimer disease-specific conformation of hyperphosphorylated paired helical filament-Tau is poly-ubiquitinated through Lys-48, Lys-11, and Lys-6 ubiquitin conjugation. J Biol Chem **281**(16): 10825–38.

Cruchaga, C., J. S. Kauwe, et al. GERAD Consortium; Alzheimer's Disease Neuroimaging Initiative (ADNI); Alzheimer Disease Genetic Consortium (ADGC), Goate AM. (2013). GWAS of cerebrospinal fluid tau levels identifies risk variants for Alzheimer's disease. Neuron **78**(2): 256–68.

De Strooper, B., R. Vassar, et al. (2010). The secretases: enzymes with therapeutic potential in Alzheimer disease. Nat Rev Neurol **6**(2): 99–107.

Dixit, R., J. L. Ross, et al. (2008). Differential regulation of dynein and kinesin motor proteins by tau. Science **319**(5866): 1086–89.

Drewes, G., A. Ebneth, et al. (1997). MARK, a novel family of protein kinases that phosphorylate microtubule-associated proteins and trigger microtubule disruption. Cell **89**(2): 297–308.

Drubin, D. G., S. C. Feinstein, et al. (1985). Nerve growth factor-induced neurite outgrowth in PC12 cells involves the coordinate induction of microtubule assembly and assembly-promoting factors. J. Cell Biol **101**: 1799–807.

Ferrer, I., G. Santpere, et al. (2008). Argyrophilic grain disease. Brain **131**:1416–32.

Flament-Durand, J., J. P. Brion JP. (1985). Ultrastructural and immunohistochemical study of neurofibrillary tangles in Alzheimer's disease. Pathol Res Pract **180**: 267.

Gillette, M. A., and Carr, S. A. (2013). Quantitative analysis of peptides and proteins in biomedicine by targeted mass spectrometry. Nat Methods **10**: 28–34.

Goedert, M., M. G. Spillantini, et al. (1989). Multiple isoforms of human microtubule-associated protein tau: sequences and localization in neurofibrillary tangles of Alzheimer's disease. Neuron **3**: 519–26.

Goedert, M., R. Jakes, et al. (1993). The abnormal phosphorylation of tau protein at Ser-202 in Alzheimer disease recapitulates phosphorylation during development. Proc Natl Acad Sci U S A **90**(11): 5066–70.

Goode, B. L., and S. C. Feinstein (1994). Identification of a novel microtubule binding and assembly domain in the developmentally regulated inter-repeat region of tau. J Cell Biol **124**: 769–82.

Grinberg, L. T., X. Wang, et al. (2013). Argyrophilic grain disease differs from other tauopathies by lacking tau acetylation. Acta Neuropathol **125** (4): 581–93.

Grundke-Iqbal, I., K. Iqbal, et al. (1986). Microtubule-associated protein tau: a component of Alzheimer paired helical filaments. J Biol Chem **261**: 6084–89.

Hardy, J. (2009). The amyloid hypothesis for Alzheimer's disease: a critical reappraisal. J Neurochem **110**(4): 1129–34.

Hasegawa, M., M. Morishima-Kawashima, et al. (1992). Protein sequence and mass spectrometric analyses of tau in the Alzheimer's disease brain. J Biol Chem **267**(24): 17047–54.

Hashiguchi, M., and T. Hashiguchi. (2013). Kinase–kinase interaction and modulation of tau phosphorylation. Int Rev Cell Mol Biol **300**: 121–60.

Holmes, B. B., S. L. DeVos, et al. (2013). Heparan sulfate proteoglycans mediate internalization and propagation of specific proteopathic seeds. Proc Natl Acad Sci U S A **110**(33): E3138–47.

Horiguchi, T., K. Uryu, et al. (2003). Nitration of tau protein is linked to neurodegeneration in tauopathies. Am J Pathol **163**: 1021–31.

Hunter, T. (2007). The age of crosstalk: phosphorylation, ubiquitination, and beyond. Mol Cell **28**(5): 730–38.

Illenberger, S., G. Drewes, et al. (1996). Phosphorylation of microtubule-associated proteins MAP2 and MAP4 by the protein kinase p110mark: phosphorylation sites and regulation of microtubule dynamics. J Biol Chem **271**(18): 10834–43.

Irwin, D. J., T. J. Cohen, et al. (2012). Acetylated tau, a novel pathological signature in Alzheimer's disease and other tauopathies. Brain **135**: 807–18.

Ishiguro, K., A. Shiratsuchi, et al. (1993). Glycogen synthase kinase 3b is identical to tau protein kinase I generating several epitopes of paired helical filaments. FEBS Lett **325**: 167–72.

Ittner, L. M., Y. D. Ke, et al. (2010). Dendritic function of tau mediates amyloid-beta toxicity in Alzheimer's disease mouse models. Cell **142**(3): 387–97.

Iyer, S. P., Y. Akimoto, et al. (2003a). Identification and cloning of a novel family of coiled-coil domain proteins that interact with O-GlcNAc transferase. J Biol Chem **278**(7): 5399–409.

Iyer, S. P., G. W. Hart. (2003b). Roles of the tetratricopeptide repeat domain in O-GlcNAc transferase targeting and protein substrate specificity. J Biol Chem **278**(27): 24608–16.

Jiang, J, W. Cun, et al. (2012) Hepatitis C virus attachment mediated by apolipoprotein E binding to cell surface heparan sulfate. J Virol **86**(13):7256–67.

Jin, M., N. Shepardson, et al. (2011). Soluble amyloid beta-protein dimers isolated from Alzheimer cortex directly induce Tau hyperphosphorylation and neuritic degeneration. Proc Natl Acad Sci U S A **108**(14): 5819–24.

Jope, R. S., and G. V. Johnson. (2004). The glamour and gloom of glycogen synthase kinase-3. Trends Biochem Sci **29**(2): 95–102.

Juhàsz, S., I. Földi, et al. (2011). Systems biology of Alzheimer's disease: How diverse molecular changes result in memory impairment in AD. Neurochem Int **58**: 739–50.

Kanaan, N. M., G. Morfini, et al. (2012). Phosphorylation in the amino terminus of tau prevents inhibition of anterograde axonal transport. Neurobiol Aging **33**(4):826.e15–30.

Katritch, V., V. Cherezov, et al. (2012). Diversity and modularity of G protein-coupled receptor structures. Trends Pharmacol Sci **33**(1): 17–27.

Keck, S., R. Nitsch, et al. (2003). Proteasome inhibition by paired helical filament-tau in brains of patients with Alzheimer's disease. J Neurochem **85**(1):115–22.

Kempf, M., and A. Clement (1996). Tau binds to the distal axon early in development of polarity in a microtubule- and microfilament-dependent manner. J Neurosci **16**(18): 5583–92.

Korolainen, M. A., T. A. Nyman, et al. (2010). An update on clinical proteomics in Alzheimer's research. J Neurochem **112**(6): 1386–414.

Kosik, K. S., C. L. Joachim, et al. (1986). Microtubule-associated protein tau is a major antigenic component of paired helical filaments in Alzheimer's disease. Proc Natl Acad Sci U S A **83:** 4044–48.

Kosik, K. S., L. D. Orecchio, et al. (1989). Developmentally regulated expression of specific tau sequences. Neuron **2:** 1389–97.

Landrieu, I., A. Leroy, et al. (2010). NMR spectroscopy of the neuronal tau protein: normal function and implication in Alzheimer's disease. Biochem Soc Trans **38**(4): 1006–11.

Landrieu, I., C. Smet-Nocca, et al. (2011). Molecular implication of PP2A and Pin1 in the Alzheimer's disease specific hyperphosphorylation of Tau. PLoS One **6**(6): e21521.

LaPointe, N. E., G. Morfini, et al. (2009). The amino terminus of tau inhibits kinesin-dependent axonal transport: implications for filament toxicity. J Neurosci Res **87:** 440–51.

Laurén, J., D. A. Gimbel, et al. (2009). Cellular prion protein mediates impairment of synaptic plasticity by amyloid-beta oligomers. Nature **457**(7233): 1128–32.

Lee, G., N. Cowan, et al. (1988). The primary structure and heterogeneity of tau protein from mouse brain. Science **239**(4837): 285–88.

Lee, V. M., B. J. Balin, et al. (1991). A68: a major subunit of paired helical filaments and derivatized forms of normal Tau. Science **251**(4994): 675–78.

Leroy, A., I. Landrieu, et al. (2010). Spectroscopic studies of GSK3{beta} phosphorylation of the neuronal tau protein and its interaction with the N-terminal domain of apolipoprotein E. J Biol Chem **285**(43): 33435–44.

Louis, J. V., E. Martens, et al. (2002). Analysis of protein phosphorylation using mass spectrometry: deciphering the phosphoproteome. Trends Biotechnol **20**(6): 261–68.

Manning, G., D. B. Whyte, et al. (2002). The protein kinase complement of the human genome. Science. **298**(5600): 1912–34.

Martin, L., X. Latypova, et al. (2011). Post-translational modifications of tau protein: implications for Alzheimer's disease. Neurochem Int **58**(4): 458–71.

Massagué, J. (2000), How cells read TGF-beta signals. Nat Rev Mol Cell Biol **1**(3): 169–78.

Mattsson, N., K. Savman, et al. (2010). Converging molecular pathways in human and neural development and degeneration. Neurosci Res **66:** 330–32.

Min, S. W., S. H. Cho, et al. (2010). Acetylation of tau inhibits its degradation and contributes to tauopathy. Neuron **67**(6): 953–66.

Mori, H., J. Kondo, et al. (1987). Ubiquitin is a component of paired helical filaments in Alzheimer's disease. Science **235**(4796): 1641–44.

Morozova, O. A., Z. M. March, et al. (2013). Conformational features of Tau fibrils from Alzheimer's disease brain are faithfully propagated by unmodified recombinant protein. Biochemistry **52**(40): 6960–67.

Morris, M., S. Maeda, et al. (2011). The many faces of tau. Neuron **70:** 410–26.

Nakamura, K., A. Greenwood, et al (2012). Proline isomer-specific antibodies reveal the early pathogenic tau conformation in Alzheimer's disease. Cell **149**(1): 232–44.

Pauwels, E. (2013). Communication: mind the metaphor. Nature **500:** 523–24.

Porzig, R., D. Singer, et al. (2007). Epitope mapping of mAbs AT8 and Tau5 directed against hyperphosphorylated regions of the human tau protein. Biochem Biophys Res Commun **358**(2): 644–49.

Prabakaran, S., G. Lippens, et al. (2012). Post-translational modification: nature's escape from genetic imprisonment and the basis for dynamic information encoding. Wiley Interdiscip Rev Syst Biol Med **4**(6): 565–83.

Qiu, C., M. Kivipelto, et al. (2009). Epidemiology of Alzheimer's disease: occurrence, determinants, and strategies toward intervention. Dialogues Clin Neurosci **11**(2): 111–28

Reitz, C., C. Brayne, et al. (2011). Epidemiology of Alzheimer disease. Nat Rev Neurol. **7**(3): 137–52.

Rhein, V., X. Song, et al. (2009). Amyloid-beta and tau synergistically impair the oxidative phosphorylation system in triple transgenic Alzheimer's disease mice. Proc Natl Acad Sci U S A **106**(47): 20057–62.

Rhinn, H., R. Fujita, et al. (2013). Integrative genomics identifies APOE ε4 effectors in Alzheimer's disease. Nature **500**(7460): 45–50.

Rosenbaum, D. M., S. G. Rasmussen, et al. (2009). The structure and function of G-protein coupled receptors. Nature **459**(7245): 356–63.

Salek, M., and O. Acuto (2012). Quantitative dynamics of phosphoproteome: the devil is in the details. Anal Chem **84**(20): 8431–36.

Schneider, A., J. Biernat, et al. (1999). Phosphorylation that detaches tau protein from microtubules (Ser262, Ser214) also protects it against aggregation into Alzheimer paired helical filaments. Biochemistry **38**(12): 3549–58.

Schweers, O., E. Schönbrunn-Hanebeck, et al. (1994) Structural studies of tau protein and Alzheimer paired helical filaments show no evidence for beta-structure. J Biol Chem **269**(39): 24290–97

Selkoe, D. J. (1991). The molecular pathology of Alzheimer's disease. Neuron. **6**: 487–98.

Serber, Z., and J. E. Ferrell, Jr. (2007), Tuning bulk electrostatics to regulate protein function. Cell **128**(3): 441–44.

Seward, M. E., E. Swanson, et al. (2013). Amyloid-β signals through tau to drive ectopic neuronal cell cycle re-entry in Alzheimer's disease. J Cell Sci **126**: 1278–86.

Siuti, N., and N. L. Kelleher. (2007). Decoding protein modifications using top-down mass spectrometry. Nat Methods **4**: 817–21.

Smet, C., A. Leroy, et al. (2004). Accepting its random coil nature allows a partial NMR assignment of the neuronal Tau protein. Chembiochem **5**(12): 1639–46.

Smet, C., J. M. Wieruszeski, et al. (2005). Regulation of Pin1 peptidyl-prolyl cis/trans isomerase activity by its WW binding module on a multi-phosphorylated peptide of Tau protein. FEBS Letts **579**(19): 4159–64.

Smet-Nocca, C., M. Broncel, et al. (2011). Identification of O-GlcNAc sites within peptides of the Tau protein and their impact on phosphorylation. Mol Biosyst **7**(5): 1420–29.

Smith, L. M., and N. L. Kelleher. (2013). Proteoform: a single term describing protein complexity. Nat Methods **10**(3): 186–87.

Sontag, J. M., V. Nunbhakdi-Craig, et al. (2012), The protein phosphatase PP2A/Bα binds to the microtubule-associated proteins Tau and MAP2 at a motif also recognized by the kinase Fyn: implications for tauopathies. J Biol Chem **287**(18): 14984–93.

Strahl, B. D., and C. D. Allis (2000). The language of covalent histone modifications. Nature **403**(6765): 41–45.

Tai, H.C., A. Serrano-Pozo, et al. (2012) The synaptic accumulation of hyperphosphorylated tau oligomers in Alzheimer disease is associated with dysfunction of the ubiquitin-proteasome system. Am J Pathol **181**(4):1426–35.

Takashima, A., K. Noguchi, et al. (1993). Tau protein kinase I is essential for amyloid beta-protein-induced neurotoxicity. Proc Natl Acad Sci U S A **90**(16): 7789–93.

Theillet, F. X., C. Smet-Nocca, et al. (2012). Cell signaling, post-translational protein modifications and NMR spectroscopy. J Biomol NMR **54**(3): 217–36.

Thomas, S. N., K. E. Funk, et al. (2012). Dual modification of Alzheimer's disease PHF-tau protein by lysine methylation and ubiquitylation: a mass spectrometry approach. Acta Neuropathol **123**(1): 105–17.

Varani, L., M. Hasegawa, et al. (1999). Structure of tau exon 10 splicing regulatory element RNA and destabilization by mutations of frontotemporal dementia and parkinsonism linked to chromosome 17. Proc Natl Acad Sci U S A **96**(14): 8229–34.

Vershinin, M., B. C. Carter, et al. (2007). Multiple-motor based transport and its regulation by Tau. Proc Natl Acad Sci U S A **104**(1): 87–92.

Vincent, I., G. Jicha, et al. (1997). Aberrant expression of mitotic cdc2/cyclin B1 kinase in degenerating neurons of Alzheimer's disease brain. J Neurosci **17**: 3588–98.

Wang, P., B. D. Lazarus, et al. (2012). O-GlcNAc cycling mutants modulate proteotoxicity in Caenorhabditis elegans models of human neurodegenerative diseases. Proc Natl Acad Sci U S A **109**(43):17669–74.

Wang, Z., N. D. Udeshi, et al. (2010), Enrichment and site mapping of O-linked N-acetylglucosamine by a combination of chemical/enzymatic tagging, photochemical cleavage, and electron transfer dissociation mass spectrometry. Mol Cell Proteom **9**(1): 153–60.

Weingarten, M. D., A. H. Lockwood, et al. (1975). A protein factor essential for microtubule assembly. Proc Natl Acad Sci U S A **72**(5): 1858–62.

Wischik, C. M., P. C. Edwards, et al. (1995). Quantitative analysis of tau protein in paired helical filament preparations: implications for the role of tau protein phosphorylation in PHF assembly in Alzheimer's disease. Neurobiol Aging **16**(3): 409–17.

Witze, E. S., W. Old, et al. (2007). Mapping protein post-translational modifications with mass spectrometry. Nat Methods **4**: 798–806.

Xu, G., J. S. Paige, et al. (2010). Global analysis of lysine ubiquitination by ubiquitin remnant immunoaffinity profiling. Nat Biotechnol **28**: 868–73.

Yin, X., N. Jin, et al. (2012). Dual-specificity tyrosine phosphorylation-regulated kinase 1A (Dyrk1A) modulates serine/arginine-rich protein 55 (SRp55)-promoted Tau exon 10 inclusion. J Biol Chem **287**(36): 30497–506.

Yuzwa, S. A., X. Shan, et al. (2012). Increasing O-GlcNAc slows neurodegeneration and stabilizes tau against aggregation. Nat Chem Biol **8**(4): 393–99.

Zempel, H., E. Thies, et al. (2010). Abeta oligomers cause localized Ca(2+) elevation, missorting of endogenous Tau into dendrites, Tau phosphorylation, and destruction of microtubules and spines. J Neurosci **30**(36): 11938–50.

Zempel, H., J. Luedtke, et al. (2013). Amyloid-β oligomers induce synaptic damage via Tau-dependent microtubule severing by TTLL6 and spastin. EMBO J **32**(22): 2920–37.

Zhang, J., S. A. Cicero, et al. (2008). Nuclear localization of Cdk5 is a key determinant in the postmitotic state of neurons. Proc Natl Acad Sci U S A **105**(25): 8772–77.

Zhang, X., I. Hernandez, et al. (2013). Diaminothiazoles modify Tau phosphorylation and improve the tauopathy in mouse models. J Biol Chem **288**(30): 22042–56.

Zheng, Y., C. Zhang, et al. (2013). Temporal regulation of EGF signalling networks by the scaffold protein Shc1. Nature. **499**(7457): 166–71.

Zheng-Fischhöfer, Q., J. Biernat, et al. (1998). Sequential phosphorylation of Tau by glycogen synthase kinase-3beta and protein kinase A at Thr212 and Ser214 generates the Alzheimer-specific epitope of antibody AT100 and requires a paired-helical-filament-like conformation. Eur J Biochem **252**(3): 542–52.

Zhou, X. Z., P. J. Lu, et al. (1999). Phosphorylation-dependent prolyl isomerization: a novel signaling regulatory mechanism. Cell Mol Life Sci **56**(9–10): 788–806.

10

Epigenetics and Network Medicine

DAWN L. DEMEO AND SCOTT T. WEISS

Introduction

Large-scale interrogation of epigenetic marks represents recent efforts to intuit contributory regulatory mechanisms that underlie human phenotypic plasticity and diversity. Whether the epigenetic marks under investigation are noncoding RNAs, histone modifications, or DNA methylation, to mention a few of the known epigenetic mechanisms, there is accumulating, convincing evidence that the epigenome in its totality is a crucial nexus between genetic variation, the environment, health, and disease (Tables 10–1A and 10–1B). Although cells generally share the same genome, different cell types, including cells within the same organ, have cell-specific epigenetic profiles. DNA methylation involves the addition of a methyl group at the C5 position of a cytosine (5mC) using DNA methyltransferase enzymes. In general, DNA methyltransferases 3a and 3b establish de novo cellular methylation patterns and DNA methyltransferase 1 maintains the methylation patterns during chromosomal replication and repair. Although it is generally supported that methylation in promoter regions is associated with decreased gene expression, and promoter demethylation with increased gene expression, rapid expansion in the number of studies with both methylation and expression data suggests that this canonical methylation—expression relationship is not absolute and is dependent on gene context. Another type of methylation event is histone protein methylation; it may be involved in transcriptional regulation. Histone methylation occurs at arginines and lysines and may relate to activation, elongation, or repression of gene expression; as with DNA, the methylation events are catalyzed by a set of arginine or lysine methyltransferases, respectively. The complexity of methylation and demethylation events, and the interplay between the different epigenetic marks, supports the relevance of placing these observations in a network context.

In the context of cellular diversity, elucidating the network characteristics of the epigenome not only affords crucial insights into the human phenotypic complexity but also provides a unique opportunity for network medicine approaches to define epigenetic drug targets (Kelly, De Carvalho et al. 2010) for neoplastic and nonneoplastic diseases. Mapping epigenetic networks will pro-

TABLE 10–1A. Epigenetic Modifications

EPIGENETIC MARK	EXAMPLE
Histone modification	Acetylation/deacetylation Methylation/demethylation Phosphorylation Sumoylation Ubiquitination
DNA	Methylation (may be gene promoter, shelf, or shore) Hydroxymethylation
RNA	Methylation (including transfer RNA [tRNA], ribosomal RNA [rRNA], and messenger RNA [mRNA])
Noncoding RNA	MicroRNA Short interfering or silencing RNA (siRNA) Piwi-interacting RNA (piRNA) Long noncoding RNA (lncRNA)

vide approaches to perhaps the most diverse and least understood networks involved in human biology.

The process of unraveling network features of human disease highlights the paramount importance of identifying disease modules within the cellular molecular interactome and then applying to these modules the layers of epigenetic perturbations that may inform phenotypic manifestations (Figure 10–1). Two limitations to comprehensive mapping of epigenetic networks have been the cost related to obtaining tissue-specific epigenetic data and a lag in methods to control the quality of data and the methods to curate and annotate them. Currently, there are ongoing national and international efforts geared toward the collection of cell- and tissue-specific epigenetic data, with the hope that these data will fuel further efforts to model epigenetic networks comprehensively. The National Institutes of Health Roadmap Epigenome Project (www.roadmapepigenomics .org), the Human Epigenome Project (www.epigenome.org), and the International Human Epigenome Consortium (ihec-epigenomes.org) are all examples of these data collection efforts. Given the cell specificity of epigenetic signatures, the most informative network approaches to epigenetics will include both organ- and cell-specific profiling.

One traditional, albeit naive, description of the encoding and regulation of epigenetic marks (such as methylation and histone modification) suggests that an environmental exposure activates the unfolding of chromatin, removes methylation marks, and exposes the gene to allow transcription and gene expression to occur. It is clear that while this scenario is sometimes true, it is a gross oversimplification and hence only part of the story. Although each epigenetic

TABLE 10–1B. Epigenetic Modifications in Human Diseases[a]

ABERRANT EPIGENETIC MARK	ALTERATION	CONSEQUENCES
Cancer		
DNA methylation	CpG island hypermethylation	Transcription repression
	CpG island hypomethylation	Transcription activation
	CpG island shore hypermethylation	Transcription repression
	Repetitive sequences hypomethylation	Transposition, recombinant genomic instability
Histone modification	Loss of H3 and H4 acetylation	Transcription repression
	Loss of H3K4me3	Transcription repression
	Loss of H4K20me3	Loss of heterochromatic structure
	Gain of H3K9me and H3K27me3	Transcription repression
Nucleosome positioning	Silencing and/or mutation of remodeler subunits	Diverse, leading to oncogenic transformation
	Aberrant recruitment of remodelers	Transcription repression
	Histone variants replacement	Diverse (promotion cell cycle/ destabilization of chromo- somal boundaries)
Neurological disorders		
DNA methylation	CpG island hypermethylation	Transcription repression
	CpG island hypomethylation	Transcription activation
	Repetitive sequences aberrant methylation	Transposition, recombinant genomic instability
Histone modification	Aberrant acetylation	Diverse
	Aberrant methylation	Diverse
	Aberrant phosphorylation	Diverse
Nucleosome positioning	Misposition in trinucleotide repeats	Creation of a "closed" chromatin domain
Autoimmune diseases		
DNA methylation	CpG island hypermethylation	Transcription repression
	CpG island hypomethylation	Transcription activation
	Repetitive sequences aberrant methylation	Transposition, recombinant genomic instability
Histone modification	Aberrant acetylation	Diverse
	Aberrant methylation	Diverse
	Aberrant phosphorylation	Diverse
Nucleosome positioning	Single-nucleotide polymorphisms in the 17q12-q21 region	Allele-specific differences in nucleosome distribution
	Histone variants replacement	Interferes with proper remodeling

[a]Examples of epigenetic variability associated with neoplastic and non-neoplastic human diseases. (Adapted with permission from Portela, A., and M. Esteller (2010). Epigenetic modifications and human disease. Nat Biotechnol **28**(10): 1057–68.)

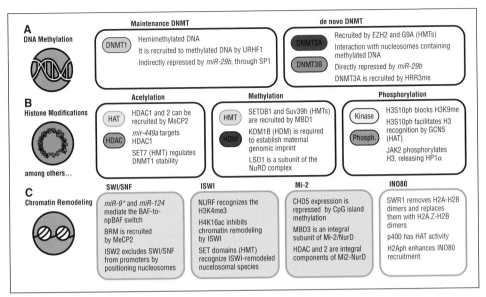

FIGURE 10–1. A (DNA methylation), B (histone modifications), and C (chromatin remodeling) demonstrate the diversity of epigenetic marks and examples of their regulation; epigenetic marks are regulated by enzymatic complexes including DNA methyltransferases (DNMT) and histone acetyltransferases (HAT). Regulation is mediated, in part, by interactions between epigenetic marks as well as genetic variation and environmental factors. The complex interplay suggested for each epigenetic mark supports the relevance of network-based approaches to unraveling the complexity associated with epigenetic variation. (Adapted with permission from Portela, A., and M. Esteller (2010). Epigenetic modifications and human disease. Nat Biotechnol **28**(10): 1057–68.)

mark studied in isolation will likely associate with specific subsets of regulatory factors, computational approaches to learning epigenetic networks, as they evolve, can be retooled and applied across the integrative genomics landscape. A number of new software tools have been described to incorporate epigenetics into gene regulatory networks by adding an epigenetic layer to existing network models (Turinsky, Turner, et al. 2011; Wang, Wang, et al. 2011; Mitra, Muller, et al. 2013; Turner, Lones, et al. 2013).

Robust advances in technology to assay the epigenome have extended the investigations of epigenetic marks from the exclusivity of cancer paradigms to a host of complex diseases including cardiovascular and pulmonary diseases, diabetes, metabolic syndrome, and autism, as well as traits such as aging and longevity.

RNA

Mechanistically, the control of chromatin activation, folding, and unfolding is a complex process. Epigenetic regulation is under the control of a variety of genomic elements, including, but probably not limited to single-nucleotide polymorphisms (SNPs), microRNAs, and a variety of noncoding RNAs. These factors inform the network of interactions that shape and maintain the totality of the epigenome. As such, integrative analytic approaches, inclusive of layers of regulatory information, are mandatory to gain insights into epigenetic plasticity and cellular specificity. With regard to epigenetics, the noncoding RNAs of greatest importance for epigenetics are likely long noncoding RNAs (lncRNAs). These lncRNAs have been implicated in a variety of genomic processes, including parent-of-origin effects, alternative splicing, and tissue-specific gene expression (Mattick 2010, 2012; Taft, Pang, et al. 2010). In addition, data suggest that lncRNAs are themselves regulated by genetic and epigenetic variation. Popadin, Gutierrez-Arcelus, and colleagues (2013) compared multiple -omics data types for multiple cell types and found that, in contrast to protein-coding genes, lncRNAs are enriched for *cis*-expression quantitative trait loci (eQTLs) and that the SNPs in these QTLs are closer to the transcription start site (TSS) in lncRNAs than for protein-coding genes. A similar trend was demonstrated for DNA methylation, for which functionally relevant DNA methylation marks appeared to be in closer proximity to the TSS of lncRNAs. Greater incorporation of these multiple -omics data types into a network context will further inform the complex features of regulation relevant to these lncRNAs.

LncRNAs are associated with chromatin-modifying complexes and histone methyltransferases and play a central role in controlling gene expression. It has been postulated that for complex transcriptional events, such as development or puberty, epigenetic regulation plays a critical role in the gene networks that are formed to guide these events. However, there is a paucity of data in which the role of epigenetic networks has been proven to be important, and there are virtually no studies that have measured these RNA elements and used them in network modeling. Clearly, as we have refined the medium- and high-throughput methodologies to gather epigenetic data, there have been nascent efforts toward aggregating the epigenetic data into a network context. What follows is a brief cross-section of the limited literature that has used epigenetic data in network models of either health or disease.

Human MicroRNA Networks

The realm of epigenetic variation includes microRNA. These small RNAs can influence gene expression in the absence of changes to genetic sequence variation. During the past decade there has been mounting evidence supporting the relevance of microRNAs in human neoplastic and non-neoplastic diseases. Key features supporting a network-based consideration of the roles for microRNA in health and disease relate to basic properties of microRNAs, including cooperativity (one gene, many influencing microRNA) and multiplicity (one microRNA, many genes). One example of microRNA playing a key regulatory role within a disease network module was provided by Parikh and colleagues, who demonstrated that miR-21 linked BMPR2, IL6, and the rho B/rho kinase pathway in pulmonary arterial hypertension (Parikh, Jin et al. 2012) (see details in Chapter 6). Since RNAs generally work in concert with other microRNAs, computational approaches to modeling microRNA-informed networks have focused on integration of multiple -omics data types.

It is very likely that microRNAs are subject to regulation, in part, by genetic sequence variation in cancer (Ryan, Robles, et al. 2010), and efforts have moved to address this type of regulation for a host of nonmalignant complex diseases. Gamazon, Ziliak, and colleagues (2012) identified a significant overlap between variants influencing microRNA and messenger RNA (mRNA), suggesting a complicated relationship between genetic variation and microRNA–mRNA relationships. Importantly microRNA eQTLs also identified by Gamazon and colleagues were enriched for SNPs previously associated with complex disease, suggesting that integration of these data with genome-wide association studies (GWAS) results may afford mechanistic understanding of disease. Although this approach is not explicitly placed in a network context, this type of integrative analysis demonstrates the dual relevance of SNP variation (for gene regulation through both microRNA and mRNA) and is highly informative. Lu, Zhang, and colleagues (2008) observed that microRNAs likely act in clustered patterns to influence disease. The authors developed microRNA-based disease networks and demonstrated that these networks present disease-specific microRNA clusters (Figure 10–2), including distinct patterns for cancer and cardiovascular diseases.

Additional approaches to modeling microRNA networks have focused on modeling the coregulation of a given gene by more than one microRNA. For example, Na and Kim (2013) developed a microRNA association network by identifying microRNAs that share target genes based on co-expression and sequence complementarity.

Recently, post-transcriptional regulation of RNA through methylation has emerged as a common modification that impacts RNA function, including splicing, intracellular trafficking, immune function, and selenoprotein incorporation. Most nitrogen, oxygen and carbon moieties in RNA are eligible for methylation in translational RNA (tRNA), ribosomal RNA, messenger RNA, and small nuclear RNA (Motorin and Helm 2011). One recent example of functional implication of RNA methylation includes the observation that variable tRNA methylation is a mechanism for regulating selenoprotein synthesis. In this accumulation of S-adenosylhomocysteine, decreased tRNA methylation results in reduced glutathione peroxidase 1 expression and increased cellular oxidative stress, a cascade of events that likely contributes to atherogenesis (Barroso,

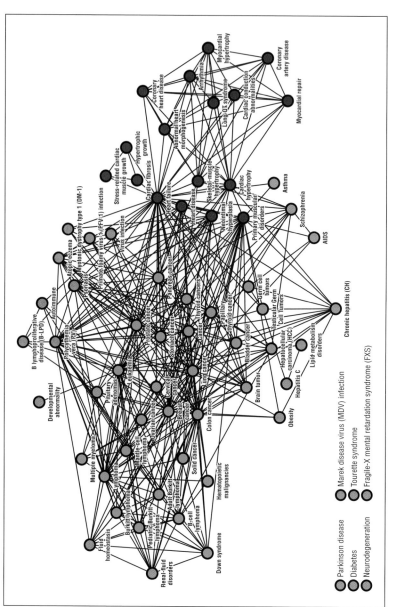

FIGURE 10–2. An example of a human miRNA disease network. Red nodes, blue nodes, and orange nodes represent cardiovascular disease, cancer, and other complex diseases, respectively. This diagrammed network was constructed by assigning an edge to two diseases if they were associated with one common microRNA. Cancers cluster together, as do cardiovascular diseases. The cancer and cardiovascular clusters are mostly disease-specific. (Adapted with permission from Lu, M., Q. Zhang, et al. (2008). An analysis of human microRNA and disease associations. PLoS One 3(10): e3420. (CC BY 3.0))

Florindo, et al. 2014). As such, accumulating evidence for a multitude of ways in which RNA modifications associate with disease supports the importance of incorporating RNA-omics into network models of common human diseases.

DNA Methylation

DNA methylation has been a frequently studied epigenetic mark with relevance for both neoplastic and other complex human diseases. Touted as an "archive" of the cumulative environment of exposures, the advantage of studying DNA methylation is, in part, borne out by the biological stability of this epigenetic mark. Network modeling of DNA methylation data may represent a fruitful approach to mining array-based genome-wide methylation data. Since one goal of modeling networks is to understand the impact on biological (phenotypic) perturbations, modeling the methylomic network in the context of common exposures (aging, smoking) may provide novel insights in this regard.

Array-based approaches to assaying the methylome have accelerated the pace of epigenetic investigation and moved the field rapidly toward considering these large datasets in the contexts of networks. For example, Mikhaylova, Zhang, and colleagues (2013) described the link between epigenomic changes and transcriptional response to allergen in mouse dendritic cells showing that the methylation pattern in allergen-naive dendritic cells of neonatal mice at risk for asthma was abnormal, but transcription was negligible until the dendritic cells were actually exposed to the allergen. Maternal asthma associated with both hypomethylation and hypermethylation, and the pathway analysis of these methylation marks indicated that about half of the differentially expressed genes interacted with known networks involved in asthma and allergy.

Sofer, Baccarelli, and colleagues (2013) looked at methylation using an Illumina chip in 141 subjects from the Normative Aging Study. They related gene-specific methylation scores to particulate air pollution levels and studied the relationship between these methylation scores and asthma pathway genes; they found that pathway genes were enriched in methylation. More recently, groups have extended network-modeling approaches to genome-wide methylation data to include a more cohesive and connected evaluation of the genome, as detailed below.

For example, eigengene networks have been applied to study the relationships between modules of gene co-methylation networks. Weighted gene co-expression network analysis (WGCNA) has been applied to DNA methylation data to identify top candidate genes based on intramodular hubs in consensus modules (Langfelder, Mischel, et al. 2013). In applying this approach, Horvath, Zhang, and colleagues (2012) addressed the identification of age-related consensus modules based on clusters of correlated CpG marks in several human tissues. The WGCNA on methylation array data from brain and blood tissue identified an age-related methylation module. Inclusion in the identified module was associated with polycomb group and CpG island status. Compared with a standard meta-analysis, the network-based approach led to a more enriched ontology, including genes associated with nervous system development and neurogenesis. In addition, this network-based approach identified module preservation between blood and brain methylation marks, suggesting that blood may be a reasonable surrogate for brain tissue, at least for aging research.

West, Beck and colleagues (2013) recently posited an approach to considering epigenetic networks including overlaying DNA methylation data with protein-protein interactome data, with a goal of improving inference about drivers of complex traits that are more robust than considering either data stream associated with the phenotype separately in a nonnetwork context. For example, human aging has been associated with significant changes in the methylome. These authors posited that age-related DNA methylation variability would demonstrate clusters in the protein–protein interactome, highlighting aging-related molecular targets and functional gene modules. Using a local greedy algorithm, they identified age-associated methylation–interactome hot spots in stem-cell differentiation pathways; these network signatures were not tissue-specific and potentially would have remained unrecognized without considering the data in a network context (West, Beck, et al. 2013). Importantly, given that best practices of network modeling of epigenetic data are still undefined, the authors benchmarked their spin glass algorithm with other module detection algorithms including jActiveModules, BioNet, and DEGAS, suggesting that their algorithm achieved robust module detection. As the field evolves, both for consideration of epigenetic interactome networks and module detection in epigenetics data as a single -omics type, multiple approaches should be considered to support the robustness of identified gene modules. An additional systems approach to overlaying DNA methylation data on the human interactome has been to examine age-associated DNA methylation variation. West, Widschwendter, and colleagues (2013) investigated the topological properties of genes with age and variable DNA methylation overlaid on a protein–protein interaction network and observed that age-associated "epigenetic drift" seems to occur in genes in the network periphery and with very low network connectivity (Figure 10–3). Extending these analyses, they observed that genes on the periphery of the network form large communities (subnetworks), suggesting that network modeling of methylation data may provide novel insights into aging and longevity (see Figure 10–3). In addition to addressing a complex phenotype such as aging, other researchers have endeavored to integrate DNA methylation and human interactome data to identify DNA methylation networks for type 2 diabetes (Liu, Wang, et al. 2014), as well as more explicitly modeling epigenome–metabolome interactions as discussed below.

Metabolomic–Epigenetic Networks

Networks of metabolomics data will likely provide novel insights into the downstream manifestations of genetic, genomic, and epigenetic variation. In this regard, DNA methylation has been suggested as one epigenetic mark that may have demonstrable impact upon human metabolism. Petersen, Zeilinger, and colleagues (2014) assessed 649 blood metabolomics traits from 1814 individuals for association with DNA methylation marks and observed seven CpG loci associated with metabotypes. In addition, they identified several subsets of CpG loci that were associated with

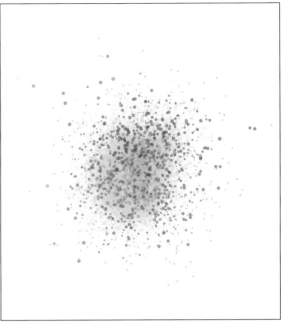

FIGURE 10–3. Age-associated epigenetic drift mapped onto the human interactome. This network diagram conveys that genes associated with variable DNA methylation with aging occupy the periphery of the network, whereas longevity genes occurred in the central part of the network. In this figure, the human protein interactome with 8969 nodes is represented with purple representing GAMPs (genes undergoing age-associated changes in promoter methylation), green representing longevity genes, and yellow representing all other genes not in these two categories. (Reprinted with permission from West, J., M. Widschwendter, et al. (2013). Distinctive topology of age-associated epigenetic drift in the human interactome. Proc Natl Acad Sci U S A 110(35): 14138–43.)

metabotypes, including 4-vinylphenol sulfate and 4-androstene-3-beta-17-beta-diol disulfate. The complexity of this approach lends itself to consideration in a network context (Figure 10–4). The approach to the integration of metabolomics and DNA methylation data did not yield findings that were as compelling as integration of genetic variation with the same metabolomics data (Suhre and Gieger 2012), but this is a promising example of the relevance of integrating of epigenetics data with additional -omics data in a network context. More studies that integrate metabolomics data with epigenetic data in a network context should extend these initial promising association findings.

Epigenetic networks are plastic and responsive to endogenous and exogenous environments. As such, from a network perspective, epigenetic marks may inform dynamic features of networks not explicitly modeled by genetic variation. This plasticity feeds forward into the potential relevance to patient care, as

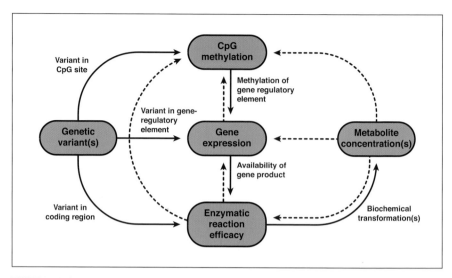

FIGURE 10–4. Schematic of the interplay between metabolomic phenotypes (metabotypes), DNA methylation, and genetic variation. Possible reactions associated with regulation are represented by the dashed lines. The complexity of the validated and proposed feedback regulation supports the relevance of network modeling of epigenetic factors to facilitate insights into the metabolome. (Adapted with permission from Petersen, A. K., S. Zeilinger, et al. (2014). Epigenetics meets metabolomics: an epigenome-wide association study with blood serum metabolic traits. Hum Mol Genet 23(2): 534–45.)

modeling the plasticity of the epigenome and epigenetic-targeted pathways offer unique pharmacoepigenetic opportunities.

Conclusion

The data available in the field of human epigenetics suggest that epigenetic control is complex, extending far beyond environmental exposures, and that network models that incorporate epigenetics will play an increasingly important role in the understanding of gene regulation. However, one of the challenges in constructing epigenetic networks is to be able to model the plasticity, epigene–epigene interactions, and the informative role of the environment. Also, the interplay between multiple epigenetic modifications, such as chromatin states and DNA methylation, adds to the complexity in modeling epigenetic networks. Epigenetic network modeling has definite challenges, not the least of which is defining the input into these network models and the relevance to their use in identifying causes of common disease (Table 10–2). However, opportunities arise from the distinct possibility to harness the plasticity of the human epigenome to develop novel therapeutics. Tools to interrogate the epigenetic marks, epigenetic data analysis, and the modeling of epigenetic networks are evolving

TABLE 10–2. How Epigenomics Is Transforming the Search for Causes of Common Human Disease[a]

EPIGENOMIC ANATOMY	POSSIBLE DISEASE LINK	NEW APPROACH TO COMMON DISEASE SEARCH
Environmentally driven epigenetic variation	Epigenome changes in absence of sequence variant	Methylome arrays, capture bisulfite sequencing, chromatin immunoprecipitation with sequencing
Regulatory site or expression	Noncoding RNAs	RNA sequencing and methods above
Key disease sequences not linked to target genes	Intrachromosomal and interchromosomal interactions	Chromatin network mapping
Regulatory sequence distant from gene	Coregulated gene clusters	Genome-scale methylation, chromatin mapping
Sequence-defined methylation	Sequence variants controlling epigenome	Linked GWAS and epigenome studies
New class of variably methylated regions (VMRs)	Sequence variants controlling epigenomic variance	New statistics for reexamining and integrating GWAS
Domain disruption, anchoring proteins	Large Organized Chromatin Modifications (LOCKs) and Lamin-associated domains (LADs)	Native chromatin whole-genome analysis

[a] Possible link between epigenetics and genetic causes of complex human diseases. (Adapted with permission from Feinberg, A. P. (2010). Epigenomics reveals a functional genome anatomy and a new approach to common disease. Nat Biotechnol **28**(10): 1049–52.)

quickly, but in many ways are the newest of the -omics to be considered in a network context. Although many statistical methods to analyze gene expression data have been modifiable and applicable to the analysis of epigenetic data, it is likely, given the diversity and plasticity of the epigenome, that the analytic approaches to and the validation of epigenetic signatures will require features that can accommodate the inherent longitudinal plasticity, and, hence, perturbability, of the epigenome. Specific tool development, with tunable parameters for modeling epigenetic network plasticity, offers the most comprehensive interrogation of these important genomic marks. Epigenetic marks, such as DNA methylation, have been suggested to provide the type of information needed to infer directed gene regulatory networks, as the epigenetic layer of information provides context to gene regulatory networks (Simcha, Younes, et al. 2013). The further development of insights into the biology of epigenetic networks will be well served by the comprehensive initiatives of the Human Epigenome Project and International Epigenome Mapping projects. One important consideration of epigenetic networks and the plasticity of epigenetic marks is that they may represent, more than other network facets, the potential of a network to be perturbed toward disease and then returned to a state that trends toward health. Continued refinement of modeling epigenetic networks promises the possibility for the development of exciting targets for treatment (Kelly, De Carvalho, et al. 2010) and potentially for prevention of disease.

References

Barroso, M., C. Florindo, et al. (2014). Inhibition of cellular methyltransferases promotes endothelial cell activation by suppressing glutathione peroxidase 1 protein expression. J Biol Chem **289**(22): 15350–62.

Feinberg, A. P. (2010). Epigenomics reveals a functional genome anatomy and a new approach to common disease. Nat Biotechnol **28**(10): 1049–52.

Gamazon, E. R., D. Ziliak, et al. (2012). Genetic architecture of microRNA expression: implications for the transcriptome and complex traits. Am J Hum Genet **90**(6): 1046–63.

Horvath, S., Y. Zhang, et al. (2012). Aging effects on DNA methylation modules in human brain and blood tissue. Genome Biol **13**(10): R97.

Kelly, T. K., D. D. De Carvalho, et al. (2010). Epigenetic modifications as therapeutic targets. Nat Biotechnol **28**(10): 1069–78.

Langfelder, P., P. S. Mischel, et al. (2013). When is hub gene selection better than standard meta-analysis? PLoS One **8**(4): e61505.

Liu, H., T. Wang, et al. (2014). Detection of type 2 diabetes related modules and genes based on epigenetic networks. BMC Syst Biol **8**(Suppl 1): S5.

Lu, M., Q. Zhang, et al. (2008). An analysis of human microRNA and disease associations. PLoS One **3**(10): e3420.

Mattick, J. S. (2010). Linc-ing long noncoding RNAs and enhancer function. Dev Cell **19**(4): 485–86.

Mattick, J. S. (2012). RNA driving the epigenetic bus. EMBO J **31**(3): 515–16.

Mikhaylova, L., Y. Zhang, et al. (2013). Link between epigenomic alterations and genome-wide aberrant transcriptional response to allergen in dendritic cells conveying maternal asthma risk. PLoS One **8**(8): e70387.

Mitra, R., P. Muller, et al. (2013). Toward breaking the histone code: bayesian graphical models for histone modifications. Circ Cardiovasc Genet **6**(4): 419–26.

Motorin, Y., and M. Helm (2011). RNA nucleotide methylation. Wiley Interdiscip Rev RNA **2**(5): 611–31.

Na, Y. J., and J. H. Kim (2013). Understanding cooperativity of microRNAs via microRNA association networks. BMC Genomics **14**(Suppl 5): S17.

Parikh, V. N., R. C. Jin, et al. (2012). MicroRNA-21 integrates pathogenic signaling to control pulmonary hypertension: results of a network bioinformatics approach. Circulation **125**(12): 1520–32.

Petersen, A. K., S. Zeilinger, et al. (2014). Epigenetics meets metabolomics: an epigenome-wide association study with blood serum metabolic traits. Hum Mol Genet **23**(2): 534–45.

Popadin, K., M. Gutierrez-Arcelus, et al. (2013). Genetic and epigenetic regulation of human lincRNA gene expression. Am J Hum Genet **93**(6): 1015–26.

Portela, A., and M. Esteller (2010). Epigenetic modifications and human disease. Nat Biotechnol **28**(10): 1057–68.

Ryan, B. M., A. I. Robles, et al. (2010). Genetic variation in microRNA networks: the implications for cancer research. Nat Rev Cancer **10**(6): 389–402.

Simcha, D. M., L. Younes, et al. (2013). Identification of direction in gene networks from expression and methylation. BMC Syst Biol **7**: 118.

Sofer, T., A. Baccarelli, et al. (2013). Exposure to airborne particulate matter is associated with methylation pattern in the asthma pathway. Epigenomics **5**(2): 147–54.

Suhre, K., and C. Gieger (2012). Genetic variation in metabolic phenotypes: study designs and applications. Nat Rev Genet **13**(11): 759–69.

Taft, R. J., K. C. Pang, et al. (2010). Non-coding RNAs: regulators of disease. J Pathol **220**(2): 126–39.

Turinsky, A. L., B. Turner, et al. (2011). DAnCER: disease-annotated chromatin epigenetics resource. Nucleic Acids Res **39**(Database issue): D889–94.

Turner, A. P., M. A. Lones, et al. (2013). The incorporation of epigenetics in artificial gene regulatory networks. Biosystems **112**(2): 56–62.

Wang, L. Y., P. Wang, et al. (2011). EpiRegNet: constructing epigenetic regulatory network from high throughput gene expression data for humans. Epigenetics **6**(12): 1505–12.

West, J., S. Beck, et al. (2013). An integrative network algorithm identifies age-associated differential methylation interactome hotspots targeting stem-cell differentiation pathways. Sci Rep **3**: 1630.

West, J., M. Widschwendter, et al. (2013). Distinctive topology of age-associated epigenetic drift in the human interactome. Proc Natl Acad Sci U S A **110**(35): 14138–43.

• 11 •

Metabolomics and Network Medicine

JESSICA LASKY-SU AND CLARY B. CLISH

Introduction

Technological advances in biology have enabled the generation of large volumes of -omics data. From these data, the emerging field of network medicine, a field still in its infancy, is attempting to understand the complex biology that connects genomics, transcriptomics, proteomics, and metabolomics to important disease states. The integration of these data using systems biology and network science approaches will lead to a better understanding of the biological mechanisms underlying the complex development of diseases. A metabolic network uses metabolic data to understand the physiological and biochemical properties of a biospecimen that results in metabolic pathways leading to a disease state. In contrast to other -omics data, relevant metabolites have diverse physicochemical properties, thereby requiring the use of a broad range of platforms to generate a comprehensive summary of the metabolic state.

In this chapter, we will provide an overview of metabolomics and its crucial role in systems biology approaches, leading to increased understanding of disease pathophysiology. Specifically, we will define metabolomics, review the current technologies used to generate metabolomics data, describe the current statistical methods and systems biology approaches used with metabolomics data alone, summarize the integrative network approaches used with metabolomics and other -omics data, and discuss the future directions of network medicine with regard to metabolomics.

The Human Metabolome Defined

The metabolome is the entire complement of low-molecular-weight molecules (molecular weight <2000 amu) in a biological sample or organism. These molecules include carbohydrates, sugars, fatty acids, lipids, nucleotides, amino acids, and short peptide chains. The total number of metabolites remains unknown and varies by biological specimen. As technology improves and sensitivity increases, the number of identified metabolites continues to increase.

Within humans, Beecher (2003) estimated approximately 2000 major metabolites. By conglomerating several metabolic profiling methods that generate metabolites from various biochemical pathways, comprehensive metabolomics data can be generated. A recent effort to catalog compounds reported to have been measured in human-derived samples as well as "expected" compounds, including drug metabolites and food-derived molecules, yielded a database with more than 40,000 entries (Wishart, Jewison, et al. 2013). Regardless of the actual number, the goal of "metabolomics" is to enable robust measurement of endogenous small molecules for the determination of metabolic phenotypes.

Measurement of the metabolome is a significant analytical challenge for a variety of reasons, several of which are described here. A key challenge is due to the differences in physical properties among compounds that constitute the metabolome. In particular, differences in polarity among groups or families of metabolites demand that different extraction procedures be used during the preparation of analytical samples. For example, nonpolar lipids such as triglycerides are most efficiently extracted using nonpolar solvents such as isopropanol or mixtures of chloroform and methanol, but these solvents are less effective for the extraction of very polar metabolites, such as glycolytic pathway intermediates. A second challenge is related to the breadth of concentration ranges at which metabolites occur in biological samples. The analytical tools most commonly used in metabolomics, nuclear magnetic resonance (NMR) spectroscopy and mass spectrometry (MS), have linear dynamic ranges for analyses that span 3 to 5 orders of magnitude, but the concentration range of metabolites in any sample will exceed this range. For example, of approximately 4000 metabolites surveyed in human serum, concentrations ranged over 11 orders of magnitude, with the most abundant metabolites such as glucose, lactate, cholesterol, and cholesteryl esters measured at millimolar concentrations and low-abundance metabolites such as prostaglandin E_1, 3,5-diiodothyronine, and cotinine N-oxide were measured at picomolar concentrations (Psychogios, Hau, et al. 2011). A third challenge arises from differences in chemical stability and, consequently, differences in rates of decomposition among metabolites, both in intact biological samples and after metabolite extraction procedures. At present, no single method in analytical technology can adequately address the diverse features of the metabolome and provide comprehensive measurements. In practice, individual metabolomics laboratories use one or more analytical methods and are capable of measuring a subset of the metabolome. Deeper coverage is often limited by the amount of biological sample that is available and practical considerations of time and cost. Nevertheless, it is possible to measure hundreds of metabolites in small-volume samples routinely and precisely. Owing to these complexities, the generation of metabolomics data is not uniform across laboratories. Therefore, laboratory precision is necessary to generate quality metabolomics data.

Technologies to Generate Metabolomics Data

Biomaterials for Metabolomics

Metabolomic data can be generated using a variety of biospecimens. Biofluids, including plasma (Vuckovic and Pawliszyn 2011), serum (OuYang, Xu, et al. 2011; Xuan, Pan, et al. 2011; Hasokawa, Shinohara. et al. 2012), saliva (Alvarez-Sanchez, Priego-Capote, et al. 2012), exhaled breath condensate (Carraro, Rezzi, et al. 2007; Montuschi, Paris, et al. 2012), and urine (Saude, Skappak, et al. 2011), are the most common specimens used, although metabolic profiling can be performed using a wide array of biologically relevant bodily tissues (Ji, Ernest, et al. 2012) as well as fecal samples (Chow, Panasevich, et al. 2014; Goedert, Sampson, et al. 2014). The number of metabolites that can be extracted and the stability of those metabolites vary by specimen. Although certain biospecimens are more relevant for specific diseases, research has shown some general consistency across metabolic profiles and various biologic specimens (Schicho, Shaykhutdinov, et al. 2012). Because no single method is capable of detecting the complete set of metabolites, several analytical techniques are required to generate more comprehensive measures of the metabolome. Metabolites are extracted from a biospecimen using separation and quantification techniques.

The analytical tools most commonly used in metabolomics are NMR spectroscopy, liquid and gas chromatography (LC, GC), and MS. Several of these techniques are used in combination to separate and quantify the analytes (LC–MS, GC–MS). A summary of the attributes of these technologies is provided in Table 11–1.

Nuclear Magnetic Resonance Spectroscopy

NMR spectroscopy takes advantage of the magnetic properties of atomic nuclei to identify metabolites in the biofluid under investigation. This method uses NMR to generate information on the structure of chemical constituents within body fluids. Specifically, when a strong magnetic field is applied, NMR measures the changes in nuclear magnetism in the atom. Each compound can be defined by a unique pattern of chemical shifts and different peak intensities (Hoffman and Ozery 2013). Some advantages of NMR are that it is fully quantitative, is

TABLE 11–1. Major Analytical Technologies Used in Metabolomics[a]

	ADVANTAGES	DISADVANTAGES
NMR	• Nondestructive • Robust • ^{13}C and ^{15}N tracer studies	• Less sensitive than MS methods • Spectral overlap • Limited breadth of metabolite coverage • Cost
GC–MS	• Cost • Breadth of coverage • Special libraries for compound Identification • Electron Ionization fragmentation can enable monitoring incorporation of stable isotopes at specific sites	• Must derivatize samples—metabolites must be volatile • Least robust technology (liner changes in GC injection port required)
LC–MS	• Sensitive • Broad coverage • Flexible • Reasonably robust	• Quality of spectral libraries does not match those for GS–MS • Moderate cost

[a]Need to use combinations of methods/technologies to achieve sufficiently broad coverage.

highly reproducible, provides minimal sample preparation, and does not destroy the biofluid being used. A distinct disadvantage of NMR is that it is less sensitive than mass spectrometry, as it measures only highly abundant compounds in the micromolar concentration range.

Mass Spectrometry

LC–MS combines the ability of chromatography to separate molecules with the ability of MS to measure the abundance of metabolites. Chromatography is a technique that is used to separate metabolites from complex mixtures (e.g., plasma or serum extracts) to facilitate quantitation. The separation of metabolites occurs through combining stationary and mobile phases. In the mobile phase, the sample is forced through a liquid that ranges in polarity from oily to water-soluble substances. This liquid will also contain stationary particles, such as silica gel (the "stationary phase"), that enable the separation of various classes of analytes, including polar analytes, ionic analytes, compounds with hydrophobic groups, small molecules, and macromolecules. GC uses similar techniques with gaseous rather than liquid substances. MS then measures the mass of ionized molecules that are used to detect and measure the abundance of metabolites. There are currently various types of MS analyzers, such as the triple quadrupole (QQQ), which can measure at low mass resolution (i.e., ±0.5 amu), has high sensitivity, and is most often used for targeted analyses. Other MS analyzers, such as the Quadrupole-time-of-flight (QTOF), Fourier transform ion cyclotron resonance (FT-ICR), and Orbitrap, have higher mass resolution but are able to generate untargeted metabolomic data.

Targeted versus Untargeted Approaches

There are two main strategies for the quantification of metabolites, the choice of which largely depends on the hypothesis being tested. A targeted metabolomics approach is typically part of a hypothesis-driven experiment. In this case, a pre-defined choice of select metabolites is quantified. Targeted metabolomics is typically limited to a set of known, chemically related metabolites. One distinct advantage of this approach is that these metabolites have been characterized previously and are often quantified using calibration approaches that are tai-lored to the metabolites being measured. As such, the metabolites are likely to be measured with optimal sensitivity. Therefore, the quantifications that are ob-tained from these targeted platforms can be compared to labeled external stan-dards that enable the verification of known metabolites. In contrast, untargeted metabolomics measures all endogenous metabolic signals in a biological sample. These methods are necessarily broader in order to capture the larger range of metabolites, but they result in reduced sensitivity. Data from the untargeted ap-proach typically result in many unidentified metabolites. Extensive data pro-cessing is then necessary to identify the unknown metabolites. The data must first be "aligned" to adjust for the differences in retention times and molecular masses, followed by peak identification and integration. Although this process is tedious, an untargeted approach allows for the identification of unknown metabolites that may, in turn, have a significant impact on disease processes. Therefore, the potential for novel scientific findings is higher, although further scrutiny of the results is necessary. Once the metabolic profiling is completed, careful bioinformatics analysis is necessary, using computer software and data-bases that identify known metabolites.

Data Cleaning and Preparation

As discussed, comprehensive metabolomics data arise from the application of various technologies using either a targeted or untargeted approach. There-fore, the data are subject to several types of biases, including differences in the accuracy of the technologies that were employed to generate the data. Data cleaning and processing can be completed using several resources, one of the most popular being MetaboAnalyst (Xia, Mandal, et al. 2012). Data processing and normalization typically begin with filtering the data, followed by several transformation procedures (most often log-normalization) that result in normalized data. Quality-control checking allows for the examination of sys-tematic errors, batch effects, sample decay, and outlying observations. Other analysis programs are also available through R, including the Metabolite Automatic Identification Toolkit (MAIT), which can identify and annotate MS peaks as well as perform initial statistical analyses (Fernandez-Albert, Llorach, et al. 2014).

Identifying unknown metabolites from untargeted metabolomic analyses presents a significant challenge to the scientific community. Metabolites are most often identified using the mass-to-charge ratio (m/z). Several databases are currently available for this identification, including the Human Metabolome DataBase (HMDB), METLIN, and Madison Metabolomics Consortium Database (MMCD), which we review here. The identification and characterization of metabolites is a necessary step in further deducing the biochemical and physiological function of a select group of metabolites. Thus, the comprehensive identification of metabolites represents a key initial step in understanding metabolic networks.

Metabolomic Databases

The Human Metabolome Database

HMDB (www.hmdb.ca) was created in an effort to help identify metabolites and link them to clinical phenotypes; it is currently the largest metabolite database worldwide (Wishart, Tzur, et al. 2007; Wishart, Jewison, et al. 2013). This electronic database contains detailed information about the metabolites found in human body specimens, with the goal of connecting chemical, clinical, and molecular data. The database contains over 40,000 annotated metabolites, including both "detected" and "expected" metabolites (metabolites known to be taken into the body but not yet identified in biofluid/tissue). For each metabolite, HMDB contains information including spectroscopic properties, relevant metabolite physiology, related enzymes and transporters, origin of the metabolite, known associations of metabolites, and disease phenotypes (Wishart, Tzur, et al. 2007; Wishart, Jewison, et al. 2013). Because many unidentified metabolites are observed through NMR and MS, HMDB also seeks to be a reference database for these metabolites. Metabolites are identified in a hierarchical manner, by subdividing them from larger "kingdoms" into more specific "classes" and finer "families." HMDB also provides information on the relevant Kyoto Encyclopedia of Genes and Genomes (KEGG) pathways for several of the metabolites, enabling further inquiry into specific biochemical pathways that may be relevant. Thus, HMDB serves as one of the primary bioinformatics tools for metabolomics research.

METLIN

METLIN (http://metlin.scripps.edu) is a public mass spectral database, in existence since 2005, and originating from Scripps Ranch; it currently contains annotation on over 65,000 metabolites, (Tautenhahn, Cho, et al. 2012) including information on mass, chemical formula, and structure. It allows for the searching of metabolites based on structure, weight, and MS/MS fragmentation patterns. Endogenous and drug metabolites are included in the database. METLIN focuses on metabolites identified through various types of MS. Reference tandem MS data are also included from known metabolites. METLIN has also cataloged individual data from various biofluids and tissues across an array of individuals and animal samples (Tautenhahn, Cho, et al. 2012).

Madison Metabolomics Consortium Database

MMCD (mmcd.nmrfam.wisc.edu) is an online database that uses NMR and MS data to identify metabolites in a biologic sample (Cui, Lewis, et al. 2008). This database contains information on metabolites collected from both electronic and other scientific resources and includes up to 50 metabolic characterizations, such as the metabolite name, chemical formula, synonym, structure, chemical, and physical properties. MMCD has capabilities that enable searching and analyzing the functionality of metabolites based on technology type (NMR, MS), structure type, or other miscellaneous characteristics. Information on the chemical formula, functional group, and experimental parameters (NMR/MS) are input into MMCD, and information on metabolites, structures, and lists of metabolites are generated.

MetaboSearch

Each of the described metabolomics databases contains only a small fraction of the total number of existing metabolites. Even combined, these databases describe only a subset of all metabolites. The program MetaboSearch was created to perform a simultaneous search across four databases (MMCD, METLIN, HMDB, and LIPID Maps [Fahy, Sud, et al. 2007; Sud, Fahy, et al. 2007]) in order to maximize the identification of unknown metabolites (Zhou, Wang, et al. 2012). The information is then compiled across the databases to generate a complete list of metabolites.

Metabolite Set Enrichment Analysis and Pathway Analyses

The absolute concentrations of metabolites can be further utilized to provide information on possible function and to provide insight into the biology underlying the observed metabolic profiles. Metabolite set enrichment analysis (MSEA) (Xia and Wishart 2010) is a technique for metabolomics data analysis that is analogous to gene set enrichment analysis (GSEA) (Subramanian, Tamayo, et al. 2005). This Web-based server is used to help interpret an array of metabolite concentrations by comparing the observed metabolite concentrations to reference compound concentration tables. MSEA includes a library of approximately predefined metabolic profiles or sets covering various metabolic pathways, diseases, biofluids, and tissue locations. Additional forms of enrichment analyses can identify metabolites that are overrepresented using several additional analytical approaches that are part of a larger Web-based analytical program, MetaboAnalyst (Xia, Mandal, et al. 2012). Individual sample profiles can also be examined by comparing the concentrations of measured metabolites in a given biofluid to the standard normal reference values in that biofluid. Identified metabolites can then be used in overrepresentation analysis. Overrepresentation analysis will use the list of previously identified metabolites to determine important underlying biological patterns represented in this group (Xia, Mandal, et al. 2012). Once enrichment analyses are performed, metabolic pathway analysis can be performed. This approach will combine the information obtained from the enrichment analyses with network methodologies to generate metabolic pathways that are important to the disease under consideration. Pathways from these approaches can be examined further using several different visualization programs, such as Cytoscape (Shannon, Markiel, et al. 2003).

Systems Biology Approaches for Metabolomics and Disease Phenotypes

Single Metabolites as Biomarkers for Disease

The first step toward developing metabolomics networks is to integrate metabolomics data with disease phenotypes. There is a long history of using metabolite(s) to define a disease state or to indicate the severity of disease. For example, diabetes mellitus is diagnosed by having a fasting blood glucose level of 126 mg/dl or greater. Measures of high-density lipoprotein (HDL) cholesterol, low-density lipoprotein (LDL) cholesterol, and triglycerides help define risk factors for coronary heart disease (Jensen, Bertoia, et al. 2014). This singular approach can be extended to all of the metabolites to generate an initial high-throughput data analysis set. Specifically, the association between each individual metabolite and the disease status can be assessed via a logistic regression model with each metabolite as a predictor variable(s) and the disease phenotype as the response variable, adjusted for relevant covariates. After this analysis is performed on all individual metabolites, a multiple testing adjustment, such as a Bonferroni correction (Dunn, 1961) or a false discovery rate (Benjamini and

Hochberg 1995), is necessary to identify significantly associated metabolites. A nested case–control study design is also often used in metabolomics research, where cases within a larger longitudinal study are compared with matched controls from the same study to assess the differences in metabolic profiles between the individuals with disease and those free from disease. This approach was used with metabolomic data from the Framingham Heart Study using 189 incident diabetic cases (identified over a 12-year period) and 189 propensity-matched control cases (Wang, Larson, et al. 2011). A paired analysis identified five metabolites that were significantly different between cases and controls. A conditional logistic regression analysis was then performed, using the five metabolites and adjusting for covariates, to predict diabetes occurrence. Odds ratios (ORs) for these metabolites ranged from 2 to 3.5 (Wang, Larson, et al. 2011). In contrast to several of the -omics data that are currently available, few metabolomics studies have independent replication of their findings. A strength of this particular study was that the key findings were independently replicated in a sample of 163 cases and controls, and four of the five top metabolites were significantly associated with incident diabetes (Wang, Larson, et al. 2011). A distinct advantage of metabolomics data is that the strength of association with disease outcome tends to be higher than what is observed with genetic data, where typical observed odds ratios are more modest (e.g., ORs <1.5 for genetic associations) (Manolio, Collins, et al. 2009). Metabolites can also be used to evaluate the association of physiological measures that are correlated with the disease of interest with quantitative molecular measures.

Metabotype

A metabolic phenotype, or metabotype, is the sum of the measured metabolites that exist in the biospecimen at a given time (Suhre and Gieger 2012). A key feature of metabotypes is that they are dynamic and can vary dramatically over time. The metabotype can be influenced by a broad range of environmental exposures, from food intake, to hormonal changes, to the intake of medications. Thus, changing any one of these exposures can significantly affect the overall metabolic state. In the context of a study design, this can be a distinct advantage, as the metabolic profile under two different environmental exposures can be compared within an individual and important differences identified.

Pharmacometabolomics

The dynamic nature of metabolites enables the study of metabolic profile changes under varying conditions relevant to disease pathogenesis or treatment. For example, the metabolic state under specific pharmacological treatments for a disease is often of interest. This "pharmacometabolomic" approach is valuable and has been successful in identifying important metabolites and biological pathways that are activated with exposure to a pharmacologic treatment. Pharmacometabolomics also enables one to differentiate the various metabolic states under different pharmacotherapies, a strategy that has been successful in identifying key metabolic differences on and off various treatments, such as resistance to aspirin treatment (Yerges-Armstrong, Ellero-Simatos, et al. 2013). A similar approach can be used to examine how specific exposures affect the metabolic state, such as physiological challenges, fasting/nonfasting states, and other environmental exposures, such as smoking. For example, studies have examined exercise-induced metabolic profiles (Lewis, Farrell, et al. 2010), differentiating the metabolic profiles at various levels of exercise-induced stress. Another approach involves assessing the metabolic profiles of cell lines that are and are not exposed to molecular agonists or antagonists, such as pharmacologic agents (Tiziani, Lodi, et al. 2009). This approach has been applied to cancer studies where NMR metabolic profiling was found to discriminate between bisphosphonate and doxorubicin effects on B16 melanoma cells (Triba, Starzec, et al. 2010). This strategy was also employed by Cao, Li, and colleagues (2013), who compared the metabolic profiles of drug-sensitive and drug-resistant breast cancer cells. Both cell lines were treated with doxorubicin (Adriamycin), which induces multiple drug resistance. Analyses revealed that the metabolic responses of the two cell lines to doxorubicin were distinct. Evidence suggested that doxorubicin modulated more metabolic pathways in the drug-sensitive breast cancer cells than in the drug-resistant cells.

Clinical trials have also integrated metabolomics data to study whether metabolic profiles differ on and off medication. In a study of patients with schizophrenia, GC–MS was performed on unmedicated individuals before and after 8 weeks of risperidone therapy. Twenty-two metabolites were identified that separated patients with schizophrenia from matched controls, and twenty metabolites were identified that differentiated patients with schizophrenia before and after treatment (Xuan, Pan, et al. 2011). This study validates that metabolic profiles vary both for diseased and nondiseased states and for individuals on and off pharmacologic treatment.

Multivariate Methods That Identify Metabolic Profiles for Disease Prediction

Although single metabolites/biomarkers are strongly related to some disease diagnoses, it is more often the case that a group of metabolites can be used to distinguish individuals with and those without disease for complex diseases. This is primarily because the state of a group of metabolites often better identifies the biochemical/metabolic pathways that are being altered physiologically by a disease. Therefore, the quantification of a vast array of diverse metabolites can be highly informative for discriminating between individuals with and those without disease. Multivariate statistical methods that incorporate high-dimensional data, such as those that incorporate all metabolites, represent powerful approaches for understanding disease attributes, ranging from discriminating between cases and controls to identifying important biochemical pathways for disease pathogenesis. Standard parametric statistical methods, such as regression analysis, are not feasible in this case because the number of individuals (n) is typically less than the number of measured metabolites (p), and, therefore, the data are inadequate for parameter estimation ($n<p$). Therefore, the high-dimensional statistical methods often applied to metabolomics data include clustering, discriminant analysis, regression models, genetic algorithms, support vector machine learning (Mahadevan, Shah, et al. 2008), and principal component analysis (Ramadan, Jacobs, et al. 2006).

Principal Component Analysis

Principal component analysis (PCA) is one of the most common data-reducing techniques used for metabolomics data that can summarize the data in fewer dimensions (Jolliffe 2002). The popularity of PCA in metabolomics is due to the fact that it is a simple nonparametric method that can project the metabolites into lower-dimensional space, revealing inherent data structure and providing a reduced dimensional representation of the original data. In this case, each principal component is a summary of metabolite contributions that are orthogonal from the other principal components and can be used as independent variables; together, these variables summarize the overall metabolic state of the individual samples.

Partial Least Square Discriminant Analysis (PLS-DA)

Various types of discriminant analysis are used with metabolomics data (Ramadan, Jacobs, et al. 2006), with partial least square discriminant analysis (PLS-DA) being the primary method currently in use. PLS-DA uses a set of correlated metabolites that is first transformed to uncorrelated variables. These uncorrelated variables are then included in a regression analysis with the case–control status as the predictor variable of interest, and the set of metabolites that most accurately predicts the case–control status is selected. Metabolic profiles have been used to discriminate between patients with and without various diseases. One such example is a study that generated metabolic profiles using serum, plasma, and urine to attempt to discriminate between patients with and without inflammatory bowel disease (IBD) (Schicho, Shaykhutdinov, et al. 2012). A total of 44 serum, 37 plasma, and 71 urine metabolites were generated using NMR. PCA and hierarchical discriminant analysis were performed to

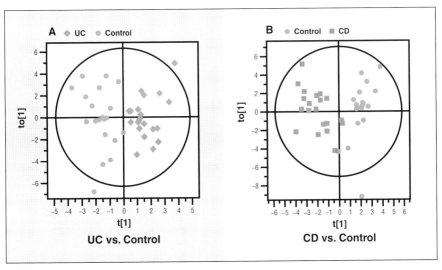

FIGURE 11–1. Quantitative metabolomic profiling of plasma by (1)H NMR spectroscopy discriminates between patients with ulcerative colitis (UC) and healthy individuals (Control) and between patients with Crohn's disease (CD) and healthy individuals. Hierarchical OPLS-DA loadings plots were obtained from scores of sub-PCA models that were separately derived from patients with Crohn's disease (CD) and ulcerative colitis (UC), and matched healthy (control) subjects. These plots represent associations between scores (tB) in plasma that were most metabolically disrupted by the inflammatory diseases. (Reprinted with permission from Schicho, R., R. Shaykhutdinov, et al. (2012). Quantitative metabolomic profiling of serum, plasma, and urine by (1)H NMR spectroscopy discriminates between patients with inflammatory bowel disease and healthy individuals. J Proteome Res 11(6): 3344–57.)

differentiate individuals with and without IBD. This study illustrated that metabolites can be used to discriminate between those with and without IBD; however, it was more difficult to differentiate individuals with Crohn's disease from those with ulcerative colitis, which would be expected, given their similar pathobiology as compared with healthy controls. Figure 11–1 summarizes the discrimination ability of PLS-DA for these IBDs as compared with control subjects. This study also illustrates that the number of metabolites that can be extracted from different biofluids varies significantly. These methods have been successfully applied to accurately distinguish between individuals with and without coronary heart disease (Brindle, Antti, et al. 2002), cardiovascular disease (Barderas, Laborde, et al. 2012), schizophrenia (Xuan, Pan, et al. 2011), IBD (Schicho, Shaykhutdinov, et al. 2012), diabetes mellitus (Wang, Larson, et al. 2011; Kim, Lee, et al. 2013), low birth weight (Ivorra, Garcia-Vicent, et al. 2012), ovarian cancer (Zhang, Wu, et al. 2012; Fong, McDunn, et al. 2013), and multiple sclerosis (Reinke, Broadhurst, et al. 2014). Analysis packages are also available, including the Metabolomics Univariate and Multivariate Analysis (MUMA) package (Team 2007), which can be used in the R statistical program, and MetaboAnalyst, which is available online (Xia, Mandal, et al. 2012).

Network Medicine and Metabolomics

Network Medicine Theory

In recent years, the field of network medicine has evolved through leveraging advances in the area of general network theory and modeling (Barabási, Gulbahce, et al. 2011). As described in Chapter 2, a fundamental principle in network medicine is the disease module hypothesis, which states that variants associated with a disease are connected. Stated another way, seemingly unrelated genes and proteins that are found to be involved in the same disease process show a high propensity to interact with each other (Hartwell, Hopfield, et al. 1999). There is considerable evidence for this principle (Hartwell, Hopfield, et al. 1999; Oti, Snel, et al. 2006; Xu and Li 2006; Goh, Cusick, et al. 2007; Wood, Parsons, et al. 2007; Hwang, Son, et al. 2008). For example, Barabási and colleagues observed 290 interactions between the products of genes associated with the same disorder, representing a 10-fold increase as compared with random expectation (Oti, Snel, et al. 2006; Goh, Cusick, et al. 2007). Two other studies found that genes linked to diseases with similar phenotypes have a significantly increased tendency to interact directly with each other (Xu and Li 2006; Hwang, Son, et al. 2008). A major implication of the network approach is that if a few disease components are identified, other disease-related components are likely to be found in their network-based vicinity. Network medicine naturally applies to metabolic networks, whose nodes are separate metabolites that are linked together when they are involved in the same biochemical reactions (Barabási, Gulbahce, et al. 2011). A group of metabolites (i.e., nodes) that are related to a disease of interest can be clustered into highly interlinked groups called modules. In a random network, each of the modules would have the same number of connections (on average); however, network theory suggests that the connections between the metabolites are not random, but rather follow a scale-free distribution (Jeong and Trembor, 2000; Barabási and Bonabeau 2003) with a small number of highly connected hubs (Barabási, Gulbahce, et al. 2011). Several publically available metabolic databases that exist, such as KEGG (Kanehisa and Goto 2000; Wixon and Kell 2000), that can be used to reconstruct the metabolic pathways and provide further insight into the functionality of these networks.

Correlation Co-expression Networks

Correlation analysis is an established approach used in systems biology. As quantitative measures, metabolites are ideally suited for correlation-based network analysis and have been used in this context (Kotze, Armitage, et al. 2013).

Pairwise correlations between metabolites can be calculated and organized into metabolic correlation networks. The correlation between metabolite concentrations varies greatly. It has been suggested that these correlations are a direct result of underlying (common or linked) enzymatic activities (Steuer, Kurths, et al. 2002). General co-expression networks based on the Pearson correlation coefficient (Zhang and Horvath 2005) can be calculated by measuring the concordance of metabolic measures. These correlation measures are used to define an adjacency matrix, which indicates the degree to which two metabolic measures are connected (Zhao, Langfelder, et al. 2010). After the general co-expression networks are generated, important modules can be identified. Hierarchical clustering and topological dissimilarity measures are used to generate clustering trees that then define different modules within the co-expression network (Yip and Horvath 2007; Langfelder, Zhang et al. 2008). These networks can be generated using weighted gene co-expression network analysis (WGCNA) (Zhao, Langfelder, et al. 2010). The WGCNA software package contains a comprehensive collection of R functions for performing various aspects of weighted correlation network analysis, including functions for network construction, module detection, gene selection, topological property calculations, data simulation, and visualization. Although WGCNA has been successfully applied in various biological contexts, (e.g., cancer, mouse genetics, yeast genetics, and analysis of brain imaging data), it has not yet been applied to metabolomics data (Carlson, Zhang et al. 2006; Ghazalpour, Doss et al. 2006; Horvath, Zhang et al. 2006; Oldham, Konopka et al. 2008).

Gaussian Graphical Models

One of the disadvantages of using correlation networks is that they cannot distinguish between direct and indirect associations (Krumsiek, Suhre, et al. 2011). Gaussian graphical models (GGMs) are able to differentiate direct and indirect effects through the use of conditional dependencies, which result in partial correlations. Determination of a direct association involves regressing one metabolite on another metabolite and ensuring that the correlation remains after adjusting for all other metabolites (Krumsiek, Suhre, et al. 2011). GGMs consider direct associations of metabolites only; thus, the observed direct effects are more likely to be robustly and strongly related to one another. GGMs were applied to a set of targeted metabolites from the German population-based cohort, the Cooperative Health Research in the Augsburg Region (KORA). A total of 1020 individuals with 151 targeted metabolites were obtained using fasting blood serum. Networks were created using standard Pearson correlations and GGMs using log-transformed metabolites. While the Pearson correlation network obtained over 5000 correlations that were significantly different from zero (after a Bonferroni adjustment),

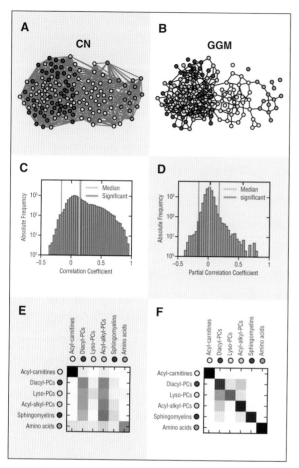

FIGURE 11–2. This figure illustrates the general differences between generating correlation networks (CNs) and Gaussian graphical model (GGM) networks. The CNs are more highly connected because they do not differentiate between direct and indirect correlations. In addition, the CNs show a bias toward a positive correlation coefficient for all metabolites. (Adapted with permission from Krumsiek, J., K. Suhre, et al. (2011). Gaussian graphical modeling reconstructs pathway reactions from high-throughput metabolomics data. BMC Syst Biol 5: 21. (CC BY 2.0))

the GGM network obtained only 417 significant partial correlations after the multiple comparison adjustment. The Pearson correlation network is, therefore, more highly connected than the GGM network (Figure 11–2A vs. 11–2B). In addition, the Pearson correlation network had a larger proportion of highly correlated metabolites, whereas the partial correlations were centered around zero (Figure 11–2C vs. 11–2D). The GGM approach was able to separate metabolites more clearly into seven known metabolite classes and remained stable when changing the samples in the dataset (Figure 11–2E vs. 11–2F) (Krumsiek, Suhre et al., 2011). The hub metabolites are also easier to identify using this approach.

Bayesian Networks

Metabolic networks can also be generated using Bayesian network methodology. Bayesian networks are based on a data structure that encodes conditional probability distributions between variables of interest using a graph composed of nodes and directed edges (Pearl 1998). In Bayesian networks, variables in the domain are modeled as random variables and represented by nodes, and directed edges between them represent a statistical dependence of the child node on the parent node. Each node is annotated with the marginal distribution of the variable conditioned on the values of its parents, and this information can be used to answer questions about the most probable values of variables in the Bayesian networks given assignments to other variables in the network. Bayesian networks have been applied to metabolomics data from an intensive care unit cohort to develop predictive models of mortality. A total of 90 subjects were enrolled in the Brigham and Women's Registry of Critical Illness (Rogers, McGeachie, et al. 2014). A metabolomic network was formed and five metabolites were found to be associated with death (sucrose, arginine, mannose, methionine, and beta-hydroxyisovalerate). This network achieved a 92% area-under-the-curve prediction of 28-day mortality. The findings were replicated in a cohort of 149 adults who were enrolled in the Community Acquired Pneumonia and Sepsis Outcome Diagnostics study and achieved 75% area-under-the-curve prediction (Rogers, McGeachie, et al. 2014).

Network Approaches to Integrate Metabolomics and Other -omics Data

Causal Pathways and Metabolomics

The central dogma of molecular biology states that DNA is transcribed into RNA, which is translated into proteins. There are approximately 21,000 genes in the human genome, which encodes many more proteins (Kiranmayi, Srinivasa Rao, et al. 2012). Metabolites result from the metabolism of these proteins. The conglomeration of endogenously synthesized small molecules or metabolites is, therefore, a direct reflection of the central dogma integrated with environmental exposures that precede disease development (Figure 11–3). An important attribute of metabolites is their close relationship to both the biological states of interest (i.e., disease status) and relevant genomic, transcriptomic, and proteomic variants causally related to the disease state. As such, metabo-profiles can be viewed as an intermediate measure that links predisposing genes and environmental exposures to a resulting disease state. Causal metabolites also typically have a stronger relationship (i.e., larger

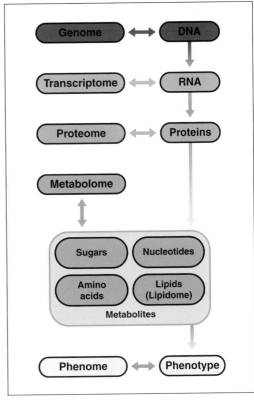

FIGURE 11–3. Schematic of -omic hierarchy.

effect size) to the underlying genetics and the disease phenotype. Thus, the integration of metabolomic data into systems biology approaches may provide a missing link between genes and disease states.

Metabolites Are Heritable

Although metabolites are influenced by environmental exposures, substantial evidence suggests that metabolites are, in part, genetically determined (Nicholson, Rantalainen et al. 2011). A study of twin pairs evaluated the longitudinal measures of plasma and urine metabolites obtained using NMR and found that many were heritable. The statistical variation of metabolites was decomposed into familial (genetic and common environment), individual-environment, and unstable components. The stable component of this variation accounted for, on average, 60% and 47% of plasma and urine metabolites, respectively (Nicholson, Rantalainen, et al. 2011). An additional study using Finnish twin pairs found that serum metabolites were largely heritable (Kettunen, Tukiainen, et al. 2012). This study concluded that the heritability of individual metabolites range widely and that some metabolites are more strongly influenced by the environment than others; however, genetic variants encode enzymes and transporter proteins that have strong influences on specific metabolites (Kettunen, Tukiainen, et al. 2012). These genetically informed metabolites (GIMs) serve as ideal intermediate links from genetic variants to disease phenotypes (Suhre and Gieger 2012). As intermediate phenotypes, GIMs tend to have larger genetic effect sizes than other disease-related phenotypes. Suhre and Gieger (2012)

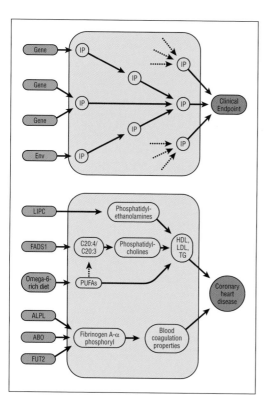

FIGURE 11–4. A, the relationship between genes, the environment, metabolites that are described as intermediate phenotypes (IPs), and the clinical outcome. Some of the IPs are related to the genes and environment while others are not explained by underlying genetics and identified environmental exposures. B, in a more concrete example, the relationship between several known genetic variants, metabolites, and coronary heart disease is depicted. This includes several known genes (*LIPC, FADS1, ALPL, ABO, FUT2*) and causal metabolites that range from blood coagulation properties to lipid profile measures that together influence the risk for coronary heart disease. (Adapted with permission from Suhre, K., and C. Gieger (2012). Genetic variation in metabolic phenotypes: study designs and applications. Nat Rev Genet 13(11): 759–69.)

summarized how metabolites can be used as GIMs both in general and for the specific example shown in Figure 11–4. Figure 11–4A illustrates how multiple genes and the environmental exposures result in various intermediate phenotypes that yield a clinical phenotype. Figure 11–4A also depicts that some of these intermediate phenotypes are not explained by either the underlying genetics or known environmental exposures. Figure 11–4B provides a concrete example showing the relationship between several known genetic variants for coronary heart disease (LIPC, FADS1, ALPL, ABO, FUT2), and causal metabolites ranging from blood-coagulation properties to lipid-profile measures that together influence the risk for coronary heart disease.

Integrating Metabolomics and Another -omics Data Type for Disease Research

Network medicine approaches can also be applied to cohorts with metabolomics data, another -omics data type, and a disease phenotype. These other -omics data types—genomics, transcriptomics, and epigenomics data—can be used in conjunction with metabolomics data and covariates to predict disease outcomes. All of these -omics data provide information at different biological levels but all explain different aspects of the underlying systems biology. Combining multiple data sources, therefore, can provide a more complete understanding of disease pathogenesis.

Metabolomics and Genomics

Genome-wide association analysis (GWAS) is a hypothesis-free approach to identify links between genetic variants and disease. However, research has shown that most genetic variants associated with complex diseases have only a modest genetic effect size (Manolio, Collins, et al. 2009). As such, an effective strategy toward identifying meaningful genetic variants for a specific disease is to use phenotypes related to the disease of interest that are more strongly related to the genetic variants of the disease. As discussed above, metabolites represent an ideal class of intermediate phenotypes that are in the causal pathway between genetic variant and disease outcome and, therefore, often have larger genetic effect sizes; thus, they are good candidates to use as intermediate phenotypes for GWAS studies (Suhre and Gieger 2012). The integration of metabolomics and GWAS data has been implemented, where each metabolite is treated as a phenotype in a GWAS analysis. This is similar to performing n GWAS analyses, where n is the total number of measured metabolites. Metabolite GWAS analyses (MGWAS) are typically performed using a regression model with the metabolite as the outcome, the single-nucleotide polymorphism (SNP) genotype as the predictor, and several covariates in the model for adjustment. These covariates often include age, sex, and genetic ancestry principal component adjustments.

MGWAS analyses were the first proposed integration of metabolomics data with another -omic dataset. Shin, Fauman, and colleagues (2014) evaluated the association of 529 blood metabolites with genome-wide SNP genotyping data in 7824 adult individuals from two European populations and identified 145 genome-wide significant metabolic loci. A network of genetic and metabolomic data was then created. GGMs were applied to connect metabolite to metabolite using partial correlation coefficients to reconstruct the metabolic pathways. The metabolites were connected to the genetic loci using the initial MGWAS results. The network summarized the relationships between nearly 400 metabolites from 60 pathways using 131 genetic loci, and is presented in Figure 11–5 (Shin, Fauman, et al. 2014).

Metabolomics and Epigenomics

In addition to identifying SNP-metabolite associations, epigenomic-metabolite associations are also relevant because DNA methylation can affect the metabolic regulation (Portela and Esteller 2010). Similar to how metabolites are integrated with SNPs, metabolites can be used as phenotypes for genome-wide epigenetic data in which the epigenetic data predict each metabolite. One of the first studies to integrate metabolites and epigenetics initially identified metabolites that were correlated with age and evaluated the association of this subset of metabolites with genome-wide epigenetic data. Through this process, a metabolite, C-glycosyl tryptophan (C-glyTrp), was identified, and the association of this metabotype was evaluated with genome-wide methylation data using 172 individuals. Three CpG-sites were associated with C-glyTrp. One of these CpG sites was found to be in the promoter of *WDR85*, and was further replicated in an independent population of 350 individuals ($\beta = -0.20$, $SE = 0.04$, $P = 2.9 \times 10^{-8}$) (Menni, Kastenmuller, et al. 2013). A second study formally coined the term *epigenome-wide association study* (EWAS) for the integration of DNA methylation and metabolomics data. This study used 649 blood metabolites as metabotypes to evaluate an association with ~450,000 CpG sites using 1814 individuals from the KORA cohort. Genome-wide significant associations were identified after adjusting for genetics suggesting that DNA methylation influences human metabolism independent of genetics.

Metabolomics and Gene Expression

Combined analyses of metabolite and gene expression data have great promise for identifying underlying regulatory networks that can link genes to the metabolome. Unfortunately, to date, few human studies have integrated metabolomics and transcriptomics data. Even when metabolomics and transcriptomics data are disparate, these two data types have been successfully combined to

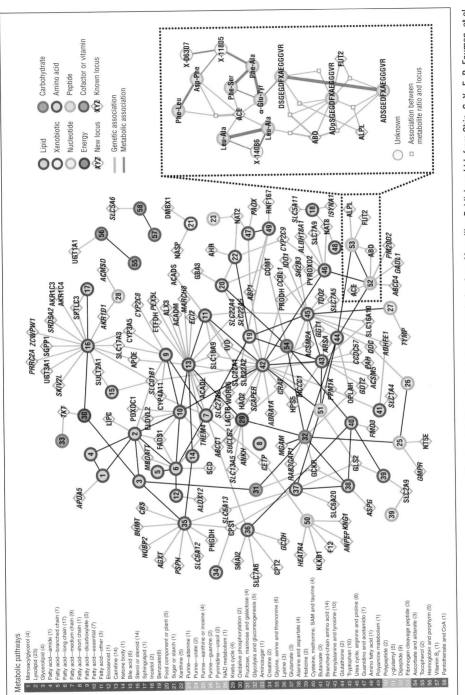

FIGURE 11–5. An atlas of genetic influences on human blood metabolites. (Reprinted with permission from Macmillan Publishers Ltd. from Shin, S. Y., E. B. Fauman, et al. (2014). An atlas of genetic influences on human blood metabolites. Nat Genet 46(6): 543–50. © 2014 Nature America, Inc.)

identify biomarkers that successfully predict disease with good accuracy (Chen, Zhu, et al. 2014). When a cohort contains expression data only, metabolomics data can also be integrated on the pathway level, as outlined in Figure 11–6. This approach was applied by Stempler, Yizhak, and colleagues (2014), who used expression data to identify high, moderate, and low differentially expressed genes between patients with Alzheimer disease (AD) and control individuals. These data were then integrated with a genome-scale computational human metabolic model to characterize the altered metabolism in AD. Metabolic modeling was also used to predict AD drug targets and biomarkers predictive of the disorder (Shlomi, Cabili, et al. 2008). The integration of expression and metabolomics data has also been performed on diseased and nondiseased cells to evaluate the major metabolic differences between six different subtypes of breast cells (Cuperlovic-Culf, Chute, et al. 2011). Metabolites with differences between cancerous and noncancerous cells as well as the estrogen-receptor-cell (+/−) status were identified. The relationship of these metabolites to differentially expressed genes was then determined, and the SCL44A1 transporter gene was implicated as a gene that affects subsequent differential expression and metabolic profiles. Additional statistical methods have been proposed to integrate these data types; one suggested approach is to use the metabolic data to generate weights that inform the subsequent gene expression analyses (Brink-Jensen, Bak et al., 2012).

Metabolomics and Proteomics

Two primary approaches have been described for integrating metabolomics and proteomics data (May, Christian, et al. 2011). The first approach is knowledge-based and relies on known metabolic databases; the second approach uses the data to inform the functionality of the pathways. Wu and Chen (2011) outlined a general approach to reconstruct metabolic networks that merges the knowledge-based and data-driven approaches. This strategy first proposes generating a "reference network" using functional annotation for metabolic enzymes that can be identified from databases such as GO, BLAST, and KEGG pathways. This network is, therefore, generated using databases of known biochemical reactions spanning a broad range of species. Enzyme functions are obtained and proteins can be annotated using programs such as BLAST (Altschul, Gish, et al. 1990). Because the genome encodes enzymes that yield metabolites, the functional annotation of metabolites is important in clarifying the reconstruction of important biochemical pathways, thereby providing an initial framework for the network. This network will differ from the "draft network," which will be derived using the metabolomics data. Differences are expected as metabolites arise from a combination of genomic and environmental influences. The reference and draft networks are then compared and discrepancies between the two iden-

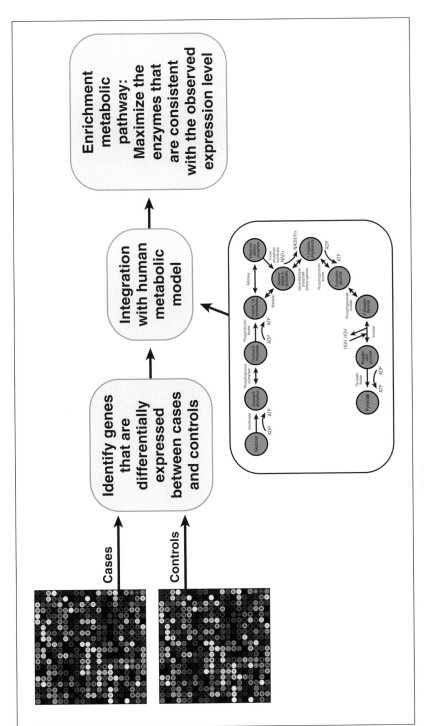

FIGURE 11–6. The integration of transcriptomic and metabolic data.

tified. The final network is generated through an iterative process that reconciles inconsistencies, expands the network by filling in the known metabolic gaps, and tests the network to determine whether the metabolites can be reproduced (Wu and Chen 2011).

Multiple -omics

Figure 11–3 summarized a general overview of the relationship between genomics, transcriptomics, proteomics, and metabolomics that result in disease outcomes (phenomics). When multiple -omics measurements are available for the same group of individual samples, the integration across these data can provide valuable insight into disease pathogenesis. The best approach by which to integrate these data, however, has yet to be determined. We now discuss several considerations for data integration.

One approach would be to incorporate all data types into one large networking model. This scenario represents the most hypothesis-free approach, in which the data drive the results. Normalization of the data across the various -omics would be necessary to ensure that the observed results are not influenced by distributional differences. Another limitation of this approach is that the number of variables used in the network would not only be extremely large, but would also vary by the type of -omics data analyzed. As such, different -omics would be artificially inflated. For example, the amount of genomic data associated with sequencing is magnitudes larger than the number of metabolites in a metabolomics sample. If all these data were pooled, the genomic data would be artificially inflated in importance with respect to the available metabolomics data. An effective strategy to correct this problem would be to filter the various data types on some predetermined basis.

A second strategy for integrating multiple -omics data is to perform sequential pairwise comparisons between the available -omics types and to then link the results together. Shin, Fauman, and colleagues (2014) used a similar approach when they first identified significant SNP-metabolite associations. They used the significant SNPs to identify *cis*-expression quantitative trait loci (eQTLs) from public repositories of four separate tissues, and then finally identified the significant *cis*-eQTLs. This approach narrows the associations in a step-by-step manner. A disadvantage of this strategy is that it does not take advantage of the power of using many -omics sources simultaneously.

A third approach would limit the data that is included in the network analysis on the basis of prior statistical or biological information. Because we are considering a disease network, limiting the input variables that are believed to be biologically relevant to the disease outcome is one approach. Variants can be selected on the basis of known biological pathways using databases. Variants can also be

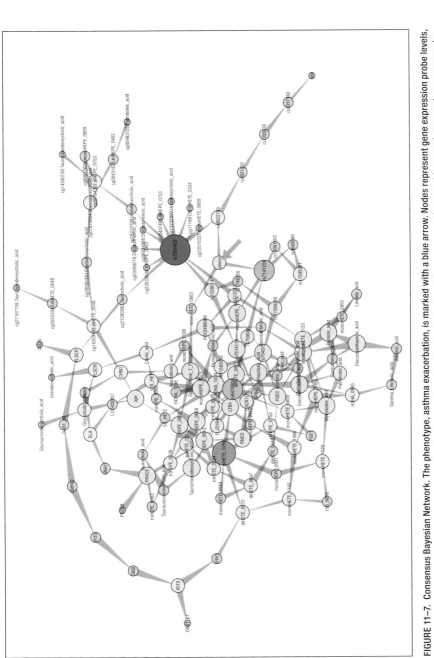

FIGURE 11-7. Consensus Bayesian Network. The phenotype, asthma exacerbation, is marked with a blue arrow. Nodes represent gene expression probe levels, CpG site methylation percents, SNP minor allele distributions, and metabolite levels. Nodes with more connections are bigger and more red; gray arrows between nodes indicate the Bayesian conditional independence of the child node given the parent nodes of the remaining nodes. Thicker arrows represent stronger statistical dependence. (Reprinted from McGeachie, M. J., H. H. Chang, et al. (2014). CGBayesNets: conditional Gaussian Bayesian network learning and inference with mixed discrete and continuous data. PLoS Comput Biol 10(6): e1003676. (CC BY 4.0))

selected on the basis of statistical association. This approach was taken by Mc-Geachie, Chang, and colleagues (2014), who studied 20 individuals with 64 lipid metabolites that were used in conjunction with genome-wide association data (Affymetrix Genome-Wide Human SNP Array 6.0), genome-wide gene expression data (Illumina Human HT-12 v4 arrays), and genome-wide methylation data (Illumina HM450 methylation arrays). Linear regression was performed with all 64 metabolites, and all of the genome-wide genetic, gene expression, and epigenetic data and the top associations were identified for each data type. Expression, SNP, and methylation probes with top associations to one or more metabolites were then included in a Bayesian network analysis. A conditional Gaussian Bayesian network (CGBN) was learned from this data using the CGBayesNets package in MATLAB version R2013b (MATLAB, MathWorks; CGBayesNets, www.cgbayesnets.com) and is presented in Figure 11–7. The resulting network differentiated asthma exacerbators and nonexacerbators with over 95% accuracy.

Conclusion

Although the field of network medicine is still in its infancy, great strides are underway to understand the complex biology that connects genomics, transcriptomics, proteomics, and metabolomics to disease outcomes. Metabolomics is an emerging -omics data type, and the generation of these data alone is complex. However, metabolites are a key link between genes and disease outcomes and, as such, provide crucial information for network biology approaches. In this chapter, we have reviewed methods for the generation of metabolomic networks and integrative metabolomics networks with other -omics data. Through several of the published findings that are summarized here, it is clear that network approaches already show great potential for providing pivotal insights into the biology underlying disease etiology that, in turn, may result in improved disease treatment and primary disease prevention.

References

Altschul, S. F., W. Gish, et al. (1990). Basic local alignment search tool. J Mol Biol. **215**(3): 403–10.

Alvarez-Sanchez, B., F. Priego-Capote, et al. (2012). Study of sample preparation for metabolomic profiling of human saliva by liquid chromatography-time of flight/mass spectrometry. J Chromatogr A **1248**: 178–81.

Barabási, A. L., and E. Bonabeau (2003). Scale-free networks. Sci Am **288**(5): 60–69.

Barabási, A. L., and N. Gulbahce, et al. (2011). Network medicine: a network-based approach to human disease. Nat Rev Genet **12**(1): 56–68.

Barderas, M. G., C. M. Laborde, et al. (2012). Metabolomic profiling for identification of novel potential biomarkers in cardiovascular diseases. J Biomed Biotechnol **2011**: 790132.

Beecher, G. R. (2003). Overview of dietary flavonoids: nomenclature, occurrence and intake. J Nutr **133**(10): 3248S–3254S.

Benjamini, Y., and Y. Hochberg (1995). Controlling the false discovery rate: a practical and powerful approach to multiple testing. J R Stat Soc **57**: 289–300.

Bonferroni, C. E. (1937). Teoria Statistica Delle Classi e Calcolo Delle Probabilitá. In Volume in onore di Riccardo Dalla Volta. Universitá di Firenze, pp. 1–62.

Brindle, J. T., H. Antti, et al. (2002). Rapid and noninvasive diagnosis of the presence and severity of coronary heart disease using 1H-NMR-based metabonomics. Nat Med **8**(12): 1439–44.

Brink-Jensen, K., S. Bak, et al. (2012). Integrative analysis of metabolomics and transcriptomics data: a unified model framework to identify underlying system pathways. PLoS One **8**(9): e72116.

Cao, B., M. Li, et al. (2013). Metabolomic approach to evaluating adriamycin pharmacodynamics and resistance in breast cancer cells. Metabolomics **9**(5): 960–73.

Carlson, M. R., B. Zhang, et al. (2006). Gene connectivity, function, and sequence conservation: predictions from modular yeast co-expression networks. BMC Genomics **7**: 40.

Carraro, S., S. Rezzi, et al. (2007). Metabolomics applied to exhaled breath condensate in childhood asthma. Am J Respir Crit Care Med **175**(10): 986–90.

Chen, K., C. Zhu, et al. (2014). Integrative metabolome and transcriptome profiling reveals discordant glycolysis process between osteosarcoma and normal osteoblastic cells. J Cancer Res Clin Oncol **140**(10): 1715–21.

Chow, J., M. R. Panasevich, et al. (2014). Fecal metabolomics of healthy breast-fed versus formula-fed infants before and during in vitro batch culture fermentation. J Proteome Res **13**(5): 2534–42.

Cui, Q., I. A. Lewis, et al. (2008). Metabolite identification via the Madison Metabolomics Consortium Database. Nat Biotechnol **26**(2): 162–64.

Cuperlovic-Culf, M., I. C. Chute, et al. (2011). 1H NMR metabolomics combined with gene expression analysis for the determination of major metabolic differences between subtypes of breast cell lines. Chem Sci **2**(11): 2263–70.

Dunn, O. J. (1961). Multiple comparisons among means. J Am Statist Assoc **56** (293): 52–64.

Fahy, E., M. Sud, et al. (2007). LIPID MAPS online tools for lipid research. Nucleic Acids Res **35**(Web Server issue): W606–12.

Fernandez-Albert, F., R. Llorach, et al. (2014). An R package to analyse LC/MS metabolomic data: MAIT (Metabolite Automatic Identification Toolkit). Bioinformatics **30**(13): 1937–39.

Fong, M. Y., J. McDunn, et al. (2013). Metabolomic profiling of ovarian carcinomas using mass spectrometry. Methods Mol Biol **1049**: 239–53.

Ghazalpour, A., S. Doss, et al. (2006). Integrating genetic and network analysis to characterize genes related to mouse weight. PLoS Genet **2**(8): e130.

Goedert, J. J., J. N. Sampson, et al. (2014). Fecal metabolomics: assay performance and association with colorectal cancer. Carcinogenesis. **35**(9): 2089–96.

Goh, K. I., M. E. Cusick, et al. (2007). The human disease network. Proc Natl Acad Sci U S A **104**(21): 8685–90.

Hartwell, L. H., J. J. Hopfield, et al. (1999). From molecular to modular cell biology. Nature **402**(6761 Suppl): C47–52.

Hasokawa, M., M. Shinohara, et al. (2012). Identification of biomarkers of stent restenosis with serum metabolomic profiling using gas chromatography/mass spectrometry. Circ J **76**(8): 1864–73.

Hoffman, R., and Y. Ozery. (2013). What is NMR? (http://chem.ch.huji.ac.il/nmr/whatisnmr /whatisnmr.html).

Horvath, S., B. Zhang, et al. (2006). Analysis of oncogenic signaling networks in glioblastoma identifies ASPM as a molecular target. Proc Natl Acad Sci U S A **103**(46): 17402–7.

Hwang, S., S. W. Son, et al. (2008). A protein interaction network associated with asthma. J Theor Biol **252**(4): 722–31.

Ivorra, C., C. Garcia-Vicent, et al. (2012). Metabolomic profiling in blood from umbilical cords of low birth weight newborns. J Transl Med **10**: 142.

Jensen, M. K., M. L. Bertoia, et al. (2014). Novel metabolic biomarkers of cardiovascular disease. Nat Rev Endocrinol **10**(11): 659–72.

Jeong, H., B. Trembor, H., et al. (2000). The large-scale organization of metabolic networks. Nature **407**: 651–54.

Ji, B., B. Ernest, et al. (2012). Transcriptomic and metabolomic profiling of chicken adipose tissue in response to insulin neutralization and fasting. BMC Genomics **13**: 441.

Jolliffe, I. T. (2002). Principal Component Analysis. New York: Springer.

Kanehisa, M., and S. Goto (2000). KEGG: Kyoto encyclopedia of genes and genomes. Nucleic Acids Res **28**(1): 27–30.

Kettunen, J., T. Tukiainen, et al. (2012). Genome-wide association study identifies multiple loci influencing human serum metabolite levels. Nat Genet **44**(3): 269–76.

Kim, O. Y., J. H. Lee, et al. (2013). Metabolomic profiling as a useful tool for diagnosis and treatment of chronic disease: focus on obesity, diabetes and cardiovascular diseases. Expert Rev Cardiovasc Ther **11**(1): 61–68.

Kiranmayi, V. S., P. V. L. N. Srinivasa Rao, et al. (2012). Metabolomics—the new omics of health care. J Clin Sci Res **3**: 131–37.

Kotze, H. L., E. G. Armitage, et al. (2013). A novel untargeted metabolomics correlation-based network analysis incorporating human metabolic reconstructions. BMC Syst Biol **7**: 107.

Krumsiek, J., K. Suhre, et al. (2011). Gaussian graphical modeling reconstructs pathway reactions from high-throughput metabolomics data. BMC Syst Biol **5**: 21.

Langfelder, P., B. Zhang, et al. (2008). Defining clusters from a hierarchical cluster tree: the Dynamic Tree Cut package for R. Bioinformatics **24**(5): 719–20.

Lewis, G. D., L. Farrell, et al. (2010). Metabolic signatures of exercise in human plasma. Sci Transl Med **2**(33): 33ra37.

Mahadevan, S., S. L. Shah, et al. (2008). Analysis of metabolomic data using support vector machines. Anal Chem **80**(19): 7562–70.

Manolio, T. A., F. S. Collins, et al. (2009). Finding the missing heritability of complex diseases. Nature **461**(7265): 747–53.

May, P., N. Christian, et al. (2011). Integration of proteomic and metabolomic profiling as well as metabolic modeling for the functional analysis of metabolic networks. Methods Mol Biol **694**: 341–63.

McGeachie, M. J., H. H. Chang, et al. (2014). CGBayesNets: conditional Gaussian Bayesian network learning and inference with mixed discrete and continuous data. PLoS Comput Biol **10**(6): e1003676.

Menni, C., G. Kastenmuller, et al. (2013). Metabolomic markers reveal novel pathways of ageing and early development in human populations. Int J Epidemiol **42**(4): 1111–19.

Montuschi, P., D. Paris, et al. (2012). NMR spectroscopy metabolomic profiling of exhaled breath condensate in patients with stable and unstable cystic fibrosis. Thorax **67**(3): 222–28.

Nicholson, G., M. Rantalainen, et al. (2011). Human metabolic profiles are stably controlled by genetic and environmental variation. Mol Syst Biol **7**: 525.

Oldham, M. C., G. Konopka, et al. (2008). Functional organization of the transcriptome in human brain. Nat Neurosci **11**(11): 1271–82.

Oti, M., B. Snel, et al. (2006). Predicting disease genes using protein-protein interactions. J Med Genet **43**(8): 691–98.

OuYang, D., J. Xu, et al. (2011). Metabolomic profiling of serum from human pancreatic cancer patients using 1H NMR spectroscopy and principal component analysis. Appl Biochem Biotechnol **165**(1): 148–54.

Pearl, J. (1998). Probabilistic reasoning in intelligent systems: networks of plausible inference. Los Altos, CA: Morgan Kaufmann.

Portela, A., and M. Esteller (2010). Epigenetic modifications and human disease. Nat Biotechnol **28**(10): 1057–68.

Psychogios, N., D. D. Hau, et al. (2011). The human serum metabolome. PLoS One **6**(2): e16957.

Ramadan, Z., D. Jacobs, et al. (2006). Metabolic profiling using principal component analysis, discriminant partial least squares, and genetic algorithms. Talanta **68**(5): 1683–91.

R Core Team (2007). R: A language and environment for statistical computing, Version 2.5.0. Vienna: R Foundation for Statistical Computing.

Reinke, S. N., D. L. Broadhurst, et al. (2014). Metabolomic profiling in multiple sclerosis: insights into biomarkers and pathogenesis. Mult Scler **20**(10): 1396–400.

Rogers, A. J., M. McGeachie, et al. (2014). Metabolomic derangements are associated with mortality in critically ill adult patients. PLoS One **9**(1): e87538.

Saude, E. J., C. D. Skappak, et al. (2011). Metabolomic profiling of asthma: diagnostic utility of urine nuclear magnetic resonance spectroscopy. J Allergy Clin Immunol **127**(3): 757–6 e1–6.

Schicho, R., R. Shaykhutdinov, et al. (2012). Quantitative metabolomic profiling of serum, plasma, and urine by (1)H NMR spectroscopy discriminates between patients with inflammatory bowel disease and healthy individuals. J Proteome Res **11**(6): 3344–57.

Shannon, P., A. Markiel, et al. (2003). Cytoscape: a software environment for integrated models of biomolecular interaction networks. Genome Res **13**(11): 2498–504.

Shin, S. Y., E. B. Fauman, et al. (2014). An atlas of genetic influences on human blood metabolites. Nat Genet **46**(6): 543–50.

Shlomi, T., M. N. Cabili, et al. (2008). Network-based prediction of human tissue-specific metabolism. Nat Biotechnol **26**(9): 1003–10.

Stempler, S., K. Yizhak, et al. (2014). Integrating transcriptomics with metabolic modeling predicts biomarkers and drug targets for Alzheimer's disease. PLoS One **9**(8): e105383.

Steuer, R., J. Kurths, et al. (2002). The mutual information: detecting and evaluating dependencies between variables. Bioinformatics **18** Suppl 2: S231–40.

Subramanian, A., P. Tamayo, et al. (2005). Gene set enrichment analysis: a knowledge-based approach for interpreting genome-wide expression profiles. Proc Natl Acad Sci U S A **102**(43): 15545–50.

Sud, M., E. Fahy, et al. (2007). LMSD: LIPID MAPS structure database. Nucleic Acids Res **35**(Database issue): D527–32.

Suhre, K., and C. Gieger (2012). Genetic variation in metabolic phenotypes: study designs and applications. Nat Rev Genet **13**(11): 759–69.

Tautenhahn, R., K. Cho, et al. (2012). An accelerated workflow for untargeted metabolomics using the METLIN database. Nat Biotechnol **30**(9): 826–28.

Tiziani, S., A. Lodi, et al. (2009). Metabolomic profiling of drug responses in acute myeloid leukaemia cell lines. PLoS One **4**(1): e4251.

Triba, M. N., A. Starzec, et al. (2010). Metabolomic profiling with NMR discriminates between biphosphonate and doxorubicin effects on B16 melanoma cells. NMR Biomed **23**(9): 1009–16.

Vuckovic, D., and J. Pawliszyn (2011). Systematic evaluation of solid-phase microextraction coatings for untargeted metabolomic profiling of biological fluids by liquid chromatography-mass spectrometry. Anal Chem **83**(6): 1944–54.

Wang, T. J., M. G. Larson, et al. (2011). Metabolite profiles and the risk of developing diabetes. Nat Med **17**(4): 448–53.

Wishart, D. S., T. Jewison, et al. (2013). HMDB 3.0—The Human Metabolome Database in 2013. Nucleic Acids Res **41**(Database issue): D801–7.

Wishart, D. S., D. Tzur, et al. (2007). HMDB: the Human Metabolome Database. Nucleic Acids Res **35**(Database issue): D521–26.

Wixon, J., and D. Kell (2000). The Kyoto encyclopedia of genes and genomes—KEGG. Yeast. **17**(1): 48–55.

Wood, L. D., D. W. Parsons, et al. (2007). The genomic landscapes of human breast and colorectal cancers. Science **318**(5853): 1108–13.

Wu, C., and C. Chen (2011). Bioinformatics for Comparative Proteomics. New York: Springer.

Xia, J., R. Mandal, et al. (2012). MetaboAnalyst 2.0—a comprehensive server for metabolomic data analysis. Nucleic Acids Res **40**(Web Server issue): W127–33.

Xia, J., and D. S. Wishart (2010). MSEA: a web-based tool to identify biologically meaningful patterns in quantitative metabolomic data. Nucleic Acids Res **38**(Web Server issue): W71–77.

Xu, J., and Y. Li (2006). Discovering disease-genes by topological features in human protein-protein interaction network. Bioinformatics **22**(22): 2800–5.

Xuan, J., G. Pan, et al. (2011). Metabolomic profiling to identify potential serum biomarkers for schizophrenia and risperidone action. J Proteome Res **10**(12): 5433–43.

Yerges-Armstrong, L. M., S. Ellero-Simatos, et al. (2013). Purine pathway implicated in mechanism of resistance to aspirin therapy: pharmacometabolomics-informed pharmacogenomics. Clin Pharmacol Ther **94**(4): 525–32.

Yip, A. M., and S. Horvath (2007). Gene network interconnectedness and the generalized topological overlap measure. BMC Bioinformatics **8**: 22.

Zhang, B., and S. Horvath (2005). A general framework for weighted gene co-expression network analysis. Stat Appl Genet Mol Biol. **4**: Article 17.

Zhang, T., X. Wu, et al. (2012). Discrimination between malignant and benign ovarian tumors by plasma metabolomic profiling using ultra performance liquid chromatography/mass spectrometry. Clin Chim Acta **413**(9–10): 861–68.

Zhao, W., P. Langfelder, et al. (2010). Weighted gene coexpression network analysis: state of the art. J Biopharm Stat **20**(2): 281–300.

Zhou, B., J. Wang, et al. (2012). MetaboSearch: tool for mass-based metabolite identification using multiple databases. PLoS One **7**(6): e40096.

12

Using Integrative -omics Approaches in Network Medicine

Shuyi Ma, John C. Earls, James A. Eddy,
and Nathan D. Price

Introduction

High-throughput experimental technologies have enabled the identification and quantification of biological components on an unprecedented scale, from genes and proteins to cells and tissues. Collectively, these technologies provide a parts list for biological systems (e.g., biochemical pathways, larger interaction networks). Efforts to understand and intervene in disease-perturbed systems through quantitative analyses of the interactions between components have embodied the emergence of network medicine. In practice, network medicine manifests as a cycle of: (1) data incorporation within networks to facilitate functional interpretation; and (2) data-driven identification, refinement, and expansion of networks and network modules. This synergistic relationship between data and networks continues to extend from genomics, transcriptomics, and proteomics to newer regimes of high-throughput measurements, including metabolomics, epigenomics, and fluxomics. Given the availability of diverse -omics data and associated network analysis tools, studies are now exploring ways to combine multiple measurement types effectively, thereby expanding the breadth, depth, and accuracy of understanding for biological systems. Such integrative -omics approaches aim to bridge between multiple different data types by leveraging network formalisms, while driving the construction and improvement of multiscale networks. The focus in this chapter is on integrative -omics analyses; therefore, we will focus primarily on analyses that are multi-omic in nature, bringing together at least two data types as sources of information. Most of these examples are necessarily in the research phase, with limited translation thus far; however, continued advances are expected to have a major impact on medicine in the future.

Background

Network formalisms provide a framework to contextualize high-throughput data, facilitating interpretation and the distillation of meaningful patterns and trends. In contrast to a more reductionist view—focusing only on the function of individual molecular players—networks describe the interactions among numerous components in a system as defined by experimentally characterized or statistically inferred associations. As such, harnessing network information has several applications to medical challenges. For example, one can incorporate and analyze high-dimensional -omics measurements (e.g., genomics, transcriptomics, proteomics, metabolomics) using a priori defined networks, facilitating associations between complex patterns of disease-induced or drug-induced molecular changes with the perturbations of biological processes. Alternatively, statistical learning within large datasets can identify previously uncharacterized relationships between network components in different health and disease settings, leading to novel hypotheses for further diagnostic and therapeutic discovery. Network formalisms also offer the advantage of being easily converted into computable models from which quantitative predictions of system behaviors can be generated, leading to testable predictions of disease mechanism and therapeutic intervention (Figure 12–1).

Numerous publicly accessible repositories of -omics data have been amassed in recent years, which form the empirical foundations for network construction (Table 12–1). These resources include publicly available databases for -omics data, as well as other repositories that provide network-connectivity information. For example, resources like Recon X and the Molecular Signatures Database provide component- and pathway-level information for metabolic and signaling networks, respectively. Notably, most network medicine studies to date have focused on a single -omics data type. These studies—particularly those dealing with genomics and transcriptomics data—are extensive and covered in other chapters of this book. However, the goals and approaches described below for integrated -omics analyses can be considered as generalized or layered extensions of selected single -omics approaches.

Efforts are now shifting to the development of methods that integrate multiple -omics types to improve biological insights; similarly, many new data-generation programs are designed to measure multiple -omics types in parallel. Rationales for multi-omic network analyses include expanded coverage of biological systems (e.g., connecting genomic perturbations with differential protein levels and shifts in metabolite concentrations), as well as reducing the weight placed on any single dataset. Importantly, several implications—such as reconciling different nomenclatures and normalizing over different measurement scales and conditions—arise when dealing with multiple -omics types. These technical implications have been previously reviewed (Arakawa and Tomita 2013) and should be the subject of continued study and development as demand for multi-omic analyses increases.

Strategies that leverage the integration of multiple -omics data types in the context of networks for medical applications can again be broadly grouped into two categories: (1) When networks already exist for a particular system, these can be used to analyze multiple -omic types in a unified context and to aid in the functional interpretation of complex patterns; and (2) Statistical tools and manual curation can be used to construct de novo networks or to expand or refine existing networks from multiple or additional data types.

Herein, we focus on the five general classes of network-based approaches to integrating multiple -omics data types. Such network-based efforts to integrate -omics data have been applied to gain insight into underlying disease mechanisms, to aid molecular disease diagnosis efforts, and to search for novel

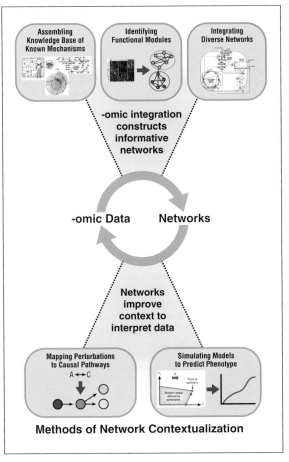

FIGURE 12–1. The synergism of integrating -omic data with networks. Integrating multiple -omics data sources facilitates the construction of more informative networks, which in turn, provide context for interpreting new information about the systems under investigation. (Some images adapted with permission from: 1) Zhang, R., M. V. Shah, et al. (2008). Network model of survival signaling in large granular lymphocyte leukemia. Proc Natl Acad Sci U S A 105(42): 16308–13, copyright (2008) National Academy of Sciences, U.S.A; 2) MacMillan Publishers Ltd: Nature (Gerstein, M. B., Kundaje A., et al. (2012). Architecture of the human regulatory network derived from ENCODE data. Nature 489(7414): 91–100), copyright (2012); 3) MacMillan Publishers Ltd: Nature Biotechnology (Orth, J. D., Thiele I., et al. (2010). What is flux balance analysis? Nat Biotechnol 28(3): 245–8), copyright (2010); 4) MacMillan Publishers Ltd: Nature (Cancer Genome Atlas Research Network (2013). Integrated genomic characterization of endometrial carcinoma. Nature 497(7447): 67–73), copyright (2013); and 5) under the Creative Commons Attribution License from Wang, Y., Eddy J. A., et al. (2012). Reconstruction of genome-scale metabolic models for 126 human tissues using mCADRE. BMC Syst Biol 6: 153. (CC BY 2.0))

therapeutic targets. Brief summaries of these five types of approaches, which will be discussed in subsequent sections, include:

TABLE 12–1. A Limited Selection of Emerging Resources to Facilitate Multi-Omic Integrative Analysis[a]

PROJECT	DESCRIPTION	AVAILABLE DATA
The Cancer Genome Atlas (Hudson, Anderson, et al. 2010) cancergenome.nih.gov	Pioneering multi-omic repository of ~20 cancers	Exome sequences; single-nucleotide polymorphisms (SNPs); methylation; messenger RNA (mRNA) and microRNA expression; clinical data
ENCyclopedia Of DNA Elements (Raney, Cline, et al. 2011) encodeproject.org/ENCODE	Attempt to identify all functional elements in human genome	Methylation; chromatin; RNA-binding proteins; transcription factor binding sites (TFBSs)
UCSC Genome Browser (Kent, Sugnet, et al. 2002) genome.ucsc.edu	Repository for genomic annotations	Genome assemblies, annotations (includes ENCODE)
Gene Expression Omnibus (Edgar, Domrachev, et al. 2002) www.ncbi.nlm.nih.gov/geo	Large public repository of gene expression and related datasets	Gene expression; genome variation; SNP; protein arrays; noncoding RNA (ncRNA)
Human Proteome Project (Legrain, Aebersold et al. 2011) www.thehpp.org	Comprehensive proteomic resource consortium	Knowledge bases, mass spectroscopy, antibody resources
Recon 2 (Thiele, Swainston, et al. 2013) humanmetabolism.org	Biochemical knowledge-base for human metabolism	The latest human metabolic network reconstruction
Molecular Signatures Database (Liberzon, Subramanian, et al. 2011) www.broadinstitute.org /msigdb	The largest collection of available gene sets	Canonical pathways; many different gene sets
Connectivity Map (Lamb, Crawford, et al. 2006) www .broadinstitute.org/cmap	Link disease to drug candidates and genetic manipulations	Pharmacologically perturbed gene expression profiles
Online Mendelian Inheritance in Man (Hamosh, Scott et al. 2005) omim.org	Catalog of human genes and genetic disorders	Knowledge base mapping genes to heritable disease

[a] *Nucleic Acids Research* has an extensive online Molecular Biology Database Collection of over 1400 databases available at http://www .oxfordjournals.org/nar/database/c/

Synthesizing multi-omics data to guide network reconstruction. Bottom-up reconstructed networks serve as a knowledge base, collecting and synthesizing information from a variety of data types to establish a holistic picture of what is known and not known about the underlying functional mechanisms for a given system. While the process of network reconstruction greatly facilitates effective surveys of existing knowledge (and identification of gaps in this knowledge), continually expanding sources of data are essential for building and refining these networks. In this section, we discuss examples of this mutually beneficial cycle as illustrated by efforts to reconstruct metabolic and transcriptional regulatory networks for medical applications.

Multi-omics data-driven inference of networks and modules. As the ability to construct knowledge-based networks can be laborious or limited by available data, statistical inference and machine learning present alternative strategies to identify functional network modules or even predict previously unknown network structures. As statistical network inference has long been a fundamental goal in systems analysis of high-throughput data, in this section, we will highlight approaches that extend these efforts to learn from multiple -omics sources.

Contextualizing statistical analysis of multi-omics data using networks. Using established networks (such as those reconstructed manually or statistically inferred) as contextual scaffolds, constraining information for statistical analyses of multiple high-throughput data types enables dimensionality reduction and provides a clearer functional interpretation of results. In this section, we will show how networks can be used to identify significant associations within and between different levels of disease -omics data and how network analysis of multi-omics data can power advanced disease-stratification approaches.

In silico mechanistic network simulations of multi-omics data. Established networks can further serve as the basis for mechanistic simulation of cellular behavior, using multi-omics data to define model inputs and parameters. Similarly, predictive mechanistic models can be directly learned from multi-omics data in an integrated network context. In this section, we will present approaches by which networks built to depict multiple levels of biological data— such as metabolic and regulatory networks—can be mathematically modeled to simulate the cellular phenotypes that emerge from multi-omics interactions.

Integrating diverse networks for expanded insight. Finally, we can integrate at a higher level networks and network models derived independently from different data types or for different biological systems to analyze higher-order and emergent effects. In this section, we will describe two examples of integrating networks and, by extension, the underlying single -omics or multi-omics information that each network respectively represents: (1) combined metabolic– regulatory networks that not only bridge mechanistic and statistical approaches, but also more directly connect environmental changes to phenotypic response; (2) studying networks across diverse cell types or even species to characterize evolutionary relationships and move towards organism- and ecosystem-level analysis.

Synthesizing Multi-omics Data to Guide Network Reconstruction

Networks help to make sense of a wide spectrum of experimental observations of underlying physiology and biochemistry. Importantly, the reconstruction of networks at the genome or cell scale typically requires compiling information from hundreds of research articles and experiments, and it forces one to reconcile the findings into a unified and quantitative hypothesis for how a cell functions. This consolidation and contextualization of knowledge provided by reconstructed networks can generate novel, testable hypotheses that can be validated through experiments, and the outcomes of these experiments can in turn expand and refine the networks. In this way, networks can be harnessed synergistically with experiments to advance knowledge of biological systems. We begin by presenting a brief overview of the knowledge-based construction of major network types that can be leveraged downstream to drive network medicine approaches.

Genome-scale metabolic networks (GSMNs) consolidate knowledge about metabolism—one of the most extensively characterized aspects of physiology—of different biological systems at the cell, tissue, or organism level to facilitate large-scale analyses and generation of novel insights. Reconstruction of such networks first requires identification and assimilation of known chemical reactions occurring in a system; reactions are then cataloged as a stoichiometric network of associations between interconverting metabolites (Figure 12–2) (Thiele and Palsson 2010). Each reaction can be linked to its catalyzing enzymes and the encoding genes via gene–protein-reaction (GPR) relationships, which are constructed from a combination of genome annotations and literature findings (Thiele and Palsson 2010). The resulting metabolic network integrates genomic and bibliomic information and provides a map that links genotype to metabolic phenotype. Reconstructed GSMNs also implicitly contain information that links together multiple -omics data types within the context of biological relationships, such as the encoding genes (genomics, transcriptomics), the enzymes (proteomics), and the metabolites (metabolomics) (Figure 12–2).

Utilizing the relationships defined by the GPR association map thus enables integration of other -omics data sources to refine metabolic networks. A common integration strategy is to apply transcriptomic or proteomic data to

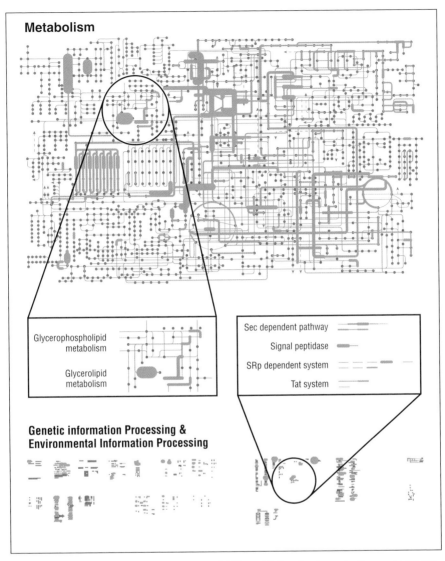

FIGURE 12–2. A genome-scale metabolic network model. The metabolic network encodes the complex set of re-actions linked by interconverting metabolites. Overlaying the reaction topology with gene–protein-reaction maps provides a mechanistic relationship between genotype and metabolic phenotype, facilitating the contextualiza-tion of multiple -omics. The highlighted network here highlights activity patterns for pathways found in the human gut microbiome (orange lines, line thickness proportional to degree of overrepresentation). (Note: Sec = Type II secretory pathway, SRp = signal recognition particle pathway, Tat = twin-arginine translocation pathway.) (Re-printed with permission from Oxford University Press (Yamada T., Letunic I., et al. (2011). iPath 2.0: Interactive Pathway Explorer. Nucleic Acids Res **39**:W412–415), copyright (2011).)

constrain a metabolic network to only the reactions that are active under a specific condition or context (Shlomi, Cabili, et al. 2008; Lewis, Schramm, et al. 2010; Zur, Ruppin, et al. 2010). In the case of human metabolism, the generic human metabolic models contain reactions from all known aspects of human metabolism across tissues (Duarte, Becker, et al. 2007; Ma, Sorokin, et al. 2007; Thiele, Swainston, et al. 2013). However, active metabolism for a particular tissue (under a particular condition) represents only a fraction of the total metabolic potential encoded in the human genome. Methods that create tissue-specific metabolic networks refine the generic human metabolic models to include preferential reactions encoded by genes that are actively expressed in tissue-specific transcriptomic data or proteomic data, as well as reactions that are required to perform known tissue-specific metabolic functions (Jerby, Shlomi, et al. 2010; Lewis, Schramm, et al. 2010; Agren, Bordel, et al. 2012; Wang, Eddy, et al. 2012). Collectively, this strategy has been leveraged to generate metabolic models that represent more than 100 tissue- and cell-line-specific metabolic models (Jerby, Shlomi, et al. 2010; Agren, Bordel, et al. 2012; Wang, Eddy, et al. 2012), which can be leveraged for context-specific and comparative studies of human metabolic phenotypes. Such studies can expand knowledge of underlying mechanism and aid in further network-model refinement.

Another system that has been intensely studied to uncover underlying mechanisms associated with genotype- and condition-dependent differences in cellular behavior is transcriptional regulation. Transcriptional regulatory networks (TRNs) associated with transcription factors have been constructed by integrating genomic sequence data with transcription factor binding information. By overlaying transcription factor binding site information extracted from e.g., genome-scale chromatin immunoprecipitation-sequencing (ChIP-seq) with gene expression correlations from transcriptomic data, genome-scale TRNs have been constructed for multiple organisms of relevance to human health, including lactic acid bacteria, which are part of the human microbiota (Ravcheev, Best, et al. 2013), as well as the microbial pathogens *Escherichia coli* (Zwir, Shin, et al. 2005; Salgado, Gama-Castro, et al. 2006), *Salmonella enterica* (Zwir, Shin, et al. 2005; Kroger, Dillon, et al. 2011), and *Mycobacterium tuberculosis* (MTB) (Galagan, Minch, et al. 2013). These regulatory networks have served as a framework to identify subnetworks associated with condition-dependent and dynamic changes in gene expression and lipid levels (Balazsi, Barabási, et al. 2005; Galagan, Minch, et al. 2013), as well as identification of virulence factors (Yoon, Ansong, et al. 2011).

The much more complex human TRN is being expansively interrogated by a suite of sequencing-based measurements, with the largest such effort being performed by the ENCODE consortium (Bernstein, Birney, et al. 2012). These

-omics datasets characterized transcription factor binding locations with genome-wide ChIP-seq and DNase I hypersensitivity footprinting for a large number of human cell lines. Additional modulations of transcription associated with noncoding RNA, histone modification, methylation, and chromosome interactions were measured by RNA sequencing (RNA-seq), ChIP-seq, reduced representation bisulfite sequencing, and complementary chromosome conformation capture techniques, respectively (Bernstein, Birney, et al. 2012). By combining transcription factor binding data, chromosomal interaction data, epigenomic data, and RNA expression data with protein–protein interaction and phosphorylation data derived from other sources, the ENCODE consortium constructed a human regulatory network for 119 transcription-associated factors across five cell lines that also incorporated the regulatory effects of distal enhancers, noncoding RNA, and phosphorylation events (Gerstein, Kundaje, et al. 2012). In examining the topology of the regulatory network, these authors found widespread combinatorial regulation patterns that differed among cell-line contexts. In addition, the authors found a large number of feed-forward loop regulatory motifs within the regulatory network. Such TRN maps will be important tools for identifying potential mechanisms underlying observed transcriptional changes in a host of disease conditions.

Signaling networks can also encapsulate multi-omics information, and are essential for including environmental inputs for truly whole-cell modeling. Genome-scale reconstructions of signaling networks are at more nascent stages than comparable reconstructions associated with metabolic and regulatory networks. Despite increasing efforts at characterizing the parts list of the signaling network, only a small fraction of signaling interactions are known (Hyduke and Palsson 2010; Prill, Saez-Rodriguez, et al. 2011). Reconstructions have typically been smaller scale, characterizing the signaling interactions of individual subsystems, including those associated with nuclear factor κB (NF-κB) (Zhang, Shah, et al. 2008; Prill, Saez-Rodriguez, et al. 2011), mitogen-activated protein kinase (MAPK) (Sachs, Perez, et al. 2005), Janus kinase—signal transducer and activator of transcription (JAK-STAT) (Papin and Palsson 2004; Zhang, Shah, et al. 2008), toll-cell receptors (Li, Thiele, et al. 2009), and the activation of cytotoxic T lymphocytes (Zhang, Shah, et al. 2008). Signaling reconstruction efforts have leveraged previous literature sources, databases, and proteomic and phosphoproteomic experiments (Sivakumaran, Hariharaputran, et al. 2003; Hyduke and Palsson 2010; Prill, Saez-Rodriguez, et al. 2011). Such networks can aid mechanistic understanding of disease-driving perturbations and drug-discovery methods that focus on kinases (Zhang, Shah, et al. 2008; Hyduke and Palsson 2010; Chen, Xu, et al. 2012).

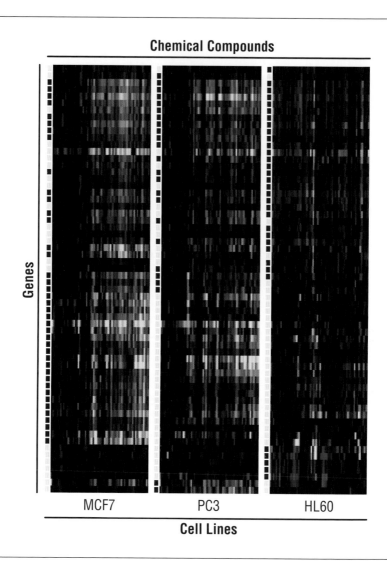

FIGURE 12–3. Biclustering can be used to find novel functions of genes. Biclustering gene expression profiles associated with different drug perturbations can identify functionally related and interacting proteins. This approach generated novel hypotheses for uncharacterized gene functionality that were experimentally validated. (Reprinted under the Creative Commons Attribution License from Iskar, M., G. Zeller, et al. (2013). Characterization of drug-induced transcriptional modules: towards drug repositioning and functional understanding. Mol Syst Biol 9: 662. (CC BY 3.0))

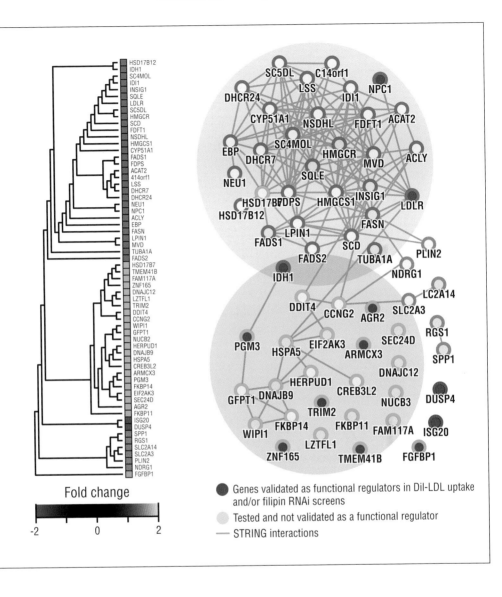

Fold change

Genes validated as functional regulators in DiI-LDL uptake and/or filipin RNAi screens

Tested and not validated as a functional regulator

— STRING interactions

Multi-omics Data-Driven Inference of Networks and Modules

Networks based on established knowledge are only partially (and, inevitably, in some cases, incorrectly) reconstructed because of our incomplete understanding of biological systems. The ability to rapidly generate networks for systems that are relatively uncharacterized, using top-down approaches primarily driven by high-throughput data, can drive the discovery of novel interactions and expand our knowledge of existing networks. To learn putative new network structures, we can leverage machine learning and inference approaches.

One statistical learning approach with applications in network medicine is biclustering. Biclustering identifies sets of biomolecules (e.g., genes) whose abundance is correlated across a given set of conditions. The term *biclustering* denotes this two-dimensional clustering of biomolecules and conditions, and it is a popular technique used to infer functional modules. One key use of biclustering is to identify potential mechanisms of drug action, which is an important step toward rational drug design. For example, this approach has recently been applied to a repository of expression profiles linked to drug perturbations, the Connectivity Map (CMAP) database. Biclustering was applied to CMAP with novel regulators of cholesterol homeostasis identified, and new mechanisms of action for existing drugs were demonstrated in vitro (Figure 12–3) (Iskar, Zeller, et al. 2013). Co-expression models found from biclustering are often used as a first step in creating data-driven networks.

Incorporating information from a variety of sources can improve the inherently low signal-to-noise ratio in large-scale biological measurements. One study used this strategy to identify dysregulated micro-RNAs that were perturbing oncogenic processes across a variety of cancers (Plaisier, Panet al. 2012). The method used was termed "framework for inference of regulation by microRNAs" (FIRM), which took a consensus approach to analyzing transcriptomic co-expression signatures, genomic sequence, and microRNA levels (Figure 12–4). The 3′ untranslated regions (UTRs) for each of the co-expressed gene sets were mined for common microRNA motifs by three orthogonal sequence analysis techniques: (1) de novo motif detection followed by hidden Markov modeling (Weeder-miRvestigator) (Pavesi, Mereghetti, et al. 2006; Plaisier, Bare, et al. 2011); (2) binding affinity probability of interaction by target accessibility (PITA) (Kertesz, Iovino, et al. 2007); and (3) sequence conservation (TargetScan) (Friedman, Farh, et al. 2009) based models. A consensus microRNA candidate set identified by FIRM was experimentally validated to regulate the targets predicted by FIRM, and functional associations (e.g., gene ontology term enrichment) subsequently linked these networks to driving several hallmarks of cancer (e.g., tissue invasion and metastasis) across many cancer types. Thus, this method provides an intriguing avenue to identify potential microRNAs for gaining network control and downstream therapeutic targeting.

Statistical inference approaches have also been harnessed to isolate driver perturbations from a set of related genes using only static data, thereby generating testable hypotheses of disease mechanisms. For example, a multi-omics Bayesian approach can identify drivers of cancer (Akavia, Litvin, et al. 2010). The study adapted a method that was previously shown to identify regulatory network modules in the model organism *Saccharomyces cerevisiae* (baker's yeast) (Lee, Pe'er, et al. 2006). This probabilistic graphical model uses a regression tree over

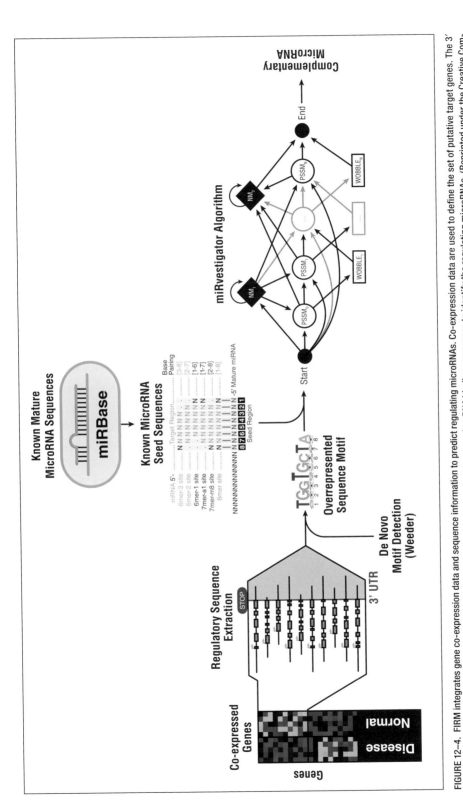

FIGURE 12–4. FIRM integrates gene co-expression data and sequence information to predict regulating microRNAs. Co-expression data are used to define the set of putative target genes. The 3′ UTR sequences from these genes are then compared with each other and against known microRNA binding sequences to identify the regulating microRNAs. (Reprinted under the Creative Commons Attribution License from Plaisier, C. L., M. Pan, et al. (2012). A miRNA-regulatory network explains how dysregulated miRNAs perturb oncogenic processes across diverse cancers. Genome Res **22**(11): 2302–14. (CC BY 3.0))

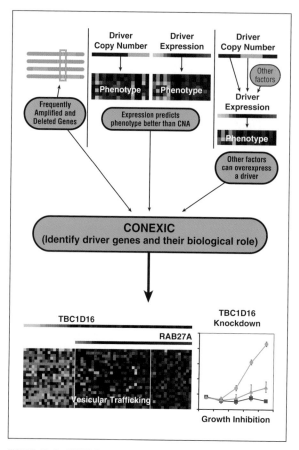

FIGURE 12–5. CONEXIC integrates mutation and expression to identify driver genes. Copy-number aberrations of putative driver genes are recursively linked to gene modules with correlated expression profiles to find the best explanation for the observed expression patterns. (Reprinted with permission from Akavia, U. D., O. Litvin, et al., (2010). An integrated approach to uncover drivers of cancer. Cell **143**(6): 1005–17, copyright (2010) with permission from Elsevier.)

sets of gene expression profiles, wherein at each level of the tree, an expression module has an identified expression driver. Their adapted method, the copy number and expression in cancer (CONEXIC) algorithm, infers the expression driver from a set of putative driver mutations identified by copy-number aberrations (Figure 12–5). Each driver's expression profile is used as a template to associate correlated gene profiles, creating gene expression modules that are putatively controlled by the driver mutation. A primary driver's expression separates the module into two submodules based on a threshold expression value. Each submodule is then recursively divided into other submodules using remaining putative driver profiles, providing a combinatorial explanation of the observed expression patterns. CONEXIC was able to isolate and experimentally validate a mutational driver in melanoma data. Such an approach could prove very useful in helping to identify specific classes of cancers with shared driver mutations and linking these back to targeted therapies.

Concurrently integrating disparate types of information adds new levels of complexity to network inference. One method developed for identifying functional modules from multi-omics data uses a joint nonnegative matrix factorization (NMF) approach to identify multidimensional modules (Figure 12–6). NMF is a machine learning technique in which the factorization of a matrix is constrained to contain only nonnegative elements. This constraint means that each observed vector is represented as an additive combination of "parts" (Lee and Seung 1999; Seung and Lee 2001). In the biological setting, these parts have

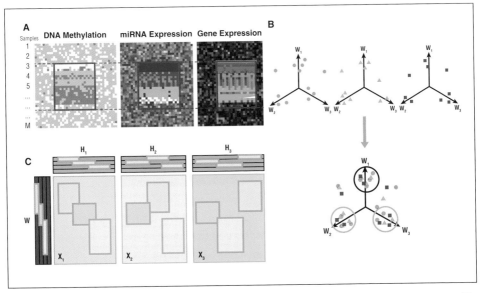

FIGURE 12–6. Nonnegative matrix factorization extracts molecules that correlate features across diverse data types. The colored matrixes in A represent three different data types. The matrixes are projected into a common feature space with appropriate scaling in B, and correlated patterns can be extracted as the joint multidimensional modules (C). X represents a matrix that can be acted on by nonnegative matrix factorization. The method factorizes X into two matrices containing values only greater than or equal to 0, denoted as W, and H, where W has the same number of rows as X and H has the same number of columns. (Reprinted with permission from Oxford University Press (Zhang, S., C. C. Liu, et al. (2012). Discovery of multidimensional modules by integrative analysis of cancer genomic data. Nucleic Acids Res **40**(19): 9379–91), copyright (2012).)

been shown to coincide with functional modules in which the defining features represent genes of canonical pathways, including, for example, the citric acid (TCA) cycle, ion transport, and functionally related genes for processes such as histone modification and membrane biosynthesis (Kim and Tidor 2003).

Multi-omics data measuring DNA methylation profiles along with mRNA and microRNA expression from The Cancer Genome Atlas (TCGA) (Hudson, Anderson, et al. 2010) were used with NMF to identify cancer-associated modules in ovarian cancer samples (Zhang, Liu, et al. 2012). In addition to sharing functional enrichment within these multidimensional modules, the modules also demonstrated multilevel synergy; that is, modules with similar gene expression patterns also shared patterns of methylation and microRNA interactions.

Contextualizing Statistical Analysis of Multi-omics Data Using Networks

Analysis of -omics data requires separating out relevant signals from a large degree of noise. Integrating heterogeneous, multi-omics measurements of completely different scales and targets further complicates the normalization required for coherent data analysis. One of the key approaches to aid in this effort is to contextualize data with biological mechanisms, which can be concisely represented by biological networks. Thus, the use of biological networks as a context for integrating multi-omics data is becoming an essential tool as -omics technologies come of age. The following survey of several multi-omics analyses demonstrates the diversity of possible approaches to integrate data as well as the potential for this type of analysis to enrich our understanding of disease.

A fundamental goal of network medicine is to identify genomic variants, linked to phenotypes, which can be used to guide treatment of disease. In particular, the analysis of combinations of genomic alterations is challenging because of the huge space of possible interactions when not conditioned on prior knowledge. The topology of GSMNs provides a useful framework for contextualizing genetic perturbations associated with disease—that is, evaluating them in the context of the biochemistry catalyzed by their respective gene products. For example, genes associated with disorders from the Online Mendelian Inheritance in Man (OMIM) database (Hamosh, Scott, et al. 2005)—ranging from coronary artery disease to Parkinson's disease—were mapped onto a GSMN of generic human metabolism (Lee, Park, et al. 2008). The study constructed a metabolic disease association network in which two disorders were linked if their associated genes catalyzed neighboring reactions in the GSMN (i.e., reactions that shared metabolites). The topology of the resulting metabolic disease association network revealed that diseases linked with neighboring reactions were significantly more likely to share comorbidity than diseases mapped to distally connected reactions, suggesting shared mechanisms and therapeutic strategies (Lee, Park, et al. 2008).

The topology of the human TRN can also serve as a framework for contextualizing disease-associated mutations. For example, overlaying nonsynonymous single-nucleotide polymorphism (SNP) mutations from the 1000 Genomes Pilot project onto the TRN revealed correlations between the number and types of transcription factor interactions and the sensitivity of the transcription factor to mutations and therapeutic interventions (Gerstein, Kundaje, et al. 2012). Moreover, mapping genome-wide association studies (GWAS)–derived significant associations from 207 different diseases onto transcription factor binding and distal chromosomal interaction data showed that inflammation-related diseases had disease-associated noncoding SNPs that were mapped to a small shared set of transcription factors (Maurano, Humbert, et al. 2012). Interestingly, these transcription factors had little overlap with the transcription factor sets that were associated with other disease classes (e.g., cancers, neuropsychiatric disorders).

Networks also provide a framework for simultaneous contextualization of multiple disparate forms of -omics data. Multiple methods of multi-omics network contextualization have been leveraged to analyze TCGA data. In one study, TCGA researchers performed an integrated analysis of endometrial carcinoma that developed four new categorical classifications based on genomic data (Kandoth, Schultz, et al. 2013). Based on these new categories, they suggested the use of their discovered genetic markers to guide the aggressiveness of treatment for endometrioid tumors. Their analyses included somatic copy-number alterations, somatic DNA mutations (from exome-sequencing analysis), gene expression, and DNA methylation and was performed using a variety of methods, both integrative and independent. We discuss two of the integrated methods used in this study in greater detail here.

The first method identifies mutual exclusivity modules (MEMo) (Ciriello, Cerami, et al. 2012). This method is based on the observation of patterns of mutual exclusivity in genetic aberrations in cancer. For example, TP53 is often mutated and MDM2 is often copy-number–amplified, but these two events rarely occur in the same tumor. This phenomenon has been observed to occur frequently in pathways; once a single gene has been altered functionally or by regulation in a pathway, other genes in the pathway remain genetically significantly unaltered relative to the background mutation rate. This phenomenon may occur because of synthetic lethality of mutually exclusive aberrations or because additional aberrations in a given pathway are not under any positive selective pressure, assuming that the initial mutation triggered the pathway-dependent perturbation required for the cancer. Based on this observation of aberrational patterns in cancer, MEMo integrates data on copy-number alterations, significant gene mutations and mRNA. This integration is performed in four steps. The first step is to generate a binary matrix that encodes significant mutational events based on existence of mutations, copy number variations, and concordant mRNA expression changes. From this matrix of significantly altered genes (SAGs), pairwise relationships are established based on an a priori–defined reference network, isolating a subnetwork that contains only interactions between SAGs. As the final step, this subnetwork is searched for groups of genes that contain mutually exclusive genetic events.

The endometrial cancer TCGA study (Kandoth, Schultz, et al. 2013) also identified pathway-distinct activation patterns with the clustering algorithm, pathway representation and analysis by direct reference on graphical models (PARADIGM) (Vaske, Benz, et al. 2010). PARADIGM integrates information from copy number, gene expression, and pathway interaction data using factor graphs (Figure 12–7). A factor graph is a graphical model that encodes the independence relationships of random variables into a belief network. These relationships are the

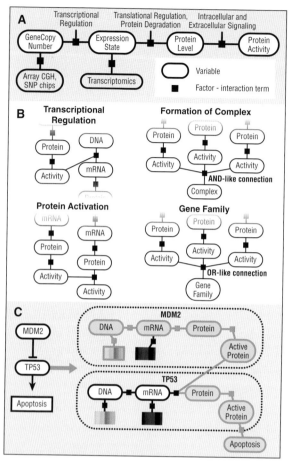

FIGURE 12–7. PARADIGM evaluates pathway-level activation based on expression and copy number of genes in the pathway. PARADIGM models diverse relationships for pathways as a factor graph, combining a priori biological knowledge for topology and inferring the strength and behavior of those relationships from observation. This process yielded aggregate pathway activity scores for systems under stress in cancer. (Note: SNP = single nucleotide polymorphism, CGH = comparative genomic hybridization, MDM2 = Mouse double minute 2 homolog)(Reprinted with permission from Oxford University Press (Vaske, C. J., S. C. Benz, et al. (2010). Inference of patient-specific pathway activities from multidimensional cancer genomics data using PARADIGM. Bioinformatics 26(12): i237–45), copyright (2010).)

"factors." This network is then trained on observed data using a technique called belief propagation, so that the strength of those relationships can be learned. PARADIGM transforms the data into a ternary representation of differential states—that is, a gene is overexpressed (1), the same (0), or underexpressed (−1), relative to a control—and it then uses domain knowledge to structure the factor graph that represents relationships of various components of the cell. Using National Cancer Institute pathway definitions, factors representing biological relationships between entities are created. The biological entities are then modeled by differential states of the observed data. The factor graph framework and simplicity of the ternary representations enable modeling of many possible combinatorial relationships, such as the relationship between copy number and gene expression contributing to an expression state, which can then be connected to protein activity. Regulatory influences of other modules are also integrated, based on the expression state from transcriptional regulators. After the PARADIGM factor graph is trained, the predicted scores for the components are clustered, giving a multi-omics partition of active, inactive and nondifferential states. A truly remarkable aspect of the successful application of PARADIGM is that, although the complexity of biology has often confounded attempts at using belief propagation, the strong delineation of relationships between genes that has emerged from -omics-based systems biology approaches and biological network information has made such whole-cell models possible. Using PARADIGM, the TCGA study found activation of WNT and deactivation of MYC pathways, consistent with the composition of the mutational information (Kandoth, Schultz, et al. 2013). The PARADIGM results further showed that different types of mutation in p53 created unique signaling patterns (Kandoth, Schultz, et al. 2013).

Linking the molecular phenotype of disease to possible drug targets is a key goal of translational systems biology and rational drug design. In the absence of techniques to directly measure these connections, statistical enrichment of functional categories can often be used to generate hypotheses regarding meaningful relationships; a category is "enriched" if observed more frequently than would be expected by chance. One approach to identify multi-omics functional and druggable modules using statistical enrichment analysis is the Expression-2Kinases (X2K) pipeline (Chen, Xu, et al. 2012), which is focused on kinases because many are known drug targets. X2K identifies modules of co-expressed genes with enriched *cis*-regulatory profiles taken from ChIP-seq/chip experiments and identifies upstream kinases that putatively regulate underlying molecular processes. X2K performs a series of enrichment analyses linking protein–DNA interactions, gene expression, protein–protein interactions, and kinase-phosphorylation.

Expanded gene regulatory networks that incorporate the effects of noncoding RNAs have been leveraged to gain insight into cancer pathophysiology, including the increasingly important goal of patient stratification. In one example, Yang, Sun, and colleagues (2013) integrated transcriptomic data from serous ovarian cancer tissue samples with microRNA, promoter methylation, and copy-number–variation data from TCGA using a multivariate linear regression model. From these data, they found a subset of genes overexpressed in the mesenchymal subtype that they predicted to be regulated by a subnetwork of 19 microRNAs. By using consensus k-means clustering of patient samples based on the expression of the genes targeted by the 19-microRNA subnetwork, the authors isolated two distinct subpopulations that differed significantly in survival outcome and tissue morphology (Yang, Sun, et al. 2013). Population 1 had higher expression of microRNA-associated genes, shorter overall survival times, and tumors that resembled collections of mesenchymal cells. In contrast, population 2 had lower expression of microRNA-associated cells, longer survival times, and tumors that contained epithelial cells. The expression values of the microRNA subnetwork–associated genes were further used to segregate 560 serous ovarian cancer samples from three other independent datasets. In each of the three validation datasets, two distinct patient subtypes with differential survival outcomes were identified based on the microRNA network–associated genes. In this study, multi-omics integration led to construction of a gene regulatory subnetwork that effectively stratified patients with serous ovarian cancer.

In Silico Mechanistic Network Simulations of Multi-omics Data

Beyond integrating and contextualizing data, the ultimate goal of many network reconstruction efforts is to enable predictive, mechanistic modeling of cellular behavior. In this way, researchers aim to simulate the effects of molecular perturbations in silico and observe the cascading effects that give rise to disease phenotypes. Importantly, such phenotypes arise from dynamic interactions across multiple types and scales of biological networks. As such, moving network modeling efforts into a more multi-omics regime will enable greater coverage of disease processes and ultimately more powerful predictions for network medicine.

Metabolic networks remain the only class of biological network reconstructed reasonably comprehensively at the genome-scale in humans. Given that metabolic networks are ultimately based on directed chemical reactions that obey the laws of mass and energy balance, they can further serve the basis for calculations to predict reaction rates (metabolic flux). These fluxes can subsequently be used to compute production and growth rates of metabolites. In flux balance analysis, the set of reactions is formulated as a stoichiometric matrix, which enumerates the ratios of metabolite participation in each reaction (Orth, Thiele, et al. 2010). A set of physically possible reaction flux rates result by enforcing a steady-state mass balance (homeostasis) and additional constraints on reaction reversibilities and maximal conversion rates. From within this space of chemically feasible reaction flux combinations, the subset of biologically relevant reaction flux profiles can be solved by optimizing an objective function. The most commonly used objective function in microbes has been to maximize the production of biomass, which serves as a proxy for maximizing growth rate (Orth, Thiele, et al. 2010). Notably, while maximal growth may be an appropriate assumption for diseases such as cancer under certain conditions (Hsu and Sabatini 2008; Kroemer and Pouyssegur 2008; Cairns, Harris, et al. 2011), the best cellular objective function to simulate many human tissues and cell types is unknown (and is likely condition-specific). Adjusting this objective function, which was developed based on microbial physiology, to better reflect human tissues is an area of active research. Integrating the GPR association map with the stoichiometric reaction framework enables simulation of the effects of different genetic perturbations on consequent reaction flux profiles and predicted growth rates (Orth, Thiele, et al. 2010). Simulations with models constructed from GSMNs can predict the effect of metabolic gene knockouts on growth under different environmental conditions. Single and combinatorial gene deletion simulations on metabolic models of many bacterial pathogens have been used to predict novel putative drug targets (Chavali, D'Auria, et al. 2012). This strategy has also been leveraged to predict drug targets for cancer (Folger, Jerby, et al. 2011).

While in silico simulations of GSMNs explicitly predict the flux (or range of possible fluxes consistent with available experimental data) through reactions in the network, these values implicitly relate to multiple levels of biological control. Metabolic flux is governed not only by enzyme abundance and posttranslational regulation (e.g., phosphorylation), but also by the abundance of metabolites and all layers of upstream and downstream regulation. Efforts are ongoing to devise effective strategies to translate flux states into insights for changes in specific -omics classes such as metabolomics, transcriptomics, and proteomics; in turn, studies have explored how best to impose condition-specific constraints on metabolic states based on different -omics measurements (Schmidt, Ebrahim, et al. 2013; Zur, Ruppin, et al. 2010). As a complement to metabolic modeling efforts, mathematical formulations of gene regulatory or signaling networks can be used to capture the interplay between the environment, the proteome, the genome, the transcriptome, and the metabolome. TRNs for human pathogens including *Mycobacterium tuberculosis* (MTB) have been leveraged to identify cascading regulatory perturbations from time-course transcriptomics data. In one study, MTB gene expression was examined in the context of the "origon"—a transcription factor and its direct and indirect regulatory targets (Balazsi, Heath, et al. 2008). When these cascade-centric subnetworks were mapped to time-course gene expression of MTB, the authors could map condition-dependent regulatory dynamics, which isolated the drivers of large-scale perturbations and suggested putative condition-specific drug targets.

Another mechanistic approach for integrating multi-omics data is emerging from Petri net modeling. Petri nets have been adopted by many fields, and as the topology and functional information of cellular interactions continues to grow, they have been applied to systems biology. Petri nets are graphical models where objects (which have initial concentrations and decay rates) are connected by transitional relationships. In the biological context, one can, for example, model the change in concentration of a protein from the nonphosphorylated to the phosphorylated state by maintaining mass through a transition in which ATP and the appropriate phosphatase are present in adequate concentrations (Figure 12–8) (Li, Pandey, et al. 2012). One study used a Petri net model to perform a flux comparative analysis of signaling pathways affected by nonsteroidal anti-inflammatory

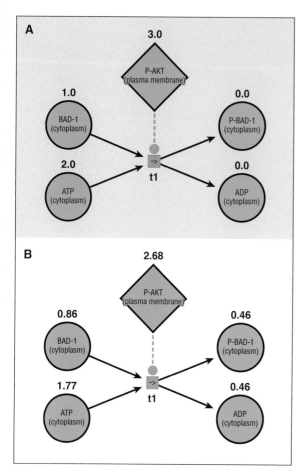

FIGURE 12–8. Example of a Petri net model of a phosphorylation reaction. Each object (green) represents a phosphorylation state of a protein, and the phosphorylation reaction is represented by the transition (orange). The concentrations of each of the model components change after the reaction transition from panel A to panel B. (Note: "P–" denotes the phosphorylated forms of the proteins, AKT = protein kinase B, BAD = Bcl-2-associated death promoter.) (Reprinted under the Creative Commons Attribution License from Li, J., V. Pandey, et al. (2012). Modeling of miRNA and drug action in the EGFR signaling pathway. PLoS One 7(1): e30140.)

drugs (NSAIDs; e.g., aspirin, ibuprofen) using mRNA and microRNA expression (Li and Mansmann 2013). A molecular model was constructed from literature on the cyclo-oxygenase pathway and its related pathways. The simulated behavior was shown to match the observed behavior of the cell under the given conditions.

Integrating Heterogeneous Networks for Expanded Insight

The networks and modules discussed thus far each inform specific aspects of a single cell, tissue, or organism. However, biological systems involve interactions of multiple networks that frequently interface across multiple tissue types or organisms (e.g., human microbiome). Preliminary efforts to integrate modeling across different network types or organisms aim to capture the emergent properties that arise from interacting networks.

A prime example of network integration is the interface of metabolic networks with transcriptional regulatory networks. The strategies developed so far, which have been effective for microbial organisms, involve harnessing the regulatory interactions between transcription factors and metabolic genes established in a transcriptional regulatory network and by defining a rule set to determine how the expression of the transcription factor affects the transcription of the target metabolic genes (Covert and Palsson 2002; Shlomi, Eisenberg, et al. 2007; Chandrasekaran and Price 2010). In one study, an integrated regulatory-metabolic model of MTB was used to simulate the effect of transcription factor knockouts on growth (Chandrasekaran and Price 2010), thereby expanding the scope of potential drug targets for further study. Intriguingly, follow-up studies have shown that linking a GSMN and a TRN can be used to refine the transcriptional regulatory interactions by enabling a much wider range of physiological data (such as growth under transcription factor knockout conditions) to be used. This process yielded substantially greater enrichment for known mechanisms than using mutual information or correlation between transcriptional regulators and their putative targets (Chandrasekaran and Price 2013).

Integration of networks across multiple organisms can yield additional insight into the emergent properties associated with their interactions. A prime application of this strategy is in the investigation of host–pathogen interactions. For example, a preliminary integrated host–pathogen metabolic network has been constructed to simulate the metabolic effects of an infection of MTB in a human alveolar macrophage (Bordbar, Lewis, et al. 2010). The resulting host–pathogen model showed improved predictions on pathogen gene essentiality compared to predictions from the MTB model without the macrophage context and led to putative drug targets.

Host–pathogen interactions have also been leveraged to gain insight into the pathophysiology of unrelated diseases. For example, a host–virus interaction network was used to recapitulate known causal genes associated with cancer (Rozenblatt-Rosen, Deo, et al. 2012). Their host–pathogen–protein interaction network, consisted of 454 interactions between 307 human proteins and 53 proteins from human papillomavirus, Epstein–Barr virus, adenovirus, and polyomavirus, which included human proteins that showed differential expression in viral ORF-transduced cell lines. The list of virally perturbed human genes was enriched for genes known to cause cancer with greater specificity than with gene lists generated by GWAS and somatic copy-number alteration studies. As we uncover more about interactions between the human body and our microbiota, integrating the networks that interact across organisms will help to expand our insight into physiology and suggest new therapeutic interventions.

Conclusion

The recent advances in high-throughput measurement technologies from large-scale efforts including TCGA (Hudson, Anderson, et al. 2010) and ENCODE (Raney, Cline, et al. 2011; Bernstein, Birney, et al. 2012) have now produced sample-specific measurements of sequencing-based multi-omics data. Integrating this wealth of data has formed the basis for the construction, refinement,

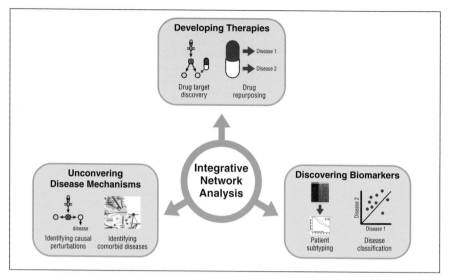

FIGURE 12–9. The medical applications of network analysis. Integrative, multi-omic network-based analyses have been used to aid the discovery of new diagnostics and therapeutics and have also shed light on previously unknown disease mechanisms. (Contains images adapted with permission from: 1) Lee, D. S., J. Park, et al. (2008). The implications of human metabolic network topology for disease comorbidity. Proc Natl Acad Sci U S A 105(29): 9880–5 , copyright (2008) National Academy of Sciences, U.S.A; and 2) Cancer Cell 23(2), Yang, D., Y. Sun, et al., Integrated analyses identify a master microRNA regulatory network for the mesenchymal subtype in serous ovarian cancer. 186–99, copyright (2013), with permission from Elsevier.)

and harnessing of networks that have yielded experimentally validated insights in biological systems. These initial network integration efforts have found patterns of disease comorbidity, identified clinically relevant subtypes in cancer, isolated disease driver genes and mechanisms associated with the interplay of multilayered regulation, and offered predictions for therapeutic targets (Figure 12–9). With the emergence of integrated personal -omics profile measurements (Chen, Mias, et al. 2012) on large populations spanning a broad spectrum of diseases, network-based integration will provide an ideal tool to build biological understanding and to develop the next generation of diagnostics and therapeutics. Thus, while integration of multiple -omics types in network medicine is a practice still very much in its infancy, it promises to emerge as a powerful approach by which to gain medical insight in the decades ahead.

References

Agren, R., S. Bordel, et al. (2012). Reconstruction of genome-scale active metabolic networks for 69 human cell types and 16 cancer types using INIT. PLoS Comput Biol 8(5): e1002518.

Akavia, U. D., O. Litvin, et al. (2010). An integrated approach to uncover drivers of cancer. Cell **143**(6): 1005–17.

Arakawa, K., and M. Tomita (2013). Merging multiple omics datasets in silico: statistical analyses and data interpretation. Methods Mol Biol **985**: 459–70.

Balazsi, G., A. L. Barabási, et al. (2005). Topological units of environmental signal processing in the transcriptional regulatory network of Escherichia coli. Proc Natl Acad Sci U S A **102**(22): 7841–46.

Balazsi, G., A. P. Heath, et al. (2008). The temporal response of the Mycobacterium tuberculosis gene regulatory network during growth arrest. Mol Syst Biol **4**: 225.

Bernstein, B. E., E. Birney, et al. (2012). An integrated encyclopedia of DNA elements in the human genome. Nature **489**(7414): 57–74.

Bordbar, A., N. E. Lewis, et al. (2010). Insight into human alveolar macrophage and M. tuberculosis interactions via metabolic reconstructions. Mol Syst Biol **6**: 422.

Cairns, R. A., I. S. Harris, et al. (2011). Regulation of cancer cell metabolism. Nat Rev Cancer **11**(2): 85–95.

Chandrasekaran, S., and N. D. Price (2010). Probabilistic integrative modeling of genome-scale metabolic and regulatory networks in Escherichia coli and Mycobacterium tuberculosis. Proc Natl Acad Sci U S A **107**(41): 17845–50.

Chandrasekaran, S., and N. D. Price (2013). Metabolic constraint-based refinement of transcriptional regulatory networks. PLoS Comput Biol **9**(12): e1003370.

Chavali, A. K., K. M. D'Auria, et al. (2012). A metabolic network approach for the identification and prioritization of antimicrobial drug targets. Trends Microbiol **20**(3): 113–23.

Chen, E. Y., H. Xu, et al. (2012). Expression2Kinases: mRNA profiling linked to multiple upstream regulatory layers. Bioinformatics **28**(1): 105–111.

Chen, R., G. I. Mias, et al. (2012). Personal omics profiling reveals dynamic molecular and medical phenotypes. Cell **148**(6): 1293–307.

Ciriello, G., E. Cerami, et al. (2012). Mutual exclusivity analysis identifies oncogenic network modules. Genome Res **22**(2): 398–406.

Covert, M. W., and B. O. Palsson (2002). Transcriptional regulation in constraints-based metabolic models of Escherichia coli. J Biol Chem **277**(31): 28058–64.

Duarte, N. C., S. A. Becker, et al. (2007). Global reconstruction of the human metabolic network based on genomic and bibliomic data. Proc Natl Acad Sci U S A **104**(6): 1777–82.

Edgar, R., M. Domrachev, et al. (2002). Gene Expression Omnibus: NCBI gene expression and hybridization array data repository. Nucleic Acids Res **30**(1): 207–10.

Folger, O., L. Jerby, et al. (2011). Predicting selective drug targets in cancer through metabolic networks. Mol Syst Biol **7**: 501.

Friedman, R. C., K. K. Farh, et al. (2009). Most mammalian mRNAs are conserved targets of microRNAs. Genome Res **19**(1): 92–105.

Galagan, J. E., K. Minch, et al. (2013). The Mycobacterium tuberculosis regulatory network and hypoxia. Nature **499**(7457): 178–83.

Gerstein, M. B., A. Kundaje, et al. (2012). Architecture of the human regulatory network derived from ENCODE data. Nature **489**(7414): 91–100.

Hamosh, A., A. F. Scott, et al. (2005). Online Mendelian Inheritance in Man (OMIM), a knowledgebase of human genes and genetic disorders. Nucleic Acids Res **33**(Database issue): D514–17.

Hsu, P. P., and D. M. Sabatini (2008). Cancer cell metabolism: Warburg and beyond. Cell **134**(5): 703–7.

Hudson, T. J., W. Anderson, et al. (2010). International network of cancer genome projects. Nature **464**(7291): 993–98.

Hyduke, D. R., and B. O. Palsson (2010). Towards genome-scale signalling network reconstructions. Nat Rev Genet **11**(4): 297–307.

Iskar, M., G. Zeller, et al. (2013). Characterization of drug-induced transcriptional modules: towards drug repositioning and functional understanding. Mol Syst Biol **9**: 662.

Jerby, L., T. Shlomi, et al. (2010). Computational reconstruction of tissue-specific metabolic models: application to human liver metabolism. Mol Syst Biol **6**: 401.

Kandoth, C., N. Schultz, et al. (2013). Integrated genomic characterization of endometrial carcinoma. Nature **497**(7447): 67–73.

Kent, W. J., C. W. Sugnet, et al. (2002). The human genome browser at UCSC. Genome Res **12**(6): 996–1006.

Kertesz, M., N. Iovino, et al. (2007). The role of site accessibility in microRNA target recognition. Nat Genet **39**(10): 1278–84.

Kim, P. M., and B. Tidor (2003). Subsystem identification through dimensionality reduction of large-scale gene expression data. Genome Res **13**(7): 1706–18.

Kroemer, G., and J. Pouyssegur (2008). Tumor cell metabolism: cancer's Achilles' heel. Cancer Cell **13**(6): 472–82.

Kroger, C., S. C. Dillon, et al. (2011). The transcriptional landscape and small RNAs of Salmonella enterica serovar Typhimurium. Proc Natl Acad Sci U S A **109**(20): E1277–86.

Lamb, J., E. D. Crawford, et al. (2006). The Connectivity Map: using gene-expression signatures to connect small molecules, genes, and disease. Science **313**(5795): 1929–35.

Lee, D. D., and H. S. Seung (1999). Learning the parts of objects by non-negative matrix factorization. Nature **401**(6755): 788–91.

Lee, D. S., J. Park, et al. (2008). The implications of human metabolic network topology for disease comorbidity. Proc Natl Acad Sci U S A **105**(29): 9880–85.

Lee, S. I., D. Pe'er, et al. (2006). Identifying regulatory mechanisms using individual variation reveals key role for chromatin modification. Proc Natl Acad Sci U S A **103**(38): 14062–67.

Legrain, P., R. Aebersold, et al. (2011). The human proteome project: current state and future direction. Mol Cell Proteomics **10**(7): M111 009993.

Lewis, N. E., G. Schramm, et al. (2010). Large-scale in silico modeling of metabolic interactions between cell types in the human brain. Nat Biotechnol **28**(12): 1279–85.

Li, F., I. Thiele, et al. (2009). Identification of potential pathway mediation targets in Toll-like receptor signaling. PLoS Comput Biol **5**(2): e1000292.

Li, J., and U. R. Mansmann (2013). Modeling of non-steroidal anti-inflammatory drug effect within signaling pathways and miRNA-regulation pathways. PLoS One **8**(8): e72477.

Li, J., V. Pandey, et al. (2012). Modeling of miRNA and drug action in the EGFR signaling pathway. PLoS One **7**(1): e30140.

Liberzon, A., A. Subramanian, et al. (2011). Molecular signatures database (MSigDB) 3.0. Bioinformatics **27**(12): 1739–40.

Ma, H., A. Sorokin, et al. (2007). The Edinburgh human metabolic network reconstruction and its functional analysis. Mol Syst Biol **3**: 135.

Maurano, M. T., R. Humbert, et al. (2012). Systematic localization of common disease-associated variation in regulatory DNA. Science **337**(6099): 1190–95.

Orth, J. D., I. Thiele, et al. (2010). What is flux balance analysis? Nat Biotechnol **28**(3): 245–48.

Papin, J. A., and B. O. Palsson (2004). The JAK-STAT signaling network in the human B-cell: an extreme signaling pathway analysis. Biophys J **87**(1): 37–46.

Pavesi, G., P. Mereghetti, et al. (2006). MoD Tools: regulatory motif discovery in nucleotide sequences from co-regulated or homologous genes. Nucleic Acids Res **34**(Web Server issue): W566–70.

Plaisier, C. L., J. C. Bare, et al. (2011). miRvestigator: web application to identify miRNAs responsible for co-regulated gene expression patterns discovered through transcriptome profiling. Nucleic Acids Res **39**(Web Server issue): W125–31.

Plaisier, C. L., M. Pan, et al. (2012). A miRNA-regulatory network explains how dysregulated miRNAs perturb oncogenic processes across diverse cancers. Genome Res **22**(11): 2302–14.

Prill, R. J., J. Saez-Rodriguez, et al. (2011). Crowdsourcing network inference: the DREAM predictive signaling network challenge. Sci Signal **4**(189): mr7.

Raney, B. J., M. S. Cline, et al. (2011). ENCODE whole-genome data in the UCSC genome browser (2011 update). Nucleic Acids Res **39**(Database issue): D871–75.

Ravcheev, D. A., A. A. Best, et al. (2013). Genomic reconstruction of transcriptional regulatory networks in lactic acid bacteria. BMC Genomics **14**: 94.

Rozenblatt-Rosen, O., R. C. Deo, et al. (2012). Interpreting cancer genomes using systematic host network perturbations by tumour virus proteins. Nature **487**(7408): 491–95.

Sachs, K., O. Perez, et al. (2005). Causal protein-signaling networks derived from multiparameter single-cell data. Science **308**(5721): 523–29.

Salgado, H., S. Gama-Castro, et al. (2006). RegulonDB (version 5.0): Escherichia coli K-12 transcriptional regulatory network, operon organization, and growth conditions. Nucleic Acids Res **34**(Database issue): D394–97.

Schmidt, B. J., A. Ebrahim, et al. (2013). GIM3E: condition-specific models of cellular metabolism developed from metabolomics and expression data. Bioinformatics **29**(22): 2900–8.

Seung, D., and L. Lee (2001). Algorithms for non-negative matrix factorization. Adv Neural Informat Proc Syst **13:** 556–62.

Shlomi, T., M. N. Cabili, et al. (2008). Network-based prediction of human tissue-specific metabolism. Nat Biotechnol **26**(9): 1003–10.

Shlomi, T., Y. Eisenberg, et al. (2007). A genome-scale computational study of the interplay between transcriptional regulation and metabolism. Mol Syst Biol **3:** 101.

Sivakumaran, S., S. Hariharaputran, et al. (2003). The Database of Quantitative Cellular Signaling: management and analysis of chemical kinetic models of signaling networks. Bioinformatics **19**(3): 408–15.

The Cancer Genome Atlas Research Network (2013). Integrated genomic characterization of endometrial carcinoma. Nature **497:** 67–73.

Thiele, I., and B. O. Palsson (2010). A protocol for generating a high-quality genome-scale metabolic reconstruction. Nat Protoc **5**(1): 93–121.

Thiele, I., N. Swainston, et al. (2013). A community-driven global reconstruction of human metabolism. Nat Biotechnol **31**(5): 419–25.

Vaske, C. J., S. C. Benz, et al. (2010). Inference of patient-specific pathway activities from multi-dimensional cancer genomics data using PARADIGM. Bioinformatics **26**(12): i237–45.

Wang, Y., J. A. Eddy, et al. (2012). Reconstruction of genome-scale metabolic models for 126 human tissues using mCADRE. BMC Syst Biol **6:** 153.

Yamada, T., I. Letunic, et al. (2011) iPath 2.0: Interactive pathway explorer. Nuc Acids Res. **39:** W412–5.

Yang, D., Y. Sun, et al. (2013). Integrated analyses identify a master microRNA regulatory network for the mesenchymal subtype in serous ovarian cancer. Cancer Cell **23**(2): 186–99.

Yoon, H., C. Ansong, et al. (2011). Systems analysis of multiple regulator perturbations allows discovery of virulence factors in Salmonella. BMC Syst Biol **5:** 100.

Zhang, R., M. V. Shah, et al. (2008). Network model of survival signaling in large granular lymphocyte leukemia. Proc Natl Acad Sci U S A **105**(42): 16308–13.

Zhang, S., C. C. Liu, et al. (2012). Discovery of multi-dimensional modules by integrative analysis of cancer genomic data. Nucleic Acids Res **40**(19): 9379–91.

Zur, H., E. Ruppin, et al. (2010). iMAT: an integrative metabolic analysis tool. Bioinformatics **26**(24): 3140–42.

Zwir, I., D. Shin, et al. (2005). Dissecting the PhoP regulatory network of Escherichia coli and Salmonella enterica. Proc Natl Acad Sci U S A **102**(8): 2862–67.

13

Cancer Network Medicine

Takeshi Hase, Samik Ghosh,
Sucheendra K. Palaniappan, and Hiroaki Kitano

Introduction

Recent advancements of cancer-molecular biology have made significant progress in understanding the hallmarks of cancer and specific treatments have been successfully developed for certain cancers; however, effective treatments for most cancer subtypes remain largely elusive. Cancers are characterized by their complexity and heterogeneity. Cancers are highly robust systems, and as such, they are able to proliferate and survive under a wide range of perturbations, for example, various anticancer therapies, naturally occurring microenvironments, and immunological responses. An important aspect in the robustness of cancers is functional redundancy (Kitano 2004), which is enabled by the heterogeneity of cancer cells and is useful for cancer cells to survive in hazardous environments (e.g., treatment with anticancer drugs or exposure to hypoxia). Almost all cancers are caused by somatic mutations (Alexandrov et al. 2013; Reimand and Bader 2013); however, the underlying biological processes are not well characterized, largely because of mutational heterogeneity (Lawrence et al. 2013); this leads to a decreased signal (driver mutations)-to-noise (passenger mutations) ratio, thereby limiting the ability of computational methods to identify causal processes.

Tumors are highly heterogeneous as a system; they are composed of diverse subpopulations of cells whose features are very different from one another. Such heterogeneity in tumors is a key to enhance their robustness through redundancy, that is, among the subpopulations in a tumor, a specific subpopulation of cells enables the tumor to maintain metastatic and proliferative ability even after anticancer treatments successfully eliminate some of the subpopulations; this feature could potentially lead to tumor redevelopment (Kitano 2004).

As mentioned in Kitano (2004), such robustness occurs at two levels of redundancy; homogeneous and heterogeneous. Homogeneous-level redundancy is built through creating copies of identical subpopulations of tumor cells. Such copies provide a storehouse of available subpopulations even when some of them are eliminated by perturbations (e.g., anticancer drugs). However, homogeneous-level redundancy is not effective against "common-mode failure," in which a hazardous perturbation is not localized and it successfully targets and eliminates all of the susceptible subpopulations. In contrast to homogeneous-level redundancy, heterogeneous-level redundancy is mediated by heterogeneous subpopulations with functional equivalence and thus may enable tumors to escape from such common-mode failure.

In tumors, genomic instability plays a key role in maintaining such heterogeneous-level redundancy and leads to various evolving genetic mutations (Lengauer et al. 1998). With advances in genomic-analysis techniques, researchers have revealed that, even within the same tumor, the subpopulations of tumor cells are immensely heterogeneous, with distinct patterns of mutations in their genome (Fisher et al. 2013). Especially, next-generation sequencing (NGS) technologies enable researchers to systematically investigate single-nucleotide polymorphisms (SNPs) and copy-number variations (CNVs) of genomic loci in various types of cancers at a genome-wide level. A large number of studies based on NGS technologies provide a huge amount evidence for genetic diversity within the same type of cancer as well as across various types of cancers (Wood et al. 2007; Consortium 2008; Ding et al. 2008; Jones et al. 2008; Parsons et al. 2008), and several bioinformatic repositories have been developed to catalog the genotypic information (Futreal et al. 2004), such as The Cancer Cell Line Encyclopedia (CCLE) (Barretina et al. 2012) and COSMIC database (Forbes et al. 2011).

A number of studies have shown that, in a large proportion of cancers, a relatively small number of genes are mutated; cases in which large numbers of genes are altered are less frequent (Garraway and Lander 2013; Vogelstein et al. 2013; Workman et al. 2013). Workman and colleagues (2013) reported that almost 140 proteins can be activated by their mutations, and these mutated proteins can then be key drivers for the initiation and progression of tumors. As mentioned in Vogelstein and colleagues (2013), tumors have several (2 to 8) driver mutations to control a certain number (~12) of important signaling pathways that are keys to regulate cell fate and survival as well as maintenance of the genome. Systematic analysis of cancer genomes using standard sets of emerging technologies provides rich data on molecular aberrations at DNA, RNA, protein, and epigenetic levels, as reported in a series of studies as part of The Cancer Genome Atlas (TCGA) project (Omberg et al. 2013; Tamborero et al. 2013; Weinstein et al. 2013; Zack et al. 2013).

Such integrated datasets provide a unique opportunity to understand commonalities, differences, and emerging themes among different cancer types as demonstrated in the Pan-Cancer analysis (PanCan) project (Ciriello et al. 2013). Leveraging data on 3299 tumors from 12 traditionally defined cancer types, Ciriello and colleagues identified clear oncogenic signatures, with inverse correlation between somatic mutations (M class) and CNVs (C class). By further classification of the M and C classes (into 31 subclasses), the authors identified similar tissues that display different traits, as well as different cancer subtypes that have the same genomic traits.

Similarly, models on cancer evolution that take both genetics (the code) and epigenetics (the gene state) into account are providing new insights into mechanisms of tumorigenesis and drug resistance (Chari and Dworkin 2013; Huang 2013; Velenich and Gore 2013). Studies have shown that viewing cancer as a disruption in an *ecosystem* of interacting cellular and microenvironmental elements, rather than an isolated cluster of mutated cells (Basanta and Anderson 2013), can provide better strategies for treatment as well as overcoming resistance (Straussman et al. 2012).

As the diverse molecular implementations of cancer have been unraveled through high-throughput sequencing of tumors and their mutations, it is becoming apparent that cancer operates at multiple levels and scales through complex interactions of genes, proteins, the epigenome, and the microenvironment. Several studies have shown the importance of a network-based systems approach in understanding and treating human diseases, particularly cancer (Blinov et al. 2004; Schadt et al. 2009; Arrell and Terzic 2010; Ghosh et al. 2011). As proposed by Barabási and colleagues (2011), cancer genes make their function together with their interacting partners including non-cancer genes. Genetic mutations of cancer genes affect not only their interacting partners but also a large number of their downstream genes through pathways embedded in a complex molecular interaction network. Therefore, molecular network analyses of cancer mutations can be the key to understanding robustness, fragilities, and disease mechanisms of cancers and, in turn, to finding novel drug targets for cancerous diseases. The molecular interaction network in a cell is represented at different levels of detail, including: (1) the genome-wide molecular interaction network (i.e., protein interaction networks and metabolic reaction networks), and (2) the detailed molecular interaction network for a specific pathway or biological mechanism (Oda et al. 2005; Le Novere et al. 2009; Matsuoka et al. 2013).

Novel small-molecule therapeutic agents that target specific genes are effective when specific mutations are present. They have opened up exciting opportunities for the treatment of cancer through higher degrees of biochemical specificity as compared with conventional chemotherapeutic agents. Well-known examples of targeted therapies include imatinib (Gleevec), which inhibits the product of the specific fusion gene product BCR-ABL in chronic myeloid leukemia (CML), and the more recent vemurafenib (Zelboraf), a BRAF kinase inhibitor that has shown significant efficacy in patients with metastatic melanoma harboring BRAFV600E mutations.

At the same time, the emerging picture of complex molecular networks underlying disease states points toward a more systems-level approach to therapy—the shift in focus from individual biomarkers to network markers of response, progression, or prognosis; and from single targeted therapies to combination drug therapies (Bozic et al. 2013; Sun et al. 2013). Hofree and colleagues (2013) introduced the concept of network-based stratification (NBS), in which patients are clustered based on mutations in similar network regions rather than on individual mutations in their genomes.

Drug-combination therapies provide a promising avenue by which to overcome unwanted off-target effects of single agents and also enhance the efficacy of a candidate compound used in combination. Developing a paradigm for combination targeted therapies is, however, substantially more complex than for traditional chemotherapeutic agents, whose lack of specificity allows relatively straightforward approaches to combinations. The ability to achieve therapeutic selectivity is a major concern in drug discovery, particularly for the treatment of cancer, metabolic diseases, and inflammatory disorders, where drug targets are present in both diseased and healthy cells. In these cases, it is essential to achieve finely tuned target modulation against the backdrop of compensatory mechanisms arising from complex interactions of molecular targets in the cell. Building a successful strategy for combinations of targeted therapies in the clinic requires the development of a systematic approach that integrates computational analysis based on molecular interaction networks and experimental studies to carefully analyze short- and long-term efficacy and safety. We refer interested readers to a review by Al-Lazikani and colleagues (2012) that further highlights the potential of drug-combination therapy for cancer and reviews the possible computational approaches to identifying optimal drug combinations.

Cancer biology is an interconnected, complex dynamic system. Network-based systems approaches accompanied by large-scale -omics experimental technologies are well poised to elucidate the complex mechanisms of the disease as well as develop new strategies for the treatment of patients, as shown schematically in Figure 13–1 (Schadt et al. 2009; Hofree et al. 2013; Weinstein et al. 2013). This chapter highlights some key aspects by which network biology-based techniques can be harnessed in this endeavor. First, we show how analyses of the human protein–protein interaction network can be used to select potential drug-target proteins for cancer. Second, as altered energy metabolism is widespread in cancer cells, we briefly explain a possible analysis strategy for metabolic reaction networks to find cancer-specific metabolic reactions. Third, we elucidate how detailed molecular networks together with dynamic modeling of their nonlinear interactions can help us understand the mechanisms underlying the efficacy of combination therapy. Finally, we discuss the potential impact of

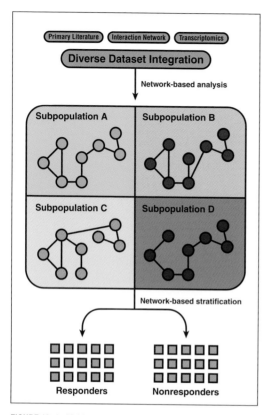

FIGURE 13–1. Multi-omics data and network-based approaches to cancer biology in clinical practice. (Reprinted by permission from Macmillan Publishers Ltd from E.E. Schadt, S.H. Friend, and D.A. Shaywitz (2009). A network view of disease and compound screening. Nat Rev Drug Disc 8(4): 285–95, copyright (2009).)

network-driven strategies integrating networks and -omics data on cancer-drug discovery and clinical practice.

Analysis of Protein–Protein Interaction Networks to Select Potential Target Proteins for Cancers

Proteins make their functions together with their interacting partners; thus, networks of protein interactions help us to investigate unknown protein functions, the role of proteins in disease mechanisms, and the discovery of novel targets for therapeutic drugs (Barabási et al. 2011; Hase et al. 2009; Hase and Niimura 2012; Vidal et al. 2011). In order to discover novel therapeutic targets for cancerous diseases, researchers studied the network metrics of protein–protein interaction networks (PINs) in humans and examined the relationships of the metrics with cancerous-disease genes and Food and Drug Administration (FDA)–approved targets for cancerous diseases.

In this section, we focus on two representative network metrics, "degree" and "modular structure" in the human PIN, and discuss their potential applications to anticancer drug design.

Degree Distribution of Oncogene and That of Genes Associated with Noncancerous Diseases

A representative network metric in a PIN is "degree" that is defined as the number of interacting partners of each protein. Knockout of a "high degree" or "hub" protein affects many proteins (e.g., interacting partners of the knockout protein) in a PIN and dramatically alters network function (Jeong et al. 2001; Yu et al. 2008). It was therefore previously postulated that as genes encode proteins with higher degrees, they have a greater chance to be disease-associated genes (Barabási et al. 2011). Several researchers have reported that the mean degree among proteins associated with diseases is significantly higher than that among the other proteins (Wachi et al. 2005; Jonsson and Bates 2006; Xu and Li 2006); yet, this is not necessarily the case for chronic complex noncancerous diseases (vide infra).

In the human PIN, genes encoding high-degree proteins tend to be "essential genes," which are defined as human genes that have orthologous genes in mice, and knockout of the orthologous genes causes embryonic lethality or postnatal lethality or sterility in mice (Liang and Li 2007). However, only a minority of disease genes are essential genes, while the remaining majority are nonessential (cf. Barabási et al. 2011). The three studies in previous paragraph (Wachi et al. 2005; Jonsson and Bates 2006; Xu and Li 2006) did not take account of this issue. Goh and colleagues (2007) investigated degree distribution of nonessential disease genes and found that they have no tendency to encode high-degree proteins. These observations indicate that most disease genes encode low- or middle-degree proteins (Feldman et al. 2008).

Goh and colleagues (2007) discussed this issue from the perspective of evolution. Because mutations of a high-degree gene disrupt functions of many interacting partners (as mentioned above), individuals with such mutations are afflicted with a dysfunctionality of important pathways that are essential to control developmental and physiological processes. Such individuals rarely survive until their reproductive years, and thus germline mutations in high-degree genes are quickly removed from the population. Therefore, proteins encoded by disease genes show a tendency to be low- and middle-degree proteins.

However, this is not the case for disease genes by somatic mutations, particularly oncogenes (Jonsson and Bates 2006). Goh and colleagues (2007) investigated the degrees of oncogenes by using information about somatic cancer genes obtained from Cancer Genome Census database (http://cancer.sanger.ac.uk/census) and found that oncogenes tend to encode high-degree proteins.

Degrees Distribution of Drug-Target Genes and Their Implications for Potential Strategies to Develop Anticancer Treatments

As for degree distribution of targets for FDA-approved drugs, most of drug-target genes encode middle- or low-degree proteins, while high-degree drug targets are very rare (Hase et al. 2009). Yao and Rzhetsky (2008) reported that degree distribution of disease genes is similar to that of drug targets and, not surprisingly, a large number of disease genes are also drug-target genes. These observations infer that potential advantageous targets exist among middle- or low-degree proteins (Hase et al. 2009). However, as the degrees of oncogenes tend to be high (as discussed above), the current therapeutic targets for cancerous disease have significantly higher degrees than those for noncancerous disease and thus tend to cause more severe adverse effects than targets for noncancerous diseases.

As discussed in Hase et al. (2009), a potential approach to solve this problem is to develop novel drug combinations targeting several low- or middle-degree proteins. Such combinations could produce synergistic antitumoral efficacy through several low- or middle-degree targets, and, at the same time, adverse events by these low- or middle-degree targets could be less severe than those by high-degree targets (e.g, targets of current anticancer drugs). However, there are a larger number of low- and middle-degree proteins in the human PIN (more than 6000) and, hence, it is considerably more difficult to select potential therapeutic targets for cancerous disease from these molecular classes (Hase et al. 2014).

Network Module–Driven Target Identification

The human PIN is a network with a modular structure, in which interaction across different modules are sparse, while those within the same module are dense (Wang and Zhang 2007). A possible strategy by which to select potential targets for cancers is to identify small modules that contain many targets for the disease of interest, because proteins in these modules could correspond to important biological functions in cancer cells. Furthermore, this strategy could be powerful in finding novel candidate targets for molecularly targeted therapies (e.g., specific kinase inhibitors), because these therapies target specific small modules embedded in the entire human PIN (Hase et al. 2014).

In this section, we briefly outline a network-guided module approach for identifying potential drug targets for cancer by Hase and colleagues (2014). To find modules that can be targeted by molecularly targeted drugs for cancers, we decomposed the genome-wide human PIN into modules and then mapped known target genes of molecularly targeted drugs for cancers on the modules.

In order to decompose the human PIN into modules, we used the Guimeráu–Amaral algorithm (Guimerá and Amaral 2005). The algorithm identified 77 modules in the network. To find modules that are targeted by molecular targeted therapeutics among the 77 modules, we mapped known drug targets of kinase inhibitors and those of monoclonal antibodies for cancerous diseases (we did not focus on particular types of cancers) on the modules and calculated fractions of drug targets to all proteins in each module. Among the 77 modules, we found that a module contains more than 60% of known drug targets of kinase inhibitors and those of monoclonal antibodies, with several proteins in the module that may be potential novel therapeutic targets (Hase et al. 2014). However, the network-decomposition technique for finding modules is limited by the size of the modules. Actually, the module having the greatest number of target genes for cancerous diseases comprises more than 2000 proteins (Figure 13–2) and, thus, still presents a challenge for selecting potential targets.

In order to address this issue, we recursively applied the module-decomposition technique in a manner similar to that proposed by Ciriello and colleagues (2013). The three steps in the method are as follows (Hase et al. 2014) (see Figure 13–2);

- Step 1. By using the Guimerá–Amaral algorithm, decompose a network (the entire human PIN or a network obtained from step 3) into several modules.
- Step 2. Map the known drug targets for kinase inhibitors or those for monoclonal antibodies in order to select a module containing the largest number of targets for these drugs.
- Step 3. Extract proteins and interactions in the selected module in step 2 to generate a network that is composed of the extracted proteins and interactions.

By applying the steps to the genome-wide human PIN a few times (see Figure 13–2), we successfully identified a small module (composed of ~200 proteins) that contains more than 40% of targets for kinase inhibitors and one for monoclonal antibodies (Hase et al. 2014). Furthermore, proteins in these modules are significantly associated with key driver pathways for proliferation and survival of cancer cells (e.g., vascular endothelial growth factor signaling). Therefore, proteins and interactions in such small modules may facilitate more efficient identification of mechanisms of drug action and novel target genes for cancerous diseases.

As mentioned above, a large proportion of targets for molecularly targeted therapeutics in cancers are distributed over a single small module. By contrast, targets of nonselective drugs for other diseases (e.g., rheumatoid arthritis) are distributed over multiple small modules and not over a single small module (Hase et al. 2014). This observation indicates that drugs of nonmolecularly targeted therapeutics do not target a single gene in a specific module but rather affect multiple genes across multiple small modules and may, therefore, have a larger number of off-target effects than molecularly targeted drugs.

In summary, modular structures and statistical features in the human PIN can be useful tools for selecting potential target proteins for cancers. With the expected explosion of genome-scale genetic mutations (e.g., SNPs, CNVs, and deep sequencing of exomes and whole genomes) from various types of cancers

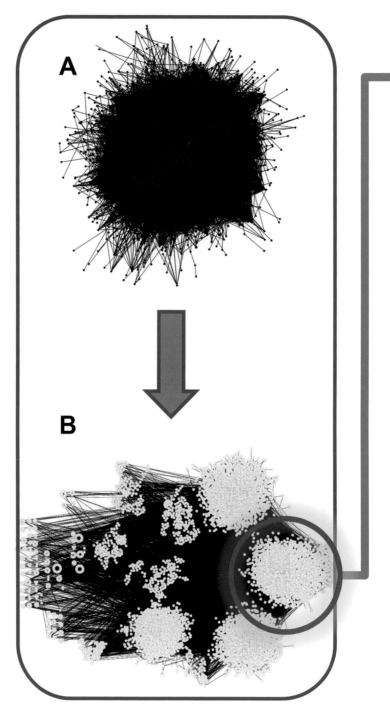

FIGURE 13–2. Schematic figure for a method to find drug-target modules in the human PIN. We recursively applied a module decomposition technique to find modules targeted molecularly by drugs for cancerous diseases (Hase et al. 2014). The network shown in A corresponds to the human PIN. We applied a module-decomposition

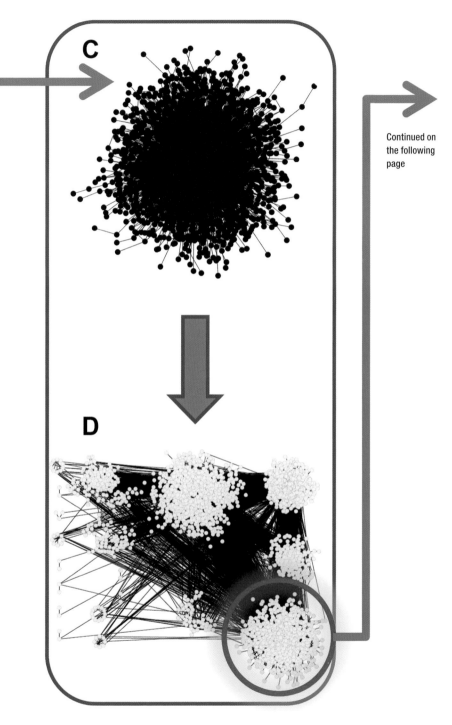

Continued on the following page

technique to this network (shown in B) and obtained a subnetwork (subnetwork circled in red in B, or C) that contains more than 60% of all drug targets of molecular-targeted drugs for cancerous diseases (first-level decomposition). Note that the size of the subnetwork (C) is still large. The smaller subnetwork in D is obtained after

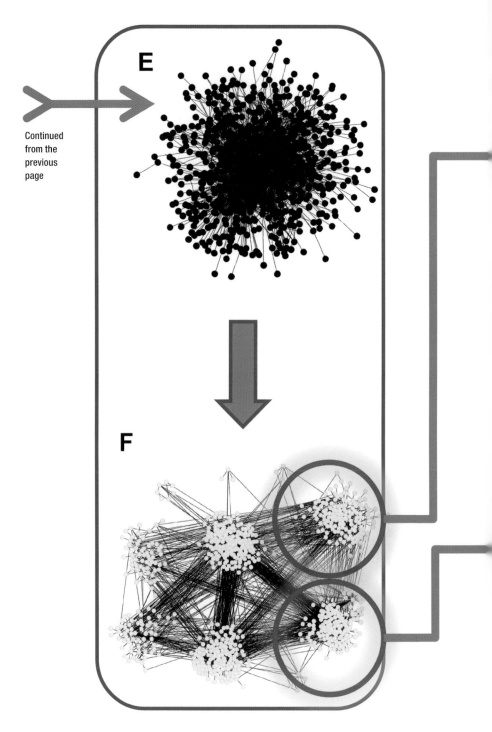

Continued from the previous page

applying module-decomposition techniques to the subnetwork in C (second-level decomposition). This network contains almost 60% of targets for molecularly targeted drugs and is composed of ~700 proteins (subnetwork circled in red in D, or E). Finally, by applying a module-decomposition technique to this subnetwork (E), we obtained two small subnetworks (small molecules), as shown in the two subnetworks circled in red in F, and in

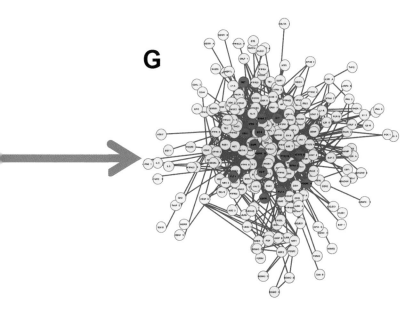

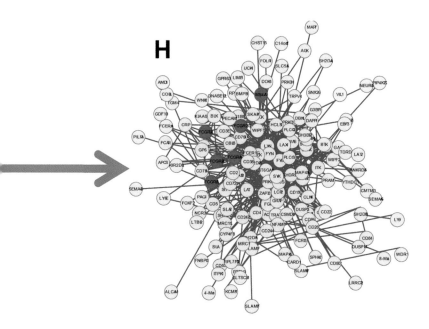

G and H) comprising 238 and 155 proteins. The two networks shown in G and H contain more than 40% and 45% of cancer-drug targets for kinase inhibitors and monoclonal antibodies, respectively (red nodes represent targets for these drugs). (Adapted from Hase et al. (2014). Identification of drug target modules in the human protein–protein interaction network. Artific Life Robot **19**;406–13. With permission of Springer.)

in the near future, an integration of PINs and these mutation data will also be promising strategies for elucidating unknown mechanisms of various types of cancers and novel targets for effective, highly specific drugs.

Cancer Metabolic Reaction Network

Abnormal metabolism is a key to understanding the initiation and development of cancers. Cancers change their metabolism in order to cope with selective pressures occurring during carcinogenesis. As mentioned in Prendergast (2013), such adaptations enable tumor cells to proliferate and satisfy high-level energy demands, as well as to escape from apoptosis and the immune system.

Several metabolic abnormalities are generally observed in various types of cancers. For example, the best-known abnormality is their preference to metabolize glucose by using aerobic glycolysis (Hsu and Sabatini 2008; Vander Heiden et al. 2009), rather than the tricarboxylic acid (TCA) cycle. Such alterations in glucose metabolism are termed the "Warburg effect" and have been accepted as hallmarks of cancer (Hanahan and Weinberg 2011). Such cancer-specific metabolic changes are essential for their proliferation and survival, and, thus, can be the Achilles' heel of cancer and exploited as anticancer targets (Hanahan and Weinberg 2011; Vander Heiden 2011).

In order to develop a successful strategy for targeting cancer metabolism, it is increasingly important to employ an integrated pipeline for data aggregation and analysis to identify cancer-specific metabolic reactions and their potential drug targets. A genome-wide human metabolic reaction network was recently published (RECOM2) and can also be a useful source for investigating mechanisms of cancer metabolism and to predict selective drug targets in cancer (Thiele et al. 2013). A computational workflow, which integrates a genome-wide metabolic network and -omics data (e.g., metabolic abundance data specific to the compounds of interest, protein abundance, gene expression, and a genome-wide PIN) will provide biological insights at a network level (Jerby and Ruppin 2012).

Several researchers developed analysis pipelines to integrate metabolic network, gene expression, and protein abundance data to infer cancer-specific metabolic reaction networks (Folger et al. 2011; Agren et al. 2012; Jerby and Ruppin 2012). These cancer-specific metabolic networks are useful resources for finding potential drug-target enzymes. For example, Folger and colleagues (2011) generated a cancer-specific metabolic network model by integrating gene expression data obtained from cancer cell lines and publicly available large-scale metabolic reaction networks. By using the network model of metabolisms in cancer and that in normal cells, they conducted a simulation study to predict the effect of single- or double-gene knockdown on the growth rate of cancer cells as well as ATP production rates of normal cells. Based on the results from the simulation, they predicted potential novel drug targets for cytostatic effects against tumor cells and synthetic lethal pairs of drug targets. These predicted pairs were in turn validated based on publicly available drug-efficacy information as well as gene expression data from the National Cancer Institute-60 cancer cell lines and 75 healthy human tissues.

Agren and coworkers (2012) also developed an interesting method, "INIT" (integrative network inference for tissues), to investigate differences in metabolism among various normal and cancer cell types. They used the INIT method to generate larger-scale metabolic networks that are activated in each of 69 normal cell types and those in each of 16 cancer cell types by integrating information of protein and metabolic abundances from different human cell types as well as tissue-specific gene expression datasets. Based on the comparative analyses of the metabolic networks in various normal and cancer cell types, they identified cancer-specific metabolic features that may be candidate therapeutic targets for cancerous diseases.

Although strategies integrating metabolic networks with expression and protein abundance data from cancer cells are powerful approaches to find cancer-specific reactions and potential drug-target genes, metabolic abundance data acquired in the presence of a candidate compound can also serve as useful resources for drug discovery. Here, we present a potential analytic pipeline that integrates the genome-wide metabolic reaction network with metabolic abundance data in the presence of a candidate compound. The pipeline could be useful for inferring reactions targeted by a candidate compound and, thus, useful for investigating mechanisms of action of the candidate.

The pipeline is based on statistical analysis of metabolomic data specific to a compound. The analysis pipeline should integrate data from multiple sources, such as metabolome abundance datasets and the genome-wide human metabolic network. In addition, the pipeline can also use other molecular network information obtained from public domain databases (e.g., protein interaction network). The key steps of the analysis pipeline are elucidated below.

1. Construction of genome-wide human metabolic networks: A genome-wide human metabolic network is available from RECON2 (Thiele et al. 2013).

2. Pattern profiling for each reaction: The key steps in the analysis pipeline are identifying a pattern profile for a reaction that indicates whether or not the reaction is triggered in a specific condition. Such pattern profiles are useful for finding cancer-specific reactions that could be targeted by anticancer drugs. For example, if a reaction from metabolite I to metabolite J has a specific profile (shown in Figure 13–3A), the reaction exists in a tumor cell not treated with

A

Reactants	Products	Tumor		Normal tissue	
		Nondrug	Drug	Nondrug	Drug
Metabolite I	Metabolite J	1	0	0	0

B

Reactants	Products	Tumor				Plasma			
		Nondrug	Low dose	Medium dose	High dose	Nondrug	Low dose	Medium dose	High dose
Metabolite A	Metabolite B	1	0	0	0	1	0	0	0
Metabolite A	Metabolite C	1	1	0	0	1	1	0	0
Metabolite B	Metabolite D	1	1	1	0	1	1	1	0
Metabolite C	Metabolite E	0	0	0	1	0	0	0	1
Metabolite C	Metabolite F	0	0	1	1	0	0	1	1
Metabolite E	Metabolite F	0	1	1	1	0	1	1	1

FIGURE 13–3. Pattern profiling for metabolic reactions under different conditions. A, Schematic example of pattern profiles that may be useful in identifying a reaction that may be sensitive to a drug for a cancer. Based on the reaction and pathway mapping, pattern profiling was performed to characterize the reactions across the four conditions. The reaction from metabolite I to metabolite J present in tumor (1, colored in orange) without compound, but absent (0, colored in blue) in the other conditions. B, Pattern profiling that can be useful to identify potential biomarker metabolites. Reactions present in some conditions (1, colored in orange), while absent in the others (0, colored in blue).

drug N, but not in a tumor cell treated with drug N or in a normal cell; this result indicates that the reaction is cancer-specific and could be inhibited by drug N. By integrating given metabolite abundance data with a genome-wide metabolic network, we can profile patterns for each reaction; that is, if two metabolites A and B have high abundance in condition 1, a reaction from metabolite A to metabolite B may exist in condition 1.

3. Network-driven analyses: Pattern profiles were employed to identify specific reactions of interest under specific conditions. For holistic analysis and interpretation, pathway-enrichment analysis was conducted for the specific reactions, and enriched pathways were visualized on the Kyoto Encyclopedia of Genes and Genomes (KEGG) pathway maps. Furthermore, to derive biological insights at the network level, different sources of information were integrated, including specific reactions, information about drug-target genes, and molecular network information (i.e., pathway from a drug-target gene to a specific reaction). Using the pipeline, information from metabolic abundance datasets was reconciled with network-level knowledge to identify potential mechanisms of action (MOA) and biomarkers for a compound, common MOA among compounds, and differences in MOA among the compounds.

Finally, we show by schematic analysis, an example of the above pipeline strategy. The example presented is for investigation of potential plasma biomarkers and drug-sensitivity analyses. Assume that a given metabolic abundance dataset contains information on metabolic abundance under no, low, medium, and high drug doses and abundances that were measured from two tissues (i.e., tumor tissue and plasma). Note that for each metabolite, its metabolic abundance was measured under eight conditions. By applying the pipeline to the metabolomic data and a genome-wide human metabolic network, we can generate 8-bit pattern profiles for each metabolic reaction (Figure 13–3B). The generated pattern profiles may be useful to find potential plasma biomarkers of the drug's effect(s).

For monitoring drug responses, plasma biomarkers are the least invasive and most convenient. Based on statistical analyses of metabolomic data, it is important to identify plasma biomarker enzymes and metabolites that may reflect changes in tumors under the four different dosage regimens. If pattern profiling for a reaction (e.g., reaction between A and B) in the tumor is the same as that in plasma, the reaction may be useful in finding common metabolic dynamics and pathways between tumor and plasma compartments. Focusing on reactions with pattern profiling as shown in Figure 13–3B can be a good strategy to find potential plasma biomarker metabolites. Such reactions (enzymes) are present only in the absence of drug in both plasma and tumor. The enzymes and metabolites associated with the enzymes can be potential plasma biomarkers.

In summary, the analytical methods integrating metabolic reaction networks and -omics data (e.g., gene expression and protein abundance data) in various types of cancer and normal tissues can be a promising strategy for uncovering mechanisms of cancer metabolism and potential target enzymes for various cancers. Furthermore, the potential analytical pipeline that integrates metabolic networks with metabolic abundance data in the presence of candidate compounds can be useful in identifying metabolic reactions that may be inhibited by the candidate compound. Such reactions may be useful for defining plasma biomarkers for the compound as well as for investigating the potential mechanism of action of the compound.

Combination Therapies

Molecular profiling of cancer can enable the development of targeted therapies based on mutation signatures for specific patient populations in addition to clinical classification of the disease. Targeted therapeutics for human diseases, such as cancer, aim to identify drug candidates that show high selectivity in the sense of targeting a specific molecule; however, owing to the underlying complexity of the molecular targets and nonlinear interactions among them, selectivity is lost in a systems sense—their efficacy is reduced by compensatory mechanisms of other pathways and molecules, preventing their use at subtoxic dosages (Lehar et al. 2009). In this respect, combination therapies attempt to leverage the underlying complexity to the advantage of treating multifactorial diseases.

Combination therapeutics have shown promising results in several case studies. Borisy and colleagues (2003) developed a high-throughput platform for systematically studying combinations of ~3000 approved drugs against various disease phenotypes. Lehar and colleagues (2009) also showed that synergistic combinations have a tendency to improve therapeutically relevant selectivity, using simulations based on bacterial metabolism as well as 94,110 multidose experiments that are relevant to various diseases. These results highlight the context-specificity of synergistic combinations, underscoring the need to employ systematic, mechanism-driven studies of combination effects. In this section, we provide an example of the role of network-driven analysis and dynamic modeling in understanding combination therapy in silico using the well-studied mitogen-activated protein kinase (MAPK) pathway and associated networks as an illustrative case study.

In the domain of small-molecule targeted therapy for cancer, several efforts have been initiated to decipher rational drug combinations for the treatment of various human carcinomas. In particular, owing to the implication of the MAPK pathway in various cancers, researchers have identified key oncogenic players and their interactions with other pathways crucial to cancer cell survival and proliferation. As reviewed by Sharma and coworkers (2007), the crucial players of the epidermal growth factor receptor (EGFR)–signal-transduction pathway involve the prosurvival arm comprising the phosphoinositide 3-kinase (PI3K)–mammalian target of rapamycin (mTOR)–Akt cascade and the pro-proliferation arm, consisting primarily of the Ras–Raf–MEK–ERK pathway. Mutations in the crucial molecules of these pathways (Ras, Raf, and PI3K) have been studied in various cancer disease subtypes (Sharma et al. 2007). The central role of these pathways in cell survival and growth, together with their complex interactions, as elucidated schematically (Figure 13–4), make them fertile areas for the development of targeted monotherapies, as well as combination therapies. Two canonical pathways, Ras–Raf–MEK–ERK (left) and PI3K–mTOR–Akt (right), are important for cell survival because they influence downstream mechanisms of activated ErbB transmembrane receptor tyrosine kinases. In this schematic figure, the blue circles represent key molecules that can be targets of molecularly targeted therapy.

A preclinical mouse model study reported that combination therapy, using rapamycin, with PD0325901, a MEK inhibitor, inhibited growth of cultured prostate cancer cells and that of androgen-independent prostate tumors (Kinkade et al. 2008). These studies conclude that such combinations might pro-

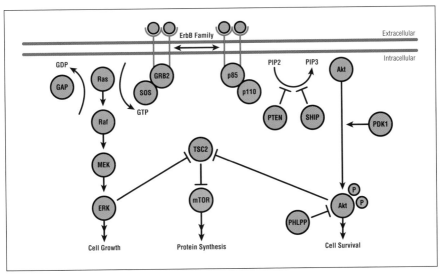

FIGURE 13–4. Canonical schematic of Ras–Raf–Mek–Erk and PI3K–mTOR–Akt pathways. Blue circles represent key molecules that can be targets of molecularly targeted therapy. ERK, extracellular signal-regulated kinase; GAP, Gap gene; GRB2, growth factor receptor-bound protein 2; MEK, MAPK/ERK kinase; mTOR, mammalian target of rapamycin; PHLPP, PH domain and leucine rich repeat protein phosphatase; PTEN, Phosphatase and Tensin Homolog Deleted from Chromosome 10; SOS, son of sevenless, TSC2 Tuberous Sclerosis Complex 2. (Adapted from Sharma et al. (2007). Epidermal growth factor receptor mutations in lung cancer. Nat Rev Cancer 7:169–81. With permission from Macmillan Publishers Ltd, copyright (2007).)

vide an effective treatment regimen for advanced prostate cancer patients in a hormone-refractory disease state.

Engelman and colleagues (2008) examined the efficacy of a dual PI3K and mammalian target of rapamycin (mTOR) inhibitor against mouse model for lung adenocarcinomas induced by p110-αH1047R expression and showed that the dual inhibitor caused significant regression of the tumors. Although tumor regression by a combination of PI3K and mTOR inhibitors was not observed in KRas (G12D) mutant strains, a combination of PI3K and MEK inhibitors (ARRY 142886) was associated with prominent synergistic effects in shrinking the KRas mutant tumors. In the case of glioblastoma cell lines (e.g., U87MG and SF-188m U251MG), Edwards and colleagues (2006) also showed that combinations of a Raf-1 inhibitor GW5074 and MEK inhibitor U0126 resulted in synergistic effects (Edwards et al. 2006).

However, context-specific synergistic effects, as highlighted by Lehar and colleagues (2009), have been reported by Smalley and Flaherty (2009), who showed that combination studies in melanoma have not successfully translated in vitro synergistic behaviors into in vivo models, partly because of inherent flaws in the existing pharmacological agents used as well as greater vulnerability of melanoma cells in vitro. Various EGFR–tyrosine kinase inhibitors

(TKIs) in combination with other agents are in different stages of development (e.g., sirolimus with gefitinib and temsirolinus with erlotinib) as reported in the work of Sharma and colleagues (2007). Further, a network-based computational and experimental study (Lee et al. 2012) highlighted the effectiveness of a systematic dose- and time-dependent approach to identifying optimal and synergistic drug combinations (see details in Chapter 14). For a specific subclass of breast cancers, it was shown that sequential pretreatment with EGFR inhibitors significantly synergized with DNA-damaging agents to increase the apoptotic response. This is attributed to the dynamic rewiring of oncogenic signaling networks and uncovering of suppressed pro-apoptotic pathways during the combination treatment.

These studies underscore the promise of combination treatments for targeted cancer therapeutics, while at the same time highlighting the need for system-level mechanistic studies to identify context specific synergistic–antagonistic effects under different genetic backgrounds.

The following sections discuss the workflow of a system-level study of the interaction dynamics of these molecular players and their impact on combination therapies targeting key components in these pathways.

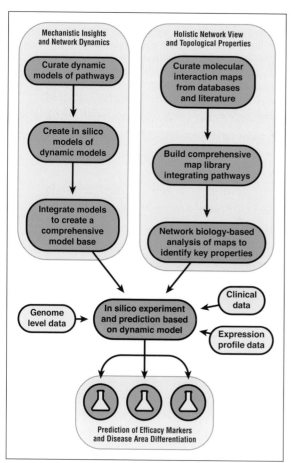

FIGURE 13–5. Schematic work flow for system-level mechanistic studies to analyze the efficacy of potential cancer treatment compounds.

Work Flow for System-Level Studies

System-level mechanistic studies are the keys to investigate drug efficacy, disease indications, and patient subpopulations. A possible workflow of a system-level mechanistic study is outlined in Figure 13–5. The workflow encompasses the core dynamic models together with a set of *in silico* experimental systems to analyze the efficacy of the compounds. The two components are built in a systematic schema integrating mechanistic knowledge and topological insights from network analysis with information from various experimental data sets.

System-Level Studies for Combination Therapies

In building a successful strategy for combinations of targeted therapies in the clinic, it is important to develop a systematic approach that integrates computational and experimental studies to analyze safety and efficacy concerns of any new candidate compound. Network biology–driven molecular-level insights can provide guidance toward the identification of specific genetic backgrounds where the combinations improve selectivity while reducing side effects.

In this section, we present an example of system-level analyses for combination therapy (combinations of a MEK inhibitor and mTOR inhibitor or PI3K inhibitor). First, we explain the genetic backgrounds that are necessary to ensure the efficacy of a compound that inhibits MEK activity. Next, we explain model construction and in silico analyses based on the model.

Genetic Backgrounds Related to Efficacy of a Compound to Inhibit MEK Activity

Mutations in upstream molecules of MEK, particularly Ras and Raf, have been associated with human cancers. KRas and BRAF mutations have been reported in 30% of all human tumors and 40% of melanomas (Hatzivassiliou et al. 2010). Moreover, a BRAF mutation at V600E can confer sensitivity to MEK inhibitors and, thus, can be a useful biomarker for cohort selection in clinical trials of compounds that inhibit MEK activity for melanoma (Solit et al. 2006).

Ras–Raf signaling, however, involves complex regulatory motifs, cross-talk and feedback both upstream and downstream of Ras–Raf. Mechanistic details of such biochemical interactions need to be captured in a systemwide network view to investigate the role of Ras–Raf mutations in melanoma, particularly in the context of selecting patient cohorts for targeted therapeutics.

Figure 13–6A illustrates the dynamic interaction involving Ras–Raf molecules upstream of MEK–ERK1–ERK2, which, under various mutation conditions, can regulate sensitivity (and resistance) to MEK inhibition. As seen in this figure, cRaf can play a critical role in MEK inhibitor sensitivity (Hatzivassiliou et al. 2010; Agren et al. 2012). Nonactivating BRAF mutations (G466E, G466V, G59R) can activate MEK–ERK signaling in a Ras-independent manner through 14–3–3. Furthermore, MEK activation can also be promoted in a Ras-dependent manner in the presence of a KRas (G12D)-driven mutation acting through co-operating oncogene BRAF (D594A) mutations, as highlighted in Figure 13–6A.

In summary, the analysis reveals several modes of MEK activation independent of BRAF(V600E)-driven mutations through signaling across other pathway components like cRaf and 14–3–3. Apart from mutational status, gene

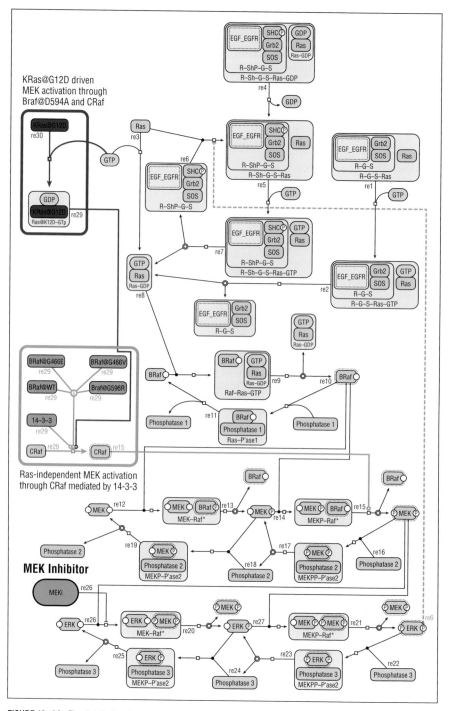

FIGURE 13–6A. The detailed molecular interaction network for BRAF signaling. This figure represents the detailed dynamic interaction network involving Ras–Raf molecules upstream of MEK–ERK1/2 under various mutation conditions.

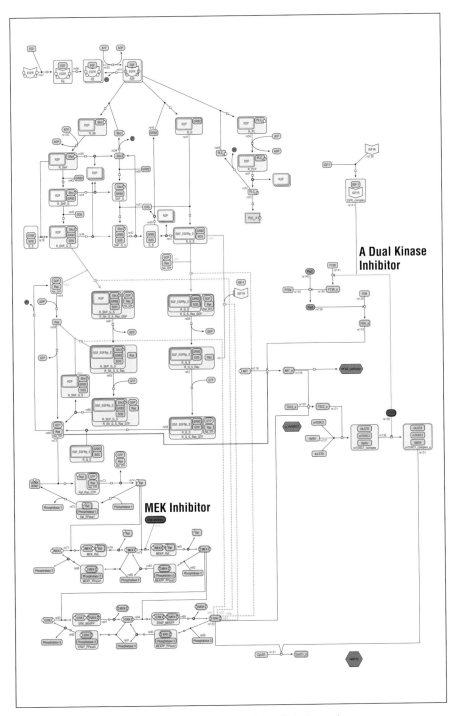

A Dual Kinase Inhibitor

MEK Inhibitor

FIGURE 13–6B. Dynamic model of the pathways capturing their genetic backgrounds.

amplification can play a role in determining sensitivity or resistance to MEK activation as analyzed in a study in melanoma cell lines (Corcoran et al. 2010). Thus, systematic genetic profiling of Ras–Raf components can facilitate selection of patient cohorts for increasing the efficacy of a MEK inhibitor in mono- or combination therapy.

In Silico Analysis of Combination Therapies: An Illustrative Case Study

In this section, we elucidate how network-driven analysis of cross-talk and feed-back loops in molecular pathways combined with dynamic modeling and simulation can provide potential hypotheses for combination therapy regimens as well as enable network-based stratification. We developed a dynamic model to capture the known biology of major interactions of the Ras–Raf–Mek–Erk pathway and PI3K–AKT–mTOR pathway as reported in the literature and existing model results. The model is based on the melanoma cell-line model that captures the mutational status of BRAF and phosphatase and tensin homolog (PTEN) molecules. Feedback loops also cross-talk between the pathways and were captured in the model, particularly the negative feedback regulation from S6K1 upstream of PI3K. Figure 13–6B shows the dynamic model of the pathways capturing their genetic backgrounds as explained in the previous section. Furthermore, in order to capture the effect of inhibitors along these pathways, the model captures the dynamics in the presence of a combination of two compounds—a MEK inhibitor and a dual kinase inhibitor that inhibits mTOR and PI3K.

The key components in the model are genetic mutations in specific cell lines as well as mathematical encapsulation of feedback control motifs. The model quantitatively captures negative feedback effects on PI3K from S6K1 as well as inhibition by the compounds. The model is constructed using CellDesigner modeling software (Funahashi et al. 2008; Le Novere et al. 2009), and stored in standardized Systems Biology Markup Language (SBML) format (Hucka et al. 2003), which allows it to be simulated by standard ordinary differential equation (ODE) solver engines supporting SBML format (Blinov et al. 2004; Hoops et al. 2006). The SBML ODE Solver Library (SOSLib) as used for the current simulation results. Based on the mathematical model, the temporal dynamics of the system are considered under different drug regimens over a 1-hour period of simulated time.

Next, we elucidate the model-based analysis obtained from combination studies involving a MEK inhibitor and a dual kinase inhibitor that can inhibit PI3K as well as mTOR. The simulation experiment shows the relative insensitivity to the dual inhibitor's dosage of the cell line in the presence of a given dose of the MEK inhibitor (low and midrange) (Figure 13–7A). As analyzed earlier, the potential release of negative feedback from S6K1 due to inhibition of its up-

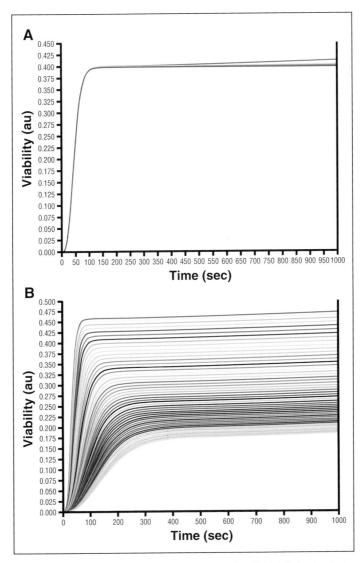

FIGURE 13–7. Results from computer simulations based on the detailed molecular interaction network in Figure 13–6. A, Simulation experiment for dose escalation of dual kinase inhibitors that inhibit PI3K and mTOR. We did the dose escalation on the dual kinase inhibitor from 0 to 25 in steps of 1, while we used one constant dosage of the MEK inhibitor. Each line represents the result of simulations under each dosage combination of the two inhibitors, and thus there are 25 lines. B, Simulation experiment for dose escalation of a compound that inhibits MEK activity. We did the dose escalation on the MEK inhibitor from 0 to 5 in steps of 0.1, while we used one constant dosage of the dual inhibitor. Each line represents the result of simulations under each dosage combination of the two inhibitors, and thus there are 50 lines.

stream mTOR can activate the PI3K driven Ras–Raf–Mek pathway, thereby decreasing the combination's efficacy for a dose escalation of the dual kinase inhibitor (Figure 13–8A).

Next, we performed in silico experiments to investigate the dynamics of the reverse process, viz., dose escalation of a compound that inhibits MEK in the presence of a given dose of the dual kinase inhibitor. As captured in Figures 13–7B and 13–8B, addition of a MEK inhibitor sensitizes the model to the dual inhibitor. It may be noted that a relatively low dose of a MEK inhibitor sensitizes the cells to the combination, even when the cells are resistant to monotherapy or using the dual kinase inhibitor. Thus, this model presents a novel mechanism whereby low doses of a MEK inhibitor can increase sensitivity to the dual kinase inhibitor for a dose at which it is ineffective as monotherapy, suggesting that a combination-drug scheduling strategy can increase efficacy without changing the toxicity profiles.

Conclusion

Cancer is a highly complex disease characterized by genomic instability, heterogeneity across and within tumors from different tissue sites or even within the same tissues of origin, and it behaves as a robust dynamic system modified by a wide range of environmental and therapeutic perturbations. With the emergence of high-throughput sequencing of whole cancer genomes as elucidated in the results of TCGA and the associated PanCan, researchers are increasingly able to obtain unprecedented insights into the molecular determinants of the disease. These genomic profiles also reveal the need to revisit the understanding of cancer and associated therapeutic strategies through a new lens beyond the traditional tissue pathology view—the lens of network medicine, in which the molecular pathology of cancer is studied and analyzed in the context of complex -omic interactions as well as between the cancer cells and their environment.

As elucidated in this chapter, computational techniques driving network-guided analytics can provide powerful tools (Ghosh et al. 2011) in understanding the complex dynamics of cancer systems as well as identifying new strategies to overcome the disease (Winslow et al. 2012). This is particularly true in developing the next generation of cancer drugs, where network-driven approaches can facilitate the discovery of targeted therapeutics, enable precise stratification of patient cohorts based on their network biomarkers, and define the optimal combination of drug regimens for patients (Dudley et al. 2011). With the advances in experimental techniques and the ever-increasing big datasets on the molecular pathology of cancer, network-driven computational

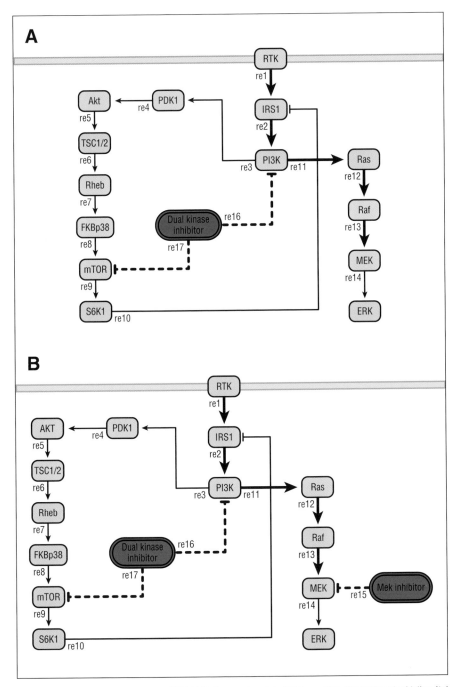

FIGURE 13–8. Role of feedback from S6K1 (p70 ribosomal protein S6 kinase 1) to PI3K (phosphatidylinositol 3-kinase) signaling pathway under monotherapy or combination therapy. A, Dynamics of the pathway under monotherapy with a dual kinase inhibitor that inhibits PI3K and mTOR (mammalian target of rapamycin). B, Dynamics of the pathway under combination therapy with a MEK (MAPK/ERK kinase) inhibitor and the dual kinase inhibitor. Bold arrows represent highly activated regulations.

techniques are uniquely poised to transform clinical oncology from the realm of intuitive medicine to personalized precision medicine (Grove 2011; Kaganovich 2012).

References

Agren, R., S. Bordel, et al. (2012). Reconstruction of genome-scale active metabolic networks for 69 human cell types and 16 cancer types using INIT. PLoS Comput Biol 8(5): e1002518.

Al-Lazikani, B., Banerji, U., et al. P. (2012). Combinatorial drug therapy for cancer in the post-genomic era. Nat Biotech 30(7): 679–92.

Alexandrov, L. B., S. Nik-Zainal, et al. (2013). Signatures of mutational processes in human cancer. Nature 500 (7463): 415–21.

Arrell, D. K., and A. Terzic (2010). Network systems biology for drug discovery. Clin Pharmacol Ther 88 (1):120–25.

Barabási, A. L., N. Gulbahce, et al. (2011). Network medicine: a network-based approach to human disease. Nat Rev Genet 12(1): 56–68.

Barretina, J., G. Caponigro, et al. (2012). The Cancer Cell Line Encyclopedia enables predictive modelling of anticancer drug sensitivity. Nature 483(7391): 603–7.

Basanta, D., and R.A. Anderson. (2013). Exploiting ecological principles to better understand cancer progression and treatment. Interface Focus 3(4): 30130020.

Blinov, M. L., J. R. Faeder, et al. (2004). BioNetGen: software for rule-based modeling of signal transduction based on the interactions of molecular domains. Bioinformatics 20(17):3289–91.

Borisy, A. A., P. J. Elliott, et al. (2003). Systematic discovery of multicomponent therapeutics. Proc Natl Acad Sci U S A 100(13): 7977–82.

Bozic, I., J. G. Reiter, et al. (2013). Evolutionary dynamics of cancer in response to targeted combination therapy. Elife 2: e00747.

Chari, S., and I. Dworkin. (2013). The conditional nature of genetic interactions: the consequences of wild-type backgrounds on mutational interactions in a genome-wide modifier screen. PLoS Genet 9(8): e1003661.

Ciriello, G., M. L. Miller, et al. (2013). Emerging landscape of oncogenic signatures across human cancers. Nat Genet 45(10): 1127–33.

Consortium, TCGA. (2008). Comprehensive genomic characterization defines human glioblastoma genes and core pathways. Nature 455(7216): 1061–68.

Corcoran, R. B., D. Dias-Santagata, et al. (2010). BRAF gene amplification can promote acquired resistance to MEK inhibitors in cancer cells harboring the BRAF V600E mutation. Sci Signal 3(149): ra84.

Ding, L., G. Getz, et al. (2008). Somatic mutations affect key pathways in lung adenocarcinoma. Nature 455(7216): 1069–75.

Dudley, J. T., R. Chen, et al. (2011). Matching cancer genomes to established cell lines for personalized oncology. Pac Symp Biocomput 2011:243–52.

Edwards, L. A., M. Verreault, et al. (2006). Combined inhibition of the phosphatidylinositol 3-kinase/Akt and Ras/mitogen-activated protein kinase pathways results in synergistic effects in glioblastoma cells. Mol Cancer Ther 5(3): 645–54.

Engelman, J. A., L. Chen, et al. (2008). Effective use of PI3K and MEK inhibitors to treat mutant Kras G12D and PIK3CA H1047R murine lung cancers. Nat Med 14(12): 1351–56.

Feldman, I., A. Rzhetsky, et al. (2008). Network properties of genes harboring inherited disease mutations. Proc Natl Acad Sci U S A 105(11): 4323–28.

Fisher, R., L. Pusztai, et al. (2013). Cancer heterogeneity: implications for targeted therapeutics. Br J Cancer 108(3): 479–85.

Folger, O., L. Jerby, et al. (2011). Predicting selective drug targets in cancer through metabolic networks. Mol Syst Biol 7: 501.

Forbes, S. A., N. Bindal, et al. (2011). COSMIC: mining complete cancer genomes in the Catalogue of Somatic Mutations in Cancer. Nucleic Acids Res **39** (Database issue): D945–50.

Funahashi, A., Y. Matsuoka, et al. (2008). CellDesigner 3.5: a versatile modeling tool for biochemical networks. Proc IEEE **96**: 1254–65.

Futreal, P. A., L. Coin, et al. (2004). A census of human cancer genes. Nat Rev Cancer **4**(3): 177–83.

Garraway, L. A., E. S. Lander. (2013). Lessons from the cancer genome. Cell **153**(1): 17–37.

Ghosh, S., Y. Matsuoka, et al. (2011). Software for systems biology: from tools to integrated platforms. Nat Rev Genet **12**(12): 821–32.

Goh, K. I., M. E. Cusick, et al. (2007). The human disease network. Proc Natl Acad Sci U S A **104**(21): 8685–90.

Grove, A. (2011. Rethinking clinical trials. Science **333**(6050):1679.

Guimerá, R., and L.A. Nunes Amaral (2005). Functional cartography of complex metabolic networks. Nature. **433**(7028): 895–900

Hanahan, D., R. A. Weinberg. (2011). Hallmarks of cancer: the next generation. Cell **144**(5): 646–74

Hase, T., and Y. Niimura. (2012). Protein-protein interaction networks: structures, evolution, and application to drug design. In: W. Cai and H. Tong, eds., Protein-Protein Interactions—Computational and Experimental Tools. Rijeka, Croatia: InTech.

Hase, T., H. Tanaka, et al. (2009). Structure of protein interaction networks and their implications on drug design. PLoS Comput Biol **5**(10): e1000550.

Hase, T., Kikuchi K., et al. (2014). Identification of drug-target modules in the human protein-protein interaction network. Artific Life Robot **19**(4): 406–13.

Hatzivassiliou, G., K. Song, et al. (2010). RAF inhibitors prime wild-type RAF to activate the MAPK pathway and enhance growth. Nature **464**(7287): 431–35.

Hofree, M., J. P. Shen, et al. (2013). Network-based stratification of tumor mutations. Nat Methods **10**(11): 1108–15.

Hoops, S., S. Sahle, et al. (2006). COPASI—a COmplex PAthway SImulator. Bioinformatics **22**(24): 3067–74.

Hsu, P. P., D. M. Sabatini. (2008). Cancer cell metabolism: Warburg and beyond. Cell **134**(5): 703–7.

Huang, S. (2013). Genetic and non-genetic instability in tumor progression: link between the fitness landscape and the epigenetic landscape of cancer cells. Cancer Metastas Rev **32**(3–4): 423–48.

Hucka, M., A. Finney, et al. (2003). The systems biology markup language (SBML): a medium for representation and exchange of biochemical network models. Bioinformatics. **19**(4): 524–31.

Jeong, H., S. P. Mason, et al. (2001). Lethality and centrality in protein networks. Nature **411**(6833): 41–42.

Jerby, L., E. Ruppin. (2012). Predicting drug targets and biomarkers of cancer via genome-scale metabolic modeling. Clin Cancer Res **18**(20): 5572–84.

Jones, S., X. Zhang, et al. (2008). Core signaling pathways in human pancreatic cancers revealed by global genomic analyses. Science **321**(5897): 1801–6.

Jonsson, P. F., and P. A. Bates. (2006). Global topological features of cancer proteins in the human interactome. Bioinformatics **22**(18): 2291–97.

Kaganovich, M. (2012). The cloud will cure cancer. (http://techcrunch.com/2012/03/29/cloud-will-cure-cancer).

Kinkade, C. W., M. Castillo-Martin, et al. (2008). Targeting AKT/mTOR and ERK MAPK signaling inhibits hormone-refractory prostate cancer in a preclinical mouse model. J Clin Invest **118**(9): 3051–64.

Kitano, H. (2004). Cancer as a robust system: implications for anticancer therapy. Nat Rev Cancer **4**(3): 227–35.

Lawrence, M. S., P. Stojanov, et al. (2013). Mutational heterogeneity in cancer and the search for new cancer-associated genes. Nature 499 (7457):214–18.

Le Novere, N., M. Hucka, et al. (2009). The systems biology graphical notation. Nat Biotechnol 2 (8):735–41.

Lee, M. J., A. S. Ye, et al. (2012). Sequential application of anticancer drugs enhances cell death by rewiring apoptotic signaling networks. Cell 149(4): 780–94.

Lehar, J., A. S. Krueger, et al. (2009). Synergistic drug combinations tend to improve therapeutically relevant selectivity. Nat Biotechnol 27(7): 659–66.

Lengauer, C., K. W. Kinzler, et al. (1998). Genetic instabilities in human cancers. Nature 396(6712): 643–49.

Liang, H., and W. H. Li (2007). Gene essentiality, gene duplicability and protein connectivity in human and mouse. Trends Genet 23(8): 375–78.

Matsuoka, Y., H. Matsumae, et al. (2013). A comprehensive map of the influenza A virus replication cycle. BMC Syst Biol 7: 97.

Oda, K., Y. Matsuoka, et al. (2005). A comprehensive pathway map of epidermal growth factor receptor signaling. Mol Syst Biol 1: 0010.

Omberg, L., K. Ellrott, et al. (2013). Enabling transparent and collaborative computational analysis of 12 tumor types within The Cancer Genome Atlas. Nat Genet 45(10): 1121–26.

Parsons, D. W., S. Jones, et al. (2008). An integrated genomic analysis of human glioblastoma multiforme. Science 321(5897): 1807–12.

Prendergast, G. C. (2013). Cancer: why tumours eat tryptophan. Nature 478(7368): 192–94.

Reimand, J., and G. D. Bader (2013). Systematic analysis of somatic mutations in phosphorylation signaling predicts novel cancer drivers. Mol Syst Biol 9: 637.

Schadt, E. E., S. H. Friend, et al. (2009). A network view of disease and compound screening. Nat Rev Drug Discov 8(4): 286–95.

Sharma, S. V., D. W. Bell, et al. (2007). Epidermal growth factor receptor mutations in lung cancer. Nat Rev Cancer 7(3): 169–81.

Smalley, K. S., and K. T. Flaherty (2009). Integrating BRAF/MEK inhibitors into combination therapy for melanoma. Br J Cancer 100(3): 431–35.

Solit, D. B., L. A. Garraway, et al. (2006). BRAF mutation predicts sensitivity to MEK inhibition. Nature 439(7074): 358–62.

Straussman, R., T. Morikawa, et al. (2012). Tumour micro-environment elicits innate resistance to RAF inhibitors through HGF secretion. Nature 487(7408): 500–4.

Sun, X., S. Vilar, et al. (2013). High-throughput methods for combinatorial drug discovery. Sci Transl Med. 5(205): 205rv1.

Tamborero, D., A. Gonzalez-Perez, et al. (2013). Comprehensive identification of mutational cancer driver genes across 12 tumor types. Sci Rep 3: 2650.

Thiele, I., N. Swainston, et al. (2013). A community-driven global reconstruction of human metabolism. Nat Biotechnol 31(5): 419–25.

Vander Heiden, M. G. (2011). Targeting cancer metabolism: a therapeutic window opens. Nat Rev Drug Discov 10(9): 671–84.

Vander Heiden, M. G., L. C. Cantley, et al. (2009). Understanding the Warburg effect: the metabolic requirements of cell proliferation. Science 324(5930): 1029–33.

Velenich, A., and J. Gore. (2013). The strength of genetic interactions scales weakly with mutational effects. Genome Biol 14(7): R76.

Vidal, M., M. E. Cusick, et al. (2011). Interactome networks and human disease. Cell 144(6): 986–98.

Vogelstein, B., N. Papadopoulos, et al. (2013). Cancer genome landscapes. Science 339(6127): 1546–58.

Wachi, S., K. Yoneda, et al. (2005). Interactome-transcriptome analysis reveals the high centrality of genes differentially expressed in lung cancer tissues. Bioinformatics 21(23): 4205–8.

Wang, Z., and J. Zhang (2007). In search of the biological significance of modular structures in protein networks. PLoS Comput Biol 3(6): e107.

Weinstein, J. N., E. A. Collisson, et al. (2013). The Cancer Genome Atlas Pan-Cancer analysis project. Nat Genet 45(10): 1113–20

Winslow, R. L., N. Trayanova, et al. (2012). Computational medicine: translating models to clinical care. Sci Transl Med 4(158): 158rv11.

Wood, L. D., D. W. Parsons, et al. (2007). The genomic landscapes of human breast and colorectal cancers. Science 318(5853): 1108–13.

Workman, P., B. Al-Lazikani, et al. (2013). Genome-based cancer therapeutics: targets, kinase drug resistance and future strategies for precision oncology. Curr Opin Pharmacol 13(4): 486–96.

Xu, J., Y. Li. (2006). Discovering disease-genes by topological features in human protein-protein interaction network. Bioinformatics 22(22): 2800–5.

Yao, L., and A. Rzhetsky. (2008). Quantitative systems-level determinants of human genes targeted by successful drugs. Genome Res 18(2): 206–13.

Yu, H., P. Braun, et al. (2008). High-quality binary protein interaction map of the yeast interactome network. Science 322(5898): 104–10.

Zack, T. I., S. E. Schumacher, et al. (2013). Pan-cancer patterns of somatic copy number alteration. Nat Genet 45(10): 1134–40.

14

Systems Pharmacology in Network Medicine

EDWIN K. SILVERMAN AND JOSEPH LOSCALZO

Introduction

Despite continued progress in understanding the molecular and cellular mechanisms of human diseases, the rate of new drug approvals to treat disease has been remarkably stagnant. An extremely small percentage of candidate drugs survive the gauntlet of drug development. These failures are not typically due to inadequacies related to pharmacokinetics; instead, most failures relate to lack of effect on the drug target in vivo, selection of the wrong drug target, or unexpected drug toxicity. Although a reductionist approach to drug discovery has worked well in some cases (e.g., the development of antiretroviral agents for the human immunodeficiency virus [HIV]), the repeated failures of this paradigm in complex diseases indicate that alternative approaches for drug development are needed. Focusing on the identification of a single key molecular target, the primary strategy of reductionist drug development, ignores the complexity of biological systems and disease pathogenesis. Systems pharmacology attempts to improve on this time-honored approach by applying systems biology and network science to identify drug targets, to understand drug action in a network context, and to predict adverse drug effects.

Systems pharmacology leverages many of the principles of network medicine that have been discussed elsewhere in this book. For example, cellular molecular networks have emergent properties that are not apparent if single molecules are studied in isolation; these emergent properties affect drug target selection, therapeutic effects, and off-target effects. Biochemical networks vary by tissue type, genetic variation, disease state, and environmental exposures; thus, understanding the relevant biological networks and their responses to pharmacological perturbations is essential for systems pharmacology. Stochastic effects play an important role in cell-to-cell variability and limit accuracy of biochemical circuits; these effects may directly affect drug efficacy. As complex diseases likely result from multiple genetic, epigenetic, and environmental factors acting in a developmental context, targeting multiple components of disease pathways may be necessary to provide effective treatment.

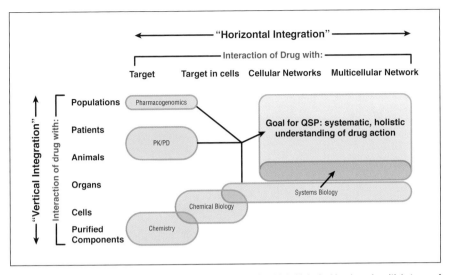

FIGURE 14–1. Overview of systems pharmacology. Integration of multiple biological levels and multiple types of networks with potential drugs can provide a holistic view of drug action in quantitative systems pharmacology (QSP). PK, pharmacokinetics; PD, pharmacodynamics. (Reprinted from Sorger, P.K., S.R.B. Allerheiligen, et al. (2011) at https://www.nigms.nih.gov/training/documents/systemspharmawpsorger2011.pdf. (CC BY-SA 3.0))

A key National Institutes of Health White Paper in 2011 by the Quantitative Systems Pharmacology Workshop Group outlined the challenges and opportunities in this field (Sorger, Allerheiligen, et al. 2011). As shown in Figure 14–1, systems pharmacology provides integration among multiple biological levels and multiple types of biological networks. In this chapter, we will consider how systems pharmacology has the potential to transform drug development and treatment, an essential goal of network medicine.

Using Network Approaches to Select Drug Targets

In conventional drug-development approaches, a single target molecule is selected, and pharmacological responses related to that molecule are assessed (Figure 14–2A) (Loscalzo 2012). Additional network connections to that molecular target are typically unknown and ignored, but they may lead to other biological effects—which may manifest as adverse events. Alternatively, systems pharmacology approaches to drug development focus on multiple molecular targets (Figure 14–2B). Some of the observed responses are desired, and others are not; however, assessment within a network context allows the desired effects to be optimized and the undesired effects to be understood—and potentially predicted.

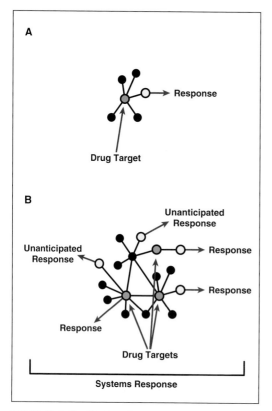

A

Response

Drug Target

B

Unanticipated
Response

Unanticipated
Response

Response

Response

Response

Drug Targets

Systems Response

FIGURE 14–2. Identification of drug targets. Comparison of a conventional drug-development approach (A) and a systems pharmacology approach (B). Nodes (black and blue) represent proteins linked to one another in a protein–protein interaction network, with drug targets in blue; yellow nodes represent responses derived from drug targets directly or indirectly (via another node). (Reprinted with permission from Loscalzo, J. (2012). Personalized cardiovascular medicine and drug development: time for a new paradigm. Circulation **125**(4): 638–45.)

Hopkins described how network approaches to pharmacology could transform drug development (Hopkins 2007). Rather than viewing drug effects on multiple targets as an unwanted problem, network pharmacology recognizes that perturbing multiple biological targets may be necessary for effective disease treatment. Many currently used drugs do have effects on multiple biological targets, including beta-lactam antibiotics and imatinib (Gleevec) (Hopkins 2007). Yildirim and colleagues found that many proteins in the cellular molecular interactome are targeted by more than one existing drug, and that most drugs target multiple proteins (Yildirim, Goh, et al. 2007). They observed that proteins which are drug targets tend to have a larger number of network connections than random proteins, but fewer network connections than proteins that are essential for survival. These network characteristics may assist in the selection of network components for drug development. Hopkins pointed out that the key challenges for network pharmacology are to select the network nodes that need to be perturbed to treat disease and to find pharmacological agents that affect those nodes (Hopkins 2008). Perturbing multiple nodes in a network can occur by using several specific pharmacological agents or by using a single pharmacological agent that impacts multiple relevant targets. More recently, Guney and colleagues developed a network proximity metric based on the closest distance between drug targets and disease-related proteins. Using this metric, they showed that although drugs only target disease genes directly in a minority of cases, drug effects tend to localize to a subset of the disease network module members (Guney, Menche, et al. 2016).

Integration of publicly available datasets like The Cancer Genome Atlas and gene pathway information in a network context can provide unique opportuni-

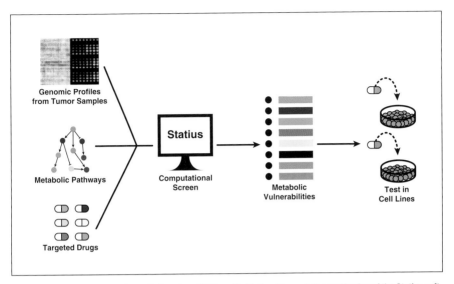

FIGURE 14–3. Identification of metabolic vulnerabilities with Statius. Shown is the application of the Statius software to the integration of multiple types of biological information and identification of potential metabolic vulnerabilities in cancer cell lines. (Reprinted from Aksoy, B. A., E. Demir, et al. (2014). Prediction of individualized therapeutic vulnerabilities in cancer from genomic profiles. Bioinformatics **30**(14): 2051–9. (CC BY 3.0))

ties for drug-target identification. In malignant tumors and cancer cell lines, Aksoy, Demir, and colleagues (2014) studied homozygous genomic deletions, which can create vulnerabilities to drugs that are damaging only to the specific malignant cells carrying those deletions. Their statistical software, called Statius, analyzes genomic deletion information along with publicly available drug-target information, metabolic isoform information, and metabolic enzyme data (Figure 14–3). They studied 4999 tumor samples and 972 cell lines, along with tissue-specific characteristics and information regarding whether those genes were essential for survival. They identified 4104 potential metabolic vulnerabilities in the cancer cells that they studied. Of those vulnerabilities, 44% were predicted to be targets of existing drugs approved by the Food and Drug Administration (FDA); however, only 8% of those drugs are currently approved for cancer treatment.

Metabolic networks have also been used to identify potential antimicrobial drug targets. Chavali, D'Auria, and colleagues (2012) noted that the increasing information regarding metabolic networks in microbial pathogens has provided opportunities for drug-target identification (Figure 14–4). In particular, flux balance analysis (FBA) has enabled more effective models based on reconstructed microbial networks. FBA, which is based on a stoichiometric matrix of coefficients describing the metabolic conversion reactions, allows identification of conditions that maximize flux through a specific targeted reaction. Additional

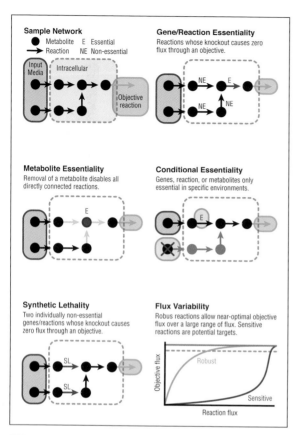

approaches leveraging metabolic networks in microbial pathogens have focused on gene essentiality (demonstration that inactivation of a specific gene prevents flux through a biochemical reaction) and flux variability (which focuses on the extent of variability for a biochemical reaction of interest). As noted in Figure 14–4, other approaches for identifying potential drug targets in metabolic networks include metabolite essentiality, conditional essentiality, and synthetic lethality.

FIGURE 14–4. Using metabolic networks to identify drug targets. Multiple strategies for drug targeting within metabolic networks are shown. (Reprinted with permission from Chavali, A. K., K. M. D'Auria, et al. (2012). A metabolic network approach for the identification and prioritization of antimicrobial drug targets. Trends Microbiol 20(3): 113–23. © 2011 Elsevier Ltd.)

Treatment Approaches Using Multiple Coordinated Drug Targets

Treatment of multiple drug targets in a time-sensitive fashion may be needed to rewire cellular molecular networks and provide effective treatment for complex diseases. Although this principle has been considered primarily in malignant diseases thus far, it is likely also relevant for nonmalignant diseases. Lee, Ye, and colleagues (2012) performed a landmark study to investigate the impact of combination drug treatment in triple-negative breast cancer (i.e., negative for the progesterone receptor, estrogen receptor, and *HER2* oncogene). They hypothesized that the order, schedule, and dose of combination chemotherapy would affect the cytotoxic effects observed in triple-negative breast cancer cell lines. In an investigation that included seven DNA-damaging drugs and eight targeted signaling inhibitors, they found that not only is the application of combination treatment important, but the sequence and timing of the administration of the multiple therapeutic agents is essential for optimal effects. Remarkably, they found that epidermal growth factor receptor (EGFR) inhibition sensitizes a subset of triple-negative breast cancer cell lines to chemotherapeutic agents that act through DNA damage if the drugs are given sequentially but not if they are given simultaneously. As shown in Figure 14–5, when an EGFR inhibitor (erlotinib) was given at least 4 hours before a DNA-damaging drug (doxorubicin), a marked increase in killing of triple-negative breast cancer cells was noted. They also assessed the impact of each chemotherapeutic regimen on the transcriptomic profile of each cell line and discovered that activity of the EGFR pathway, rather than EGFR gene expression itself, was key. They performed functional studies of apoptotic pathways and found that EGFR inhibition causes rewiring of the oncogenic signature with increased apoptosis through a caspase-8-mediated mechanism. All of the breast cancer cell lines (including both triple-negative and nonnegative) were not responsive to this ordered drug treatment combination, demonstrating the impact of disease heterogeneity on ther-

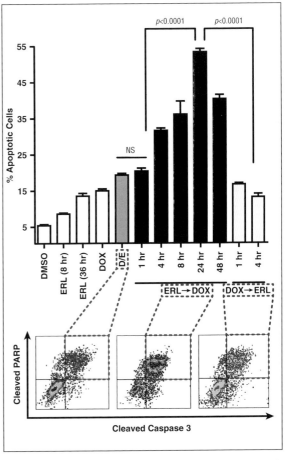

FIGURE 14–5. Impact of timing of coadministration of chemotherapeutic agents. Administration of EGFR inhibitor at least 4 hours before doxorubicin (DOX) provides increased cytotoxic effects in triple-negative breast cancer cells. DMSO, dimethyl sulfoxide; ERL, erlotinib; D/E, doxorubicin and erlotinib added at same time; ERL→DOX, erlotinib administered before doxorubicin; DOX→ERL, doxorubicin administered before erolitinib; NS, not significant; PARP, poly-ADP-ribose polymerase. (Reprinted with permission from Lee, M. J., A. S. Ye, et al. (2012). Sequential application of anticancer drugs enhances cell death by rewiring apoptotic signaling networks. Cell **149**(4): 780–94. © 2012 Elsevier Inc.)

apeutic responses. Since oncogenic signaling networks have multiple levels of feedback, single protein measurements were not able to predict cellular responses to drugs accurately; this is likely also true for complex nonmalignant diseases.

Approaches to understanding cellular molecular network structure and control may assist in the design of rational multidrug regimens for complex diseases. Sturm, Orton, and colleagues (2010) used both mathematical models and

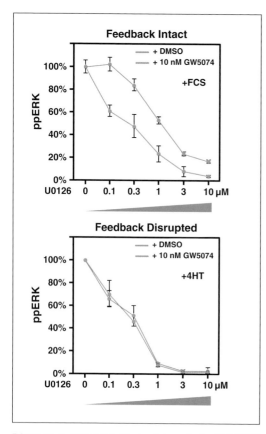

FIGURE 14–6. Differential effects of drugs in the ERK–MAPK pathway. Cooperative effects of a MEK inhibitor (U0126) and a Raf-1 inhibitor (GW5074) on phosphorylated ERK (ppERK) production are noted only when the feedback system is intact (top) and not when it is disrupted with 4-hydroxy-tamoxifen (4HT) (bottom). DMSO, dimethyl sulfoxide; FCS, fetal calf serum. (Reprinted with permission from Sturm, O. E., R. Orton, et al. (2010). The mammalian MAPK/ERK pathway exhibits properties of a negative feedback amplifier. Sci Signal 3(153): ra90.)

experimental validation to demonstrate that the extracellular signal-regulated kinase (ERK)–mitogen-activated protein kinase (MAPK) signaling pathway, which is a key regulator of multiple biological processes, has properties of a negative feedback amplifier. This negative feedback amplifier behavior is created by combining negative feedback loops with a three-tiered cascade of kinases that amplifies biological signals. Negative feedback amplifiers provide resistance to perturbations of the amplifier. These investigators found that this property leads to less effective inhibition when component members of the pathway are targeted than when related external targets are used. Thus, a methyl ethyl ketone (MEK) inhibitor, which targets the ERK–MAPK pathway directly, is less effective at inhibiting this pathway than an EGFR inhibitor; however, when the negative feedback amplifier is pharmacologically disabled, the MEK inhibitor provides potent inhibition of phosphorylated kinase ERK (ppERK) production. In addition to using external targets, an alternative pharmacological strategy is to inhibit the negative feedback amplifier in conjunction with ERK–MAPK inhibition. As shown in Figure 14–6, inhibiting the negative feedback amplifier with a Raf-1 inhibitor (GW5074) provided increased sensitivity to a MEK inhibitor (U0126) only when the feedback system was intact. This study demonstrates that careful biological delineation of regulatory networks can direct the selection of pharmacological targets and suggest biologically effective drug combinations (rational polypharmacy).

Although the use of multidrug combination treatments for both malignant and nonmalignant diseases is appealing, it remains uncertain as to how best to construct such therapeutic regimens.

Garmaroudi and colleagues (2016) developed one such approach using a targeted system in the nitric oxide-guanylyl cyclase pathway. They defined 13 reactions in that pathway whose kinetic constants are known and used a deterministic ODE model together with combinatorial inhibition of single, paired, and triple reactions to determine the optimal combination of reactions to inhibit in order to optimize cyclic GMP production. The computationally identified combination was then tested experimentally, confirming its benefits. Zhang, Birtwistle, and colleagues (2014) proposed another approach for developing multidrug cancer chemotherapy regimens that uses both pharmacokinetic and enhanced pharmacodynamic modeling methods. They demonstrated the application of this approach using the vascular endothelial growth factor receptor (VEGFR2) pathway, which is essential for tumor angiogenesis. Their procedure begins by building a biochemical network based on the scientific literature using ordinary differential equations; their VEGFR2 model included 40 biochemical reactions. Next, a set of parameter estimates (rate constants and protein abundances) is selected from the literature, and the dynamic responses of the network to variation in the levels of different component signaling molecules are assessed. Although the authors recognize the challenges of selecting appropriate parameter values (i.e., the five intracellular protein concentrations and the true intracellular rate constants), they contend that systems biology models are typically not sensitive to a moderate degree of parameter misspecification. An approach known as global Sobal sensitivity analysis is then used to select the molecular targets most likely to be susceptible to pharmacological perturbation within the biochemical network. In addition to sunitinib, which binds directly to the VEGFR active site, four other chemotherapeutic agents were selected. Finally, optimization-based control methods are used to develop specific combination drug regimens over a 28-day chemotherapy cycle. Thus, in a regimen that included daily sunitinib treatment, one of the other chemotherapeutic agents (bevacizumab, an inhibitory antibody which binds VEGF) was excluded from the final regimen. An intriguing aspect of this method is that the therapeutic components can be modified based on specific genomic or other unique characteristics of the individual patient's tumor. For example, including a mutation that removed phosphatidylinositol-3,4,5-triphosphate 3-phosphatase (PTEN) led to marked dosage adjustments for all five of the selected chemotherapeutic agents, including a high dose of bevacizumab on day 1. Although extensive validation will be required, these examples of this framework demonstrate that systems biology methods have the potential to guide the development and selection of combination chemotherapy regimens. Taken together, these and other approaches suggest that rational polypharmacy developed through systems pharmacology holds promise for successful therapeutics.

Using -omics Approaches to Select Drug Targets
and as Indicators of Drug Efficacy

When analyzed in a network context, -omics data have the potential to assist in the selection of drug targets. For example, Zeidan-Chulia, de Oliveira, and colleagues (2014) performed a focused gene expression analysis of genes involved in Alzheimer's disease, as well as NOTCH, WNT, and apoptosis pathways, in cerebellar brain tissue samples from patients with autism; they found that a high percentage of these genes (31%) showed differential expression in autistic brains. They generated a network of genes in these four pathways using the STRING database with Cytoscape, and they identified the central components of this network. They next evaluated 47 drugs that have been used or proposed for use in autism. Based on the number of genes in the network targeted by these drugs—especially for the genes that were centrally located in the network and that showed differential expression in autistic brain tissue—they contend that rapamycin and magnesium are the most promising candidates for the treatment of autism.

Although advances in dealing with batch effects and other contributors to noisy data in gene expression analysis have led to improvements in concordance between transcriptomic analyses of similar cellular and tissue samples, there are still substantial challenges in identifying likely drug targets based on gene expression analysis. Haibe-Kains, El-Hachem, and colleagues (2013) compared gene expression profiles and drug response assays in two large pharmacogenomic studies of cancer cell lines, the Cancer Genome Project and the Cancer Cell Line Encyclopedia. They focused on the overlapping set of 15 anticancer drugs and 471 cell lines that were studied in both projects. They found generally high correlations in the genome-wide gene expression measurements performed in the overlapping cell lines from these two studies, despite the use of different versions of the Affymetrix GeneChip. However, when they compared drug sensitivity measurements for the 15 anticancer drugs in the 471 common cell lines, they noted generally poor correlations between the drug responses measured in these two studies. There were multiple study design differences between these two investigations in the drug sensitivity measurements, including assay types, drug concentrations, and summary statistics, that likely contributed to these inconsistencies. Owing to these irreproducible drug sensitivity measurements, poor correlations between the gene expression and drug sensitivity measures were observed in these two studies. The authors contend that improvements in the approaches and standards used for drug sensitivity measurements will be needed in order for transcriptomic analysis to be useful for drug response prediction.

Wang and Loscalzo (2016) used a protein-protein interactome-based analysis to explore the relationships between drug targets, diseases, and drug target interactors to identify novel applications of drugs to diseases for which they were not developed (i.e., drug repurposing) and to identify potential off-target toxicities of drugs. Using myocardial infarction as a case study, they developed a bipartite network of myocardial infarction disease proteins and drug targets and derived 12 drug-target disease modules that give novel insights into therapeutic strategies for this disease. They also indicated that this approach can be generalized to any disease or drug compilation.

In addition to transcriptomics, other -omics approaches, like proteomics, may be important tools for identifying the patients most likely to have a beneficial treatment response and/or to understand drug efficacy (or lack thereof). Individual protein biomarkers have already been used to stratify patients for clinical trials; for example, selection of subjects based on C-reactive protein (CRP) levels was performed in the Justification for the Use of Statins in Prevention: an Intervention Trial Evaluating Rosuvastatin (JUPITER) randomized clinical trial, which demonstrated that rosuvastatin provided marked risk reduction for vascular events among individuals with elevated CRP levels (Ridker, Danielson, et al. 2008). Larger scale proteomics analyses in clinical trials have been reported in small study populations, including assessment of the impact of different diets on peripheral blood mononuclear cell protein levels in a subset of LIPGENE study participants (Diet, Genomics, and Metabolic Syndrome: An Integrated Nutrition, Agro-food, Social, and Economic Analysis) (Rangel-Zuniga, Camargo, et al., 2015). In addition, proteome-wide analysis of a letrozole-resistant breast cancer cell line identified several potentially relevant biological pathways involved in letrozole-resistant breast cancer (Tilghman, Townley, et al. 2013). Aromatase inhibitors like letrozole are frequently used in postmenopausal breast cancer treatment regimens, but aromatase resistance limits their therapeutic utility. Therefore, Tilghman and colleagues performed quantitative proteomic analysis of 1743 proteins in a comparison between two different breast cancer cell lines: a control cell line that had been transfected with the aromatase gene and this same cell line that had been exposed to letrozole in xenograft culture for more than 1 year in ovariectomized nude mice. Trypsin digestion followed by mass spectrometry identified 863 proteins with significantly different levels of expression between these two cell lines. Pathway analysis of proteins with differential expression levels (Figure 14–7) revealed multiple proteins related to the actin cytoskeleton. The authors speculated that Rho-ROCK signaling could be mediating the observed changes in cell motility, and treating the cells with a ROCK inhibitor partially reversed the defect in cell migration. Although this study is limited by the relatively small fraction of the proteome that

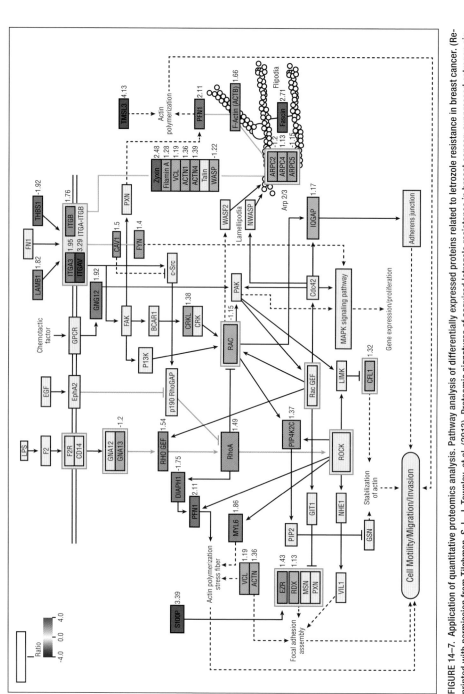

FIGURE 14–7. Application of quantitative proteomics analysis. Pathway analysis of differentially expressed proteins related to letrozole resistance in breast cancer. (Reprinted with permission from Tilghman, S. L. I. Townley, et al. (2013). Proteomic signatures of acquired letrozole resistance in breast cancer: suppressed estrogen signaling and increased cell motility and invasiveness. Mol Cell Proteomics 12(9): 2440–55.)

was investigated, it demonstrates the potential of proteomic studies to provide insights into drug resistance—and the identification of molecular targets to reverse drug resistance.

If -omics measurements are going to be useful tools for patient stratification or clinical outcomes in pharmacological trials, developing standards for the application of -omics data in clinical trials will be essential. Following an Institute of Medicine report on this topic, the National Cancer Institute conducted a workshop that led to 30 specific recommendations regarding biological specimens, assay requirements, data analysis, clinical trial design, and ethical/legal/social issues that need to be addressed in order for -omics measurements to guide clinical trials (McShane, Cavenagh, et al. 2013a, b). Biological specimen issues included consideration of whether the sample type, quantity, and handling requirements that were used in the research studies that identified the specific -omics measure could realistically be obtained in a clinical trial. Assay requirements include quality metrics, such as accuracy, precision, sensitivity, and specificity, as well as the development of standard operating procedures for the performance of these assays. Careful assessments of the data analysis approaches used to implicate the -omics measurement are required, including consideration of whether model overfitting (a common challenge when the number of parameters modeled exceeds the number of samples measured) could be involved. If an -omics assay is proposed for use in the guidance of treatments in a clinical trial, FDA approval may be required.

Understanding Off-Target Effects of Drugs in a Network Context

In addition to the development of more effective therapeutic regimens, another goal of systems pharmacology is to understand and minimize off-target drug effects. Bioinformatic analysis of large, publicly available datasets may provide useful insights regarding adverse drug events. Automated filtering of pharmacoepidemiology data by Bauer-Mehren, van Mullingen, and colleagues (2012) showed the power of combining medical informatics and bioinformatics to identify and understand adverse drug events. These investigators used a two-staged approach of signal filtering and signal substantiation to identify relationships between drugs and adverse drug reactions. Their signal filtering is based on text mining of previously reported relationships between a drug and an adverse reaction. Their signal substantiation procedure attempts to provide insight into the biological mechanisms for the adverse event by assessing for similarities in proteins related to both the drug and the adverse event or by determining whether drug metabolites are related to the adverse event either directly or through their biological network partners. The authors' goal is to find shared biological pathways for the drug and the clinical event of interest. They applied their approach to the risk of a prolonged electrocardiographic QT interval (a harbinger of sudden cardiac death), which has been associated with some anti-psychotic medications, among many other drug classes. For haloperidol, which has a high risk of QT prolongation, close connections of both the drug and the clinical event to the HERG protein (a potassium channel encoded by *KCNH2*) were identified. This biochemical mechanism had been previously reported, and *KCNH2* mutations have been associated with some cases of the genetically determined long-QT syndrome. Novel mechanistic relationships identified with these bioinformatic approaches become testable hypotheses for focused experimentation.

Large bioinformatics databases of reported drug adverse events, created by the FDA and other governmental regulatory agencies, are typically based on self-report by physicians, pharmaceutical companies, and patients; thus, they are susceptible to multiple types of bias. Tatonetti, Ye, and colleagues (2012) noted that relevant biases in these databases include underreporting of adverse events by clinicians; effects of diagnostic indication (e.g., hyperglycemia is often reported with antidiabetic agents but likely relates to the underlying diabetes rather than the drug); medications that are frequently co-administered with the drug of interest; and patient characteristics such as age and sex. They developed a method based on propensity score analysis, which matches patients who are taking a medication of interest to other patients who are not taking that medi-cation; their approach limited the effects of many of the biases noted above in adverse event reports, including effects of unmeasured factors. Using this ap-proach, they created a database of predicted drug–drug interactions, and they found a potential interaction between thiazide diuretics and serotonin reuptake inhibitors on QT prolongation.

By describing the network of genes and proteins affected by a drug of interest, systems pharmacology has the potential to make systematic predictions re-garding likely off-target effects of new drugs. Huang, Wu, and colleagues (2011) demonstrated the utility of including information based on biological pathways (gene ontology) or protein–protein interaction networks (PPI) in predicting ad-verse drug effects. Their overall procedure, shown in Figure 14–8, begins with known drug-target interactions, which are expanded to include related genes based on gene ontology (GO) or PPI (from the HAPPI (Human Annotated and Predicted Protein Interaction) database) information. Adverse drug reaction information related to this expanded set of targets is analyzed to select a set of key features; either statistical (logistic regression) or machine learning (sup-port vector machine) approaches are then used to generate a predictive model of likely adverse events. Tenfold cross-validation is used to test model performance. Using cardiotoxicity as a key adverse drug effect, these authors demonstrated that inclusion of either GO or PPI network information leads to significant improvements in prediction accuracy. For example, use of PPI information with support vector machine analysis increased the area under the curve for the prediction of adverse cardiotoxic drug reactions as compared with no network information from 0.579 to 0.771. In their analyses, support vector machine models typically performed better than logistic-regression models.

As noted above, drug combinations will likely form the basis for many systems pharmacology therapeutic regimens. A study by Zhao and colleagues suggested that utilization of specific combinations of drugs may also be able to limit adverse drug effects. Zhao, Nishimura, and colleagues (2013) used the FDA Adverse Event Reporting System (FAERS) database to

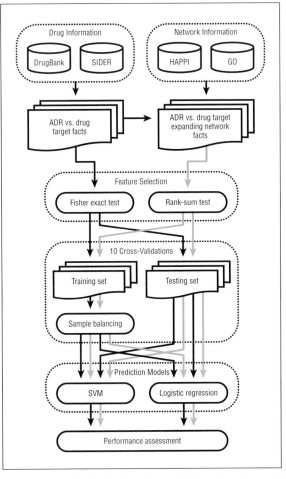

FIGURE 14–8. Prediction of off-target drug effects using pathway and network approaches. Approach to the integration of the protein–protein interaction network (HAPPI) or gene ontology (GO) along with drug (Drug-Bank) and drug adverse effects (SIDER) information to predict off-target drug effects. ADR, adverse drug reactions; SVM, support vector machines. (Reprinted from Huang, L. C., X. Wu, et al. (2011). Predicting adverse side effects of drugs. BMC Genomics 12(Suppl 5): S11. (CC BY 2.0))

confirm that rosiglitazone, a drug used to treat diabetes mellitus, is associated with a significantly increased risk of cardiovascular events, including myocardial infarction (MI) and stroke. They also used the FAERS database to identify drugs that were associated with a reduction in rosiglitazone-related MIs and found that co-administration of exenatide (another antidiabetic drug) reduced the rate of rosiglitazone-related MIs from 34.0% to 2.1%. Although the FAERS data are subject to a variety of biases, this exenatide effect was robust to adjustment for a range of potential confounding variables. Zhao, Nishimura, and colleagues then used cell biological networks based on gene regulatory and protein–protein interaction information related to the known rosiglitazone target (peroxisome proliferator–activated receptor gamma) to implicate thrombosis as a likely biological process for the rosiglitazone–exenatide interaction. They also identified plasminogen activator inhibitor-1 (PAI-1) as a potential molecular mediator for this interaction. Murine studies in spontaneously diabetic (*db/db*) mice confirmed that exenatide leads to a reduction in PAI-1 levels when co-administered with rosiglitazone, along with differences in blood clot characteristics (clot formation time and maximum clot firmness). Although this rosiglitazone–exenatide relationship will need to be confirmed in prospective clinical trials, this work demonstrates the potential utility of bioinformatic and network medicine approaches to identify combinations of drugs that can minimize adverse drug effects.

Conclusion

Systems pharmacology and network medicine have the potential to transform drug development. As shown in Figure 14–9, traditional drug development for a disease is focused on the selection of a single key molecular target, which is studied in cellular and animal model systems (Silverman and Loscalzo 2013). Human clinical trials follow a prescribed regulatory pathway from safety to dose

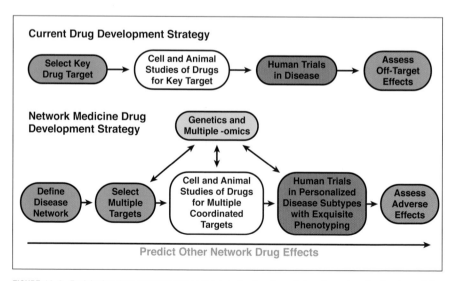

FIGURE 14–9. Envisioning drug development in the era of network medicine. Current and network medicine approaches to drug development for complex diseases are compared. (Reprinted with permission from Silverman, E. K., and J. Loscalzo (2013). Developing new drug treatments in the era of network medicine. Clin Pharmacol Ther **93**(1): 26–8.)

determination and efficacy. Off-target effects are often not identified until late in the drug-development process, and they can lead to abandonment of an otherwise promising therapeutic agent. A drug-development pipeline based on network medicine and systems pharmacology would begin by defining the disease network module within the cellular molecular interactome, with the selection of multiple molecular targets that would be studied in a coordinated manner in cellular and animal models. Genomic and other types of -omics information would be used to tailor therapeutic regimens and provide readouts of drug efficacy. As Chen and Butte (2013) point out, the rapidly expanding array of publicly available -omics data will provide an invaluable resource in network medicine drug development. Human clinical trials would involve comprehensive phenotyping using imaging and novel phenotyping approaches to identify subsets of patients within heterogeneous complex diseases that are most likely to benefit from the therapeutic regimen. This detailed phenotyping will be an essential feature of successful systems pharmacology approaches as better and more direct links between perturbed molecular pathways and precise phenotypes will improve the therapeutic efficacy of drug-development strategies. Adverse drug effects would be predicted largely based on network relationships—and potentially mitigated by carefully selected drug combinations—rather than unexpected and unwelcome surprises. However, realization of this goal will likely require a major change in philosophy and approach throughout much of the pharmaceutical industry. Perhaps a first step would be to use -omics data as early readouts of likely drug efficacy, since the decision about whether to move forward with a drug in early stages is expensive and difficult.

References

Aksoy, B. A., E. Demir, et al. (2014). Prediction of individualized therapeutic vulnerabilities in cancer from genomic profiles. Bioinformatics 30(14): 2051–59.

Bauer-Mehren, A., E. M. van Mullingen, et al. (2012). Automatic filtering and substantiation of drug safety signals. PLoS Comput Biol 8(4): e1002457.

Chavali, A. K., K. M. D'Auria, et al. (2012). A metabolic network approach for the identification and prioritization of antimicrobial drug targets. Trends Microbiol 20(3): 113–23.

Chen, B., and A. J. Butte (2013). Network medicine in disease analysis and therapeutics. Clin Pharmacol Ther 94(6): 627–29.

Garmaroudi, F. S., D. E. Handy, et al. (2016). Systems pharmacology and rational polypharmacy: nitric oxide-cyclic GMP signaling pathway as an illustrative example and derivation of the general case. PLoS Comput Biol 12(3): e1004822.

Guney, E., J. Menche, et al. (2016). Network-based *in silico* drug efficacy screening. Nature Communications 7:10331.

Haibe-Kains, B., N. El-Hachem, et al. (2013). Inconsistency in large pharmacogenomic studies. Nature 504(7480): 389–93.

Hopkins, A.L. (2007). Network pharmacology. Nature Biotechology 25(10): 1110–11.

Hopkins, A.L. (2008). Network pharmacology : the next paradigm in drug discovery. Nature Chemical Biology 4(11): 682–90.

Huang, L. C., X. Wu, et al. (2011). Predicting adverse side effects of drugs. BMC Genomics 12(Suppl 5): S11.

Lee, M. J., A. S. Ye, et al. (2012). Sequential application of anticancer drugs enhances cell death by rewiring apoptotic signaling networks. Cell 149(4): 780–94.

Loscalzo, J. (2012). Personalized cardiovascular medicine and drug development: time for a new paradigm. Circulation 125(4): 638–45.

McShane, L. M., M. M. Cavenagh, et al. (2013a). Criteria for the use of omics-based predictors in clinical trials. Nature 502(7471): 317–20.

McShane, L. M., M. M. Cavenagh, et al. (2013b). Criteria for the use of omics-based predictors in clinical trials: explanation and elaboration. BMC Med 11: 220.

Rangel-Zuniga, O.A., A. Camargo, et al. (2015). Proteome from patients with metabolic syndrome is regulated by quantity and quality of dietary lipids. BMC Genomics 16: 509.

Ridker, P. M., E. Danielson, et al. (2008). Rosuvastatin to prevent vascular events in men and women with elevated C-reactive protein. N Engl J Med 359(21): 2195–207.

Silverman, E. K., and J. Loscalzo (2013). Developing new drug treatments in the era of network medicine. Clin Pharmacol Ther 93(1): 26–28.

Sorger, P. K., S. R. B. Allerheiligen, et al. (2011). Quantitative and Systems Pharmacology in the Post-genomic Era: New Approaches to Discovering Drugs and Understanding Therapeutic Mechanisms. An NIH White Paper by the QSP Working Group available at https://www.nigms.nih.gov/training/documents/systemspharmawpsorger2011.pdf, pp. 1–47.

Sturm, O. E., R. Orton, et al. (2010). The mammalian MAPK/ERK pathway exhibits properties of a negative feedback amplifier. Sci Signal 3(153): ra90.

Tatonetti, N. P., P. P. Ye, et al. (2012). Data-driven prediction of drug effects and interactions. Sci Transl Med 4(125): 125ra31.

Tilghman, S. L., I. Townley, et al. (2013). Proteomic signatures of acquired letrozole resistance in breast cancer: suppressed estrogen signaling and increased cell motility and invasiveness. Mol Cell Proteomics 12(9): 2440–55.

Wang, R. S., and J. Loscalzo (2016). Illuminating drug action by network integration of disease genes: A case study of myocardial infarction. Mol Biosyst 12(5): 1653–66.

Yildirim M.A., K.-I. Goh, et al. (2007). Drug-target network. Nature Biotechnology 25(10): 1119–26.

Zeidan-Chulia, F., B. H. de Oliveira, et al. (2014). Altered expression of Alzheimer's disease-related genes in the cerebellum of autistic patients: a model for disrupted brain connectome and therapy. Cell Death Dis 5: e1250.

Zhang, X. Y., M. R. Birtwistle, et al. (2014). A general network pharmacodynamic model-based design pipeline for customized cancer therapy applied to the VEGFR pathway. CPT Pharmacometrics Syst Pharmacol 3: e92.

Zhao, S., T. Nishimura, et al. (2013). Systems pharmacology of adverse event mitigation by drug combinations. Sci Transl Med 5(206): 206ra140.

15

Systems Approaches to Clinical Trials

ELLIOTT M. ANTMAN

Introduction

In 1965, Gordon Moore predicted that, with unit costs falling, there would be a dramatic increase in the number of transistors that could be squeezed onto a silicon chip (Moore 1965). The explosion of technological advances in electronics and computer hardware validated Moore's prediction and led to contemporary smartphones and tablet devices. The same pattern has not been seen in the development of novel technologies designed to improve human health. While some successes are being reported in the development of new medical devices, the biomedical literature is replete with articles describing a steady decrease in the number of new drugs introduced into clinical medicine despite extensive commitment of vast research and development (R&D) financial resources. Scannell and colleagues have even pointed out a negative slope in the numbers of new drugs per billion dollars (U.S.) of R&D spending between 1950 and 2010—a situation opposite to the slope Moore described; hence they named it Eroom's law (writing "Moore" backward).

Possible approaches to changing the slope of Eroom's law include: (1) developing new approaches to target discovery, identification, and validation (Lindsay 2003; Rawlins 2004; Fox, Farr-Jones, et al. 2006; Orloff, Douglas, et al. 2009); (2) capitalizing on the benefits of a team approach through consortia of academic centers; (National Center for Advancing Translational Sciences); (3) enhancing industry–academic relationships (National Center for Advancing Translational Sciences; Allison 2012); (4) utilizing creative approaches to regulatory science (Buckman, Huang, et al. 2007; Lesko 2007; Lumpkin, Eichler, et al. 2012); and (5) using biological insights to improve the design of clinical trials (Antman, Weiss, et al. 2012). Advances in systems biology, systems pharmacology, and computational biology—all essential elements of Network Medicine—position biomedical investigators especially well to act on the first and last approach noted above; this chapter will focus on the last approach, improvements in clinical trial design. Expanding on concepts originally introduced more broadly in a review on systems pharmacology, pharmacogenetics, and clinical trial design in network medicine, (Antman, Weiss, et al. 2012), this chapter will address how insights derived from a network medicine approach may inform clinical trial designs to develop new treatments for human disease more efficiently.

Network Medicine and Clinical Trial Design

Modeling and Simulation

Application of a network medicine approach to drug development now allows investigators to adopt the "learn and confirm" approach introduced by Sheiner, Beal, and colleagues (1989). In the first major learn–confirm cycle, Sheiner notes that investigators learn what dose is tolerated in normal subjects (phase 1) and confirm that such a dose shows early promising efficacy findings in patients with the disease of interest (phase 2A). This is followed by the second-more complex learn–confirm cycle in which additional exploration of the efficacy–safety balance is performed in patients (phase 2B) before a large confirmatory, registration-pathway trial is undertaken (phase 3). The goal is to incorporate all of the information that affects a patient's response along the prognostic factor axis and all of the controllable aspects of a drug regimen along another axis to define a therapeutic response surface in which benefit is maximized and risk is minimized (Figure 15–1) (Sheiner, Beal, et al. 1989). Incorporating the detailed findings from genetics, -omics research, data on post-translational processing, and epigenetics greatly enhances our understanding of the prognostic-factor axis. Merging such information with data from systems biology and systems pharmacology enhances our understanding of the perturbations of a network imposed by a drug regimen and permits a holistic model of the therapeutic response surface (Lee, Chu, et al. 2011; van der Graaf 2012). A contemporary construct that builds on the learn–confirm model and incorporates the new concepts discussed above is model-based drug development (Figure 15–2) (Miller, Ewy, et al. 2005; Lalonde, Kowalski, et al. 2007; Milligan, Brown, et al. 2013), an approach that uses a process of continually updating a model to refine decision making (Zineh and Woodcock 2013).

Model-based drug development relies heavily on clinical pharmacology and pharmacometrics (van der Graaf 2012; Zineh and Woodcock 2013). The latter refers to the science of mathematical modeling to characterize and predict a drug's pharmacokinetic and pharmacodynamic behavior (van der Graaf 2012). An example from the development of a drug for the management of type 2 diabetes mellitus will illustrate many of the principles involved in this model-based approach. While fasting plasma glucose (FPG) is often used as a short-term biomarker of glycemic control, the use of glycated hemoglobin (HbA_{1c}) is preferable as a biomarker for long-term glycemic control. A mechanistic model de-

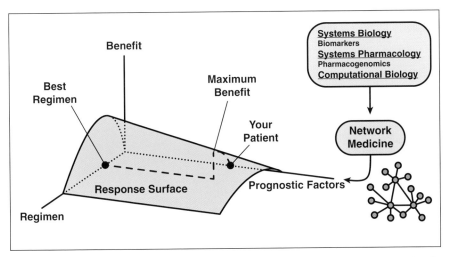

FIGURE 15–1. Using biologic insights to optimize selection of therapeutics. The therapeutic response surface for a given drug relates patient prognostic factors (such as sex, age, and weight) and dose regimen (amount and timing) to benefit, the net utility of efficacy, and toxicity. A plane perpendicular to the prognostic axis at the value of "your" patient intersects the surface forming a curve (as shown). The optimal regimen for a given patient is that corresponding to the maximum of this curve on the benefit axis (here, the value on the maximum benefit position on the surface). Biologic insights from systems biology and systems pharmacology, coupled with advances in computational biology, all contribute to a network view of disease and how the network might be perturbed by an intervention (bottom right). These insights allow contemporary investigators to develop a holistic model of the therapeutic response surface. (Adapted with permission from Sheiner, L.B. (1997). Learning versus confirming in clinical drug development. Clin Pharmacol Ther **61**(3): 275–91.)

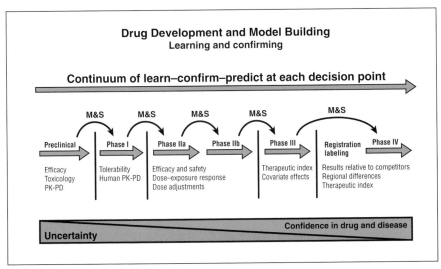

FIGURE 15–2. Model-based drug development. Modeling and simulation (M&S) are performed before each decision point to quantitatively assess the risk of moving forward. The drug and disease model is continuously updated to include new information acquired during drug development. PK, pharmacokinetics; PD, pharmacodynamics. (Adapted with permission from Lalonde, R. L., K. G. Kowalski, et al. (2007). Model-based drug development. Clin Pharmacol Ther **82**(1): 21–32.)

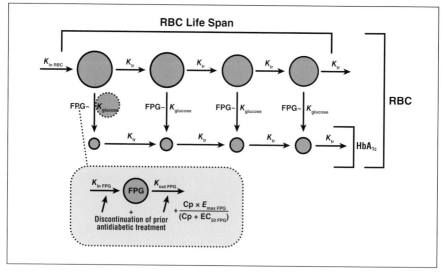

FIGURE 15–3A. Schematic representation of the mechanism-based model for the FPG–HbA$_{1c}$ relationship. In the plasma, the concentration (Cp) versus FPG effect is described by a sigmoidal E_{maxFPG} function including E_{maxFPG}, the maximum effect on K_{outFPG} the first-order degradation rate constant of FPG and EC$_{50FPG}$, the plasma concentration achieving half-maximal effect on E_{maxFPG}. Red blood cell (RBC) maturation is described by K_{inRBC}, a zero-order rate constant of RBC release in blood circulation, and K_{tr}, a first-order transit rate constant between each maturation stage. The FPG model includes a zero-order production rate constant of FPG and a glycosylation rate $K_{glucose}$ of RBCs to yield HbA$_{1c}$. FPG, fasting plasma glucose; HbA$_{1c}$, glycated hemoglobin. (Adapted with permission from Hamren, B., E. Bjork, et al. (2008). Models for plasma glucose, HbA1c, and hemoglobin interrelationships in patients with type 2 diabetes following tesaglitazar treatment. Clin Pharmacol Ther **84**(2): 228–35.)

scribing the interplay between release and aging of red blood cells (RBCs), the impact of a dual peroxisome proliferator–activated receptor (PPAR) α/γ agonist on FPG, and the rate of glycoslyation of the hemoglobin in RBCs over their lifespan is shown in Figure 15–3A. This construct uses a one-compartment model with first-order absorption and elimination to describe the drug plasma concentration, an E_{max} model of its effects on FPG, and a first-order transit rate constant between four stages of RBC maturation (Hamren, Bjork, et al. 2008; Karlsson, Vong, et al. 2013). The nonlinear mixed-effects model shown in Figure 15–3A can be used to test the null hypothesis of no drug effect versus the alternative hypothesis of a drug effect—a useful tool during the proof-of-concept (POC) phase of drug development (Karlsson, Vong, et al. 2013). This example of a network medicine approach and a pharmacometrics model is more efficient than a classical POC design with a placebo and active arm (Karlsson, Vong, et al. 2013). The pharmacometrics model yielded a smaller sample size by a factor of 8.4 for a power of 80% as compared with a standard *t*-test–based power calculation (see Figure 15–3B) (Karlsson, Vong, et al. 2013).

Modeling and simulation (Fusaro, Patil, et al. 2013) are contemporary tools from network medicine that can be used to design clinical trials. Warfarin, a commonly used oral anticoagulant, requires regular monitoring of a patient's blood coagulation status using the international normalized ratio (INR). Adjusting the dose of warfarin requires an integrated assessment of a subject's demographics, genotype (for metabolizing warfarin [CYP2C9] and the functionality of their vitamin K epoxide reductase subunit 1 [VKORC1]), and concomitantly administered medications. Since the percent of time the INR is in the therapeutic range (TTR) is a metric used to judge the quality of warfarin therapy, an algorithm for warfarin management is clinically desirable. Although several algorithms have been proposed, it is useful to assess their relative efficacy in producing a high TTR value.

Fusaro, Patil, and colleagues (2013) simulated a population treated with warfarin by creating "clinical avatars" using Bayesian modeling. A total of 200,000 avatars were created and used to conduct a series of clinical trial

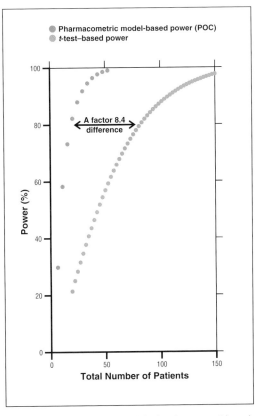

FIGURE 15–3B. Power of clinical trial using pharmacometric modeling. Power curve comparison between the pharmacometric model–based power (orange circles) and the *t*-test based power (blue circles), for the proof-of-concept scenario. The difference in study size was 8.4-fold (10 vs. 84 total number of patients) in favor of the pharmacometric approach. (Reprinted with permission from Karlsson, K. E., C. Vong, et al. (2013). Comparisons of analysis methods for proof-of-concept trials. CPT: Pharmac Syst Pharmacol **2**: e23.)

simulations (1000 replicates) to evaluate the CoumaGen and Wilson algorithms for warfarin-dose adjustment. The simulation framework accurately reproduced the data reported previously from the actual CoumaGen trial, and the investigators were able to improve the estimated TTR by modifying the CoumaGen algorithm using the Wilson algorithm for days 3 to 90 (Figure 15–4). The systems-based clinical trial simulation framework developed by Fusaro and colleagues lays the foundation for extending clinical trial simulations to a range of medical fields for refinement of dosing regimens in various populations before embarking on logistically complex and expensive phase 3 trials.

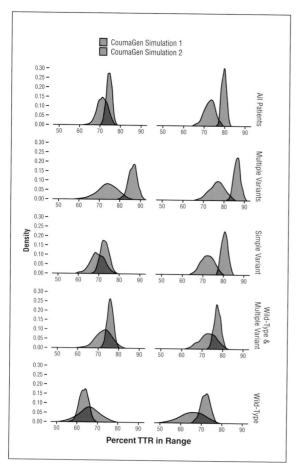

FIGURE 15–4. Clinical trial simulation using pharmacogenomic data. Density plots of the primary outcomes (therapeutic range [TTR]) for each study arm, standard clinical and pharmacogenetic, stratified by genotype subsets for the CoumaGen Simulation 1 and 2 studies. There is less variance in CoumaGen Simulation 2 as compared with Simulation 1 because of differences in protocol designs. Genotype subsets are ordered from extensive metabolizer (wild-type) to poor metabolizer (multiple variants) status and illustrate the sensitivity of the model to predicting changes in TTR corresponding to known genetic factors. (Reprinted with permission from Fusaro, V. A., P. Patil, et al. (2013). A systems approach to designing effective clinical trials using simulations. Circulation 127(4): 517–26.)

Another example from the cardiovascular field demonstrates how statistical modeling of clinical pharmacology findings can be used to guide dose selection. Edoxaban is an orally active factor Xa inhibitor that was investigated for prevention of embolic strokes in patients with atrial fibrillation. Prior to embarking on a phase 3, registration-pathway trial, 15 studies were done to explore a range of doses in an array of phase 1 to phase 2b settings (Salazar, Mendell, et al. 2012). The data from these studies were used to construct a population pharmacokinetic model, including drug interactions (P-glycoprotein inhibitor effect). Interrogation of the exposure–safety relationship showed that increasing edoxaban exposure was significantly associated with a higher incidence of bleeding. A logistic-regression model was used to examine the relationship between the minimum concentration of edoxaban at steady state ($C_{min,ss}$) and the incidence of all bleeding events (Figure 15–5). Based on the modeling in Figure 15–5, a phase 3 trial of edoxaban was designed to test an edoxaban regimen that would be expected to have no worse bleeding than a warfarin control and another edoxaban regimen that would be estimated to have at least a 10% lower incidence of bleeding as compared with warfarin (Salazar, Mendell, et al. 2012). Since once-daily dosing of edoxaban appeared to be associated with less bleeding than twice-daily regimens (see Figure 15–5), the regimens taken for-

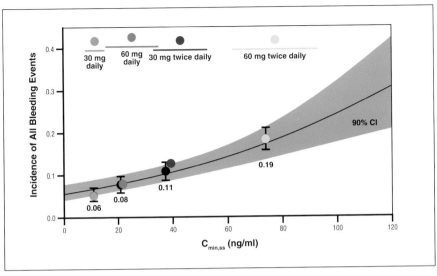

FIGURE 15–5. Regression modeling of phase 2 data to plan phase 3 trial. Goodness-of-fit of logistic-regression model. The solid black line represents the logistic model prediction and the blue shaded area represents the 90% confidence interval (CI). Horizontal colored bars represent the 10th to 90th percentiles of the minimum concentration at steady state ($C_{min,ss}$) by treatment group. The colored symbols represent the incidence of bleeding events by edoxaban treatment group and are plotted at the median $C_{min,ss}$ for each treatment group. Black squares and whiskers represent the computed median and ±1 standard error of incidence of bleeding events for each quartile of $C_{min,ss}$ across all four dosages. (Reprinted with permission from Salazar, D. E., J. Mendell, et al. (2012). Modelling and simulation of edoxaban exposure and response relationships in patients with atrial fibrillation. Thromb Haemost **107**(5): 925–36.)

ward in the phase 3 trial were 60 mg once daily and 30 mg once daily (Ruff, Giugliano, et al. 2010). Based on a population pharmacokinetic model, 50% reductions in the 60-mg and 30-mg doses were built into the phase 3 protocol for patients with diminished renal function or for those who were receiving drugs that are strong P-glycoprotein inhibitors (Ruff, Giugliano, et al. 2010; Salazar, Mendell, et al. 2012).

Network medicine can also focus on drug combinations in drug development. The classic list of drug interactions (additive, synergistic, antagonistic) is an oversimplification and does not account for the variation in interactions that can be observed with different doses (Yeh and Kishony 2007). The use of isobolograms and response surfaces allows one to summarize drug interactions when the targets of the drugs are serially aligned in a single pathway or are in parallel pathways; network analysis may lead to identification of unexpected interactions (Tallarida 2006; Lehar, Zimmermann, et al. 2007; Yeh and Kishony 2007; Cokol, Chua, et al. 2011). Network analyses of signaling pathways may help define new approaches to treatment with standard drugs. For example, administering chemotherapeutic agents sequentially rather than simultaneously may sensitize cells to their anticancer effects by rewiring signal networks (Lee, Ye, et al. 2012) (see details in Chapter 14).

Conceptual Framework for Adaptations to Clinical Trials

Figure 15–6A shows the basic structure of a clinical trial. Subjects who fulfill the enrollment criteria are randomly assigned according to a prespecified allocation ratio to the treatment arms under investigation and followed for the occurrence of the primary endpoint. In the conventional frequentist approach, the sample size is set prior to enrollment of subjects and the trial is completed without modification (see Figure 15–6A). By its very nature, this simple classical design is characterized by uncertainty about the relative efficacy and safety of the treatment regimens. At the design stage of the trial, limited information exists about the treatment effect of the test intervention and information about the parameters needed to describe it accurately may be sparse. The frequentist approach is generally familiar to the clinical community and may lead to three erroneous conclusions, especially if the findings are read in an unnuanced fashion: (1) A p value of <0.05 indicates a true difference between treatments; (2) The more "significant" the p value is, the greater the difference between treatments; and (3) A "statistically significant" difference equates to a "clinically significant" difference (Rawlins 2004).

The FDA introduced a Critical Path Initiative in 2004 to encourage adapting clinical trials to improve the likelihood of a successful trial (Buckman, Huang et al. 2007; European Medicines Agency and Committee for Medicinal Products for Human Use 2007; Food and Drug Administration, Center for Drug Evaluation and Research (CDER) et al. 2011). The concept of adapting an ongoing trial to evolving data in order to identify patients expected to respond more favorably to the test therapy is appealing to sponsors and investigators. Adaptations to clinical trials may also ameliorate the "pipeline problem" and accelerate the delivery of new treatments to fulfill unmet medical needs (Lindsay 2003; Miller, Ewy, et al. 2005; Lesko 2007; Peck 2010).

Adaptations to clinical trials can occur at one or more of the three major levels shown by the arrows in Figure 15–6B and may involve one or more of the elements shown at each level. The types of adaptations may also be different during the exploratory and confirmatory stages of drug development. (FDA CDER et al. 2011). Regulatory guidance documents indicate that when the information flows from a source external to the trial and provokes an adaptation, it is referred to as a *reactive revision* (see Figure 15–6C) (FDA CDER et al. 2011). The term *adaptive design* is used when investigators prospectively plan to adapt the trial based on interim data internal to the trial (see Figure 15–6D). Important unplanned findings that arise on review of interim data may provoke an adaptation to the trial, as

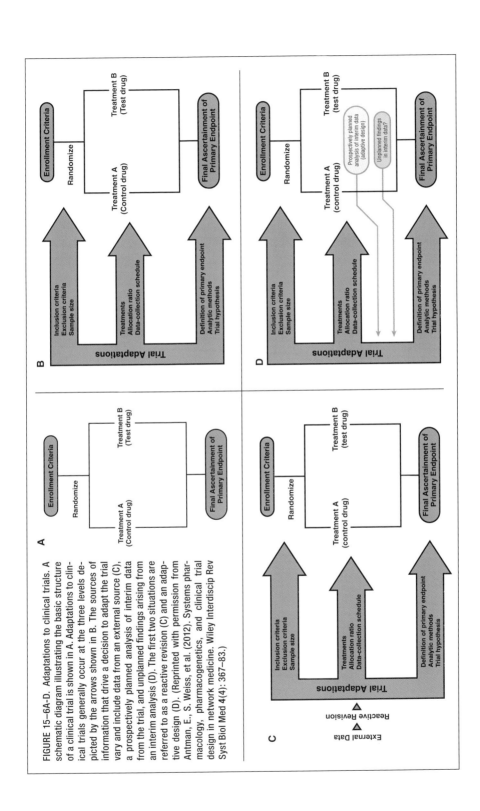

FIGURE 15–6A–D. Adaptations to clinical trials. A schematic diagram illustrating the basic structure of a clinical trial is shown in A. Adaptations to clinical trials generally occur at the three levels depicted by the arrows shown in B. The sources of information that drive a decision to adapt the trial vary and include data from an external source (C), a prospectively planned analysis of interim data from the trial, and unplanned findings arising from an interim analysis (D). The first two situations are referred to as a reactive revision (C) and an adaptive design (D). (Reprinted with permission from Antman, E., S. Weiss, et al. (2012). Systems pharmacology, pharmacogenetics, and clinical trial design in network medicine. Wiley Interdiscip Rev Syst Biol Med 4(4): 367–83.)

well. Such findings are anticipated to occur more frequently as fields such as systems biology and systems pharmacology mature (see Figure 15–6D).

Examples of Adaptations to Clinical Trials
EXPLORATORY PHASE

Dose-Ranging Assessment

Prior to the start of the exploratory phase, the true position and shape of the dose–response relationship for a drug is unknown (Huang and Temple 2008). Therefore, an important initial goal of dose ranging is to identify the "no effect" and the "maximally tolerated" doses. In an adaptive dose-finding trial, small cohorts of subjects are enrolled to frame the region of interest—the steeply rising midportion of the dose–response curve (Figure 15–7). It is inefficient and costly to enroll too many subjects at the doses on the flat portions of the sigmoidal shape of the curve (see Figure 15–7).

An example from a study of antithrombotic therapy for acute myocardial infarction illustrates the principles of an adaptive dose-finding phase 2 study that was based on the concept of networking between the coagulation system and the processes of platelet activation and aggregation. Anticoagulant and antiplatelet agents are typically used in combination, but the ideal combination reperfusion regimen is uncertain. Thus, during the exploratory phase of development of combination reperfusion therapy with reduced-dose fibrinolytics plus glycoprotein IIb/IIIa inhibitors, a sequential probability ratio test (SPRT) was used to quickly screen candidate drug regimens that appeared promising for restoring antegrade flow in a totally thrombotically occluded culprit coronary artery (Antman, Giugliano, et al. 1999). The source for designing the SPRT was historical data showing that ~50% of patients achieve full antegrade flow (Thrombolysis in Myocardial Infarction [TIMI] grade III flow) with a front-loaded 100-mg alteplase regimen at 90 minutes. The TIMI 14 study tested the glycoprotein IIb/IIIa inhibitor abciximab in combination with varying doses of fibrinolytics as part of the combination regimen, using an open-label angiographic trial format. The prespecified SPRT boundaries were 30% (H_0) and 50% (H_a) TIMI III flow with type I and II error rates of 0.0001% and 10%, respectively, for the abciximab-alone group, and boundaries of 60% (H_0) and 80% (H_a) TIMI III flow with type I and II error rates of 1% and 2.5%, respectively, for groups in which abciximab was combined with a fibrinolytic agent (Antman, Giugliano, et al. 1999). The objectives of this SPRT structure were to quickly screen for ineffective dose regimens (<<50% TIMI III flow) and identify promising regimens (>>60% TIMI III flow) that might be tested further. It was estimated that 35 to 70 patients per treatment group would provide sufficient information to identify regimens that

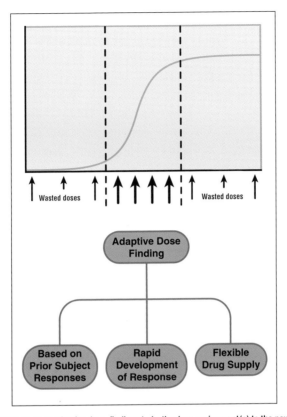

FIGURE 15–7. In an adaptive dose-finding study, the dose assignment(s) to the next sub-ject, or next cohort of patients, is based on responses of previous subjects, and the dose assignment is chosen to maximize the information about the dose–response curve, ac-cording to some predefined objective metric (e.g., variability in parameter estimates). In a traditional dose-finding trial, selecting a few doses may not adequately represent the dose–response relationship, leading many patients to be allocated to "noninformative," or "wasted," doses, as shown. In adaptive dose finding, the strategy is to include initially only a few patients on many doses to explore the dose–response relationship and then to allocate the dose range of interest to a greater number of patients. This strategy reduces the allocation of patients to noninformative doses. Compared with fixed randomization, this approach has the ethical advantage that fewer subjects are assigned doses that are too high or too low; it can also avoid additional, separate trials that might be necessary when fixed dose-finding trials do not adequately define the dose range. Adaptive dose-finding trials also require an infrastructure that allows the rapid communication of re-sponses from trial sites to a central unblinded analysis center and of adaptive dose as-signments to the trial sites. Randomization software capable of rapidly computing the dynamic allocation of doses to subjects is also mandated by adaptive trials because prespecified randomization lists will not work. In addition, a flexible drug-supply process is required because demand for doses is not fixed in advance, but rather evolves as infor-mation on responses at various doses is gathered as the trial progresses. (Modified with permission from Orloff, J., F. Douglas, et al. (2009). The future of drug development: ad-vancing clinical trial design. Nat Rev Drug Discov 8(12): 949–57. © 2009 Macmillan Pub-lishers Limited.)

were likely to be considered candidates for additional testing. A total of 14 different reperfusion regimens were evaluated during the dose-finding phase using a 1:1 allocation ratio. During further dose exploration, 3 of the reperfusion regimens were tested with one patient randomly assigned to the control regimen for every two patients randomly assigned to an experimental regimen. While the adaptive design to dose ranging in trials like TIMI 14 was useful for identifying a candidate combination reperfusion regimen, it cannot substitute for a large clinical endpoint study. A confirmatory phase 3 study powered for clinical endpoints identified a serious safety concern of excessive bleeding, limiting the clinical applicability of combination reperfusion therapy (Antman, Giugliano, et al. 1999; Antman, Gibson et al. 2000; Topol 2001).

New approaches and insights into target discovery and validation present investigators with the opportunity to define a dose–response relationship in a more sophisticated fashion (Lindsay 2003). In conventional dose-ranging studies with broadly cytotoxic cancer agents, the 3+3 design is commonly used to limit the toxicity rate to ≤33% (Ivy, Siu, et al. 2010). The 3+3 design begins with 3 patients at an initial dose level. Enrollment at the next-higher dose level may occur if no patients exhibit dose-limiting toxicity. If one patient exhibits dose-limiting toxicity, the design calls for 3 more patients to be enrolled at the dose for which a possible signal of concern has arisen. When dose-limiting toxicity is estimated to be 33%, the next-lower dose tested is recommended for phase 2 testing; however, since new molecularly targeted cancer agents are less likely to be generally cytotoxic, more aggressive dose-ranging studies have been proposed for testing such drugs. Accelerated dose-titration schemes that have been proposed include: (1) a rapid initial dose-escalation phase; (2) intrapatient dose-escalation; and (3) statistical analysis of a dose-toxicity model and a continual Bayesian reassessment method that specifies a target level of toxicity, the number of patients per cohort, a mathematical model of dose toxicity, and formal stopping rules (Sheiner, Beal, et al. 1989; Simon, Freidlin, et al. 1997; Ishizuka and Ohashi 2001).

Enrichment Strategies

Another approach taken during the exploratory phase is to identify patients who are more likely to have a beneficial response based on a biomarker measurement. A clinically useful biomarker is one that impacts clinical outcomes and lies along the causal pathway between the disease and clinical outcomes (Fleming and DeMets 1996). Biomarkers may be indicators of the presence or absence of disease (i.e., lie quite proximal to "disease" along the disease-outcomes continuum). From a drug-development perspective, a biomarker is a druggable target itself or identifies the presence of a druggable target. The utility of a biomarker is further defined by whether it is a valid surrogate that explains all, or an important component, of the effect of the intervention on outcomes (Fleming and DeMets 1996; Institute of Medicine 2010).

Examples of biomarker-based clinical trial designs are shown in Figure 15–8 (Freidlin, McShane, et al. 2010). In the biomarker-stratified design, all patients are randomly assigned to the treatments being tested regardless of biomarker status. The biomarker-enrichment design randomly assigns only patients who are biomarker-positive in order to direct the patient to a particular treatment. When selecting one of the biomarker-based design strategies, consideration should be given to the regulatory implications of the findings (Zineh and Woodcock 2013). If an enrichment strategy is used, regulatory authorities may require that the drug indication be linked to a companion diagnostic test—especially if there is a >90% prevalence of diagnostic positivity.

The principles depicted in Figure 15–8 are exemplified in the field of cancer therapeutics, in which targeted molecular agents are being developed based on the complex molecular aspects of tumor biology. An example of the enrichment design is the development of the BRAF inhibitor, PLX4032, in patients with malignant melanoma who have the BRAF V600E mutation (Chapman, Hauschild, et al. 2011). Metastatic melanoma is an aggressive cancer; standard therapies include high-dose interleukin-2 and dacarbazine, which produce only limited rates of response (10% to 20%) (Flaherty, Puzanov, et al. 2010). BRAF is the most frequently mutated protein kinase in human malignancies. A BRAF mutation is seen in 40% to 60% of mela-

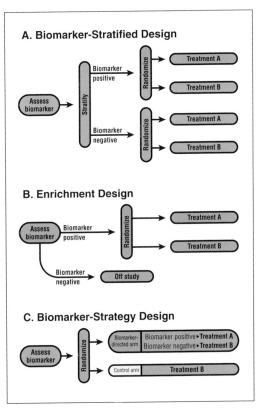

FIGURE 15–8. Clinical trial designs using biomarker measurements. A, Biomarker-stratified design, in which all patients are randomly assigned regardless of biomarker status, with the random assignment and analysis plan stratified by the biomarker status. Sometimes, a standard (nonstratified) randomization can be used (with the analysis plan stratified by the biomarker) when postrandomization biomarker evaluation is feasible. B, Enrichment design, in which the biomarker is evaluated on all patients, but random assignment is restricted to patients with specific biomarker values. C, Biomarker-strategy design, in which patients are randomly assigned to an experimental treatment arm that uses the biomarker to direct therapy or to a control arm that does not. Some biomarker-strategy designs evaluate biomarkers only in patients randomly assigned to the biomarker-directed arm. (Reprinted with permission from Freidlin, B., L. M. McShane, et al. (2010). Randomized clinical trials with biomarkers: design issues. J Natl Cancer Inst 102(3): 152–60.)

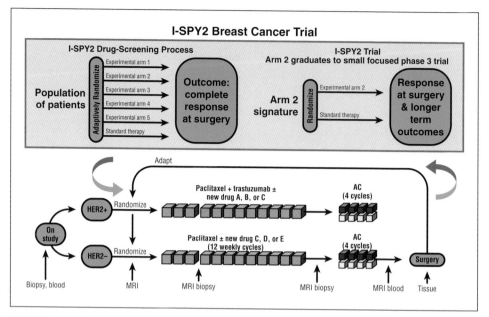

FIGURE 15–9. I-SPY 2 Trial Design Top, I-SPY2 schema. On the left side is shown the screening process, attempting to pair experimental arms with patient subsets. The example shows five experimental arms being compared with standard therapy as a control. Randomization is adaptive in that patients who are doing better on a particular therapy are assigned that therapy with higher probability (downward directed curved arrow). On the right side is shown the case in which experimental arm 2 has shown sufficient benefit within a particular patient subset, its so-called signature, that it graduates into a small phase 3 confirmatory trial in that subset (upward directed curved arrow). Bottom, For HER2+ patients in the study, some new drugs with specific anti-HER2 activity may be administered in lieu of trastuzumab: anthracycline (AC) (e.g., doxorubicin) and cyclophosphamide. HER2, human epidermal growth factor receptor 2; I-SPY 2, investigation of serial studies to predict your therapeutic response with imaging and molecular analysis 2; MRI, magnetic resonance imaging. (From Berry, D. A., R. S. Herbst, et al. (2012). Reports from the 2010 Clinical and Translational Cancer Research Think Tank meeting: design strategies for personalized therapy trials. Clin Cancer Res 18(3): 638–44.)

nomas, and the majority are the V600E mutations (substitution of glutamic acid for valine at the amino acid 600 position) (Flaherty, Puzanov, et al. 2010). PLX4032 is a potent inhibitor of the BRAF V600E mutation. A phase 2 study using the biomarker-enrichment design was conducted by restricting enrichment to patients with melanoma who had the BRAF V600E mutation as ascertained by a polymerase-chain-reaction assay (Flaherty, Puzanov, et al. 2010). PLX4032 induced complete or partial tumor regression in 81% of patients, with the duration of response ranging from 2 to 18 months.

The I-SPY2 trial is a multidimensional biomarker-strategy trial of neoadjuvant chemotherapy for women with large primary cancers of the breast (Berry, Herbst, et al. 2012). The trial uses three types of biomarkers: (1) standard FDA-approved biomarkers to establish patient eligibility and to form the basis for a stratified randomization (Figure 15–9); (2) qualifying biomarkers that are not yet FDA-approved but are evaluated for assessing therapeutic response; and

(3) exploratory biomarkers that will be assessed by the analysis of well-characterized blood and tissue specimens (Barker, Sigman, et al. 2009).

As illustrated in Figure 15–9, patients are assigned to various treatments using a stratification scheme based on the signature profile for the following standard biomarkers: hormone receptor status (+/−), human epidermal growth factor receptor 2 (HER2) status (+/−), and MammaPrint score (Barker, Sigman, et al. 2009). The treatment arm design allocates HER2(+) patients to paclitaxel plus trastuzumab and HER2(−) patients to paclitaxel alone for 12 weekly cycles. Both treatment arms then receive doxorubicin plus cyclophosphamide. New drugs (e.g., agents A to E in Figure 15–9) are candidates for testing provided they have been shown to be safe in relevant phase 1 studies.

From the array of standard biomarkers noted above, 14 profiles of interest have been identified. A Bayesian adaptive randomization scheme is used in I-SPY2 to "learn" as the trial proceeds which particular profile predicts a response to specific treatment regimens (Barker, Sigman, et al. 2009; Berry, Herbst, et al. 2012). The primary endpoint is pathological complete response (see Figure 15–9) (Berry, Herbst, et al. 2012). The Bayesian structure is targeted to identify an agent that is estimated to have an 85% probability of success in a future randomized phase 3 trial of 300 patients (Berry, Herbst, et al. 2012). Experimental arms are treated in a dynamic fashion, with agents being added or dropped as dictated by the Bayesian model. Integral to the I-SPY2 trial is a sophisticated bioinformatics support structure to provide the computational backbone for processing clinical data, pathological results, biomarker profile, and -omics data.

The I-SPY2 trial illustrates key features necessary for an adaptive dose-finding trial (see Figure 15–7): an analytic plan based on the response in subjects enrolled previously (Bayesian in this case), the rapid development of the endpoint of interest (pathological complete response as shown in Figure 15–9), and a flexible drug supply to expeditiously incorporate new regimens into the randomization scheme (Orloff, Douglas, et al. 2009). It is also an excellent example of industry–academic collaboration and is viewed quite favorably by regulatory authorities (Esserman and Woodcock 2011). It should be recognized that the phase 2 nature of I-SPY2 is an important foundation for a seamless transition to a definitive phase 3 trial using the regimens that "survive" the modeling in phase 2 (see Figure 15–9) (Berry, Herbst, et al. 2012).

Efficacy and safety assessments may be incorporated in an adaptively designed phase 2 trial. K-134, a selective phosphodiesterase 3 (PDE3) inhibitor, has vasodilatory effects and more pronounced antiplatelet effects than cilostazol (Lewis, Connor, et al. 2011). Three doses of K-134 (25, 50, and 100 mg twice daily) were compared with placebo or cilostazol (100 mg twice daily) in patients with stable claudication (Lewis, Connor, et al. 2011). The statistical design was engineered to eliminate one of the K-134 regimens if adverse effects or intolerability occurred at an unacceptable rate. The safety endpoints were resting tachycardia (heart rate >120 bpm) and ischemia on treadmill testing, and a cutoff of 20% of the population exhibiting these endpoints was used; the tolerability endpoint (40% population cutpoint) was discontinuation of the study drug for any reason. Interim analyses were designed with 80% two-tailed confidence intervals for each endpoint based on logistic dose–response models. The 25-mg dose was dropped because of a recommendation from the data monitoring committee. The investigators estimated that the design described above prevented approximately 43 subjects from being assigned to a rejected dose if a conventional fixed design had been used (Lewis, Connor, et al. 2011).

CONFIRMATORY PHASE

The confirmatory phase of drug development builds on the dose-ranging exploration and safety data acquired in phase 1 and phase 2 trials. Since the end goal of drug development is to bring a new therapy into clinical use, sponsors must provide evidence to regulatory authorities that their product is safe and effective. Traditionally, from the perspective of the FDA, this has required submission of the findings from two "adequate and well-controlled" studies. Several shifts have occurred in that regulatory posture, including a willingness on the part of regulatory authorities to accept data from a single large randomized trial, preferably with a broad representation of the population; and interest in pursuing a seamless transition from phase 2 to phase 3 in the process of drug development (Gallo, Chuang-Stein, et al. 2006; Bretz, Koenig, et al. 2009; FDA CDER et al. 2010a; Chow and Corey 2011; Tournoux-Facon, De Rycke, et al. 2011). In a seamless design approach, the final analysis of the dose(s) carried forward involves data from both phase 2 and phase 3 studies (Bretz, Branson, et al. 2009). Since a seamless design involves multiple "looks" at the data on the doses of interest, it is important for investigators to include statistical adjustments to project the overall type I error (Bretz, Branson, et al. 2009; Dmitrienko, D'Agostino, et al. 2013). To deal with this constraint, it has been proposed that seamless designs be divided into inferentially seamless designs, in which data from both stages of a development program are used, and operationally seamless designs, in which only data from subjects enrolled after the selection decision was made are involved (Orloff, Douglas, et al. 2009). Seamless designs are of particular interest as we enter the era of network medicine (Loscalzo and Barábasi 2011). Many of the concepts described in previous chapters will inform the early and mid-phases of drug development, will form the logical basis for adaptive designs of clinical trials, and potentially, will result in a greater use of a seamless transition to the confirmatory phase.

While a seamless approach is attractive, several challenges are illustrated by the following example. The long-acting β_2-adrenoceptor agonist indacaterol was studied in patients with chronic obstructive pulmonary disease. The development program consisted of a first-stage adaptive design in which four doses of indacaterol (75, 150, 300, and 600 mcg) were compared with placebo over 2 weeks (Barnes, Pocock, et al. 2010). There were 111 to 115 subjects in each of the indacaterol arms. The prespecified efficacy criteria for the indacaterol arms compared the forced expiratory volume in 1 second (FEV_1) to the highest value of: (1) the difference between tiotropium and placebo, (2) the difference between formoterol and placebo, or (3) 120 ml. Additional efficacy criteria compared the area under the curve in 1 to 4 hours (AUC_{1-4h}) for FEV_1 to the highest value of: (1) the difference between tiotropium and placebo or (2) the difference between formoterol and placebo. All four indacaterol doses exceeded the prespecified efficacy criterion for FEV_1 and doses of 150 mcg or higher exceeded the FEV_1 AUC_{1-4h} criterion. The frequency of adverse events leading to withdrawal and to serious adverse events was similar across the four indacaterol arms. Since the 150-mcg and 300-mcg doses fulfilled the efficacy criteria for both FEV_1 and FEV_1 AUC_{1-4h}, those two doses were taken forward to the second stage of drug development and continued to show significant benefit against the reference efficacy criteria at 26 weeks. Review of the new drug application by the FDA observed that, in fact, all doses of indacaterol were superior to placebo and had a similar effect size (Chowdhury, Seymour, et al. 2011). Since concerns exist about toxicity from long-term use of long-acting β-agonists in patients with asthma, additional dose-ranging and safety analyses were requested by the FDA. These follow-up studies showed a pattern suggesting a plateau of the dose–response (bronchodilator) effect of indacaterol at a dose of 75 µg or higher by 2 weeks. Additional studies conducted by the sponsor and modeling studies to support a dose of 150 µg did not, in the opinion of the FDA or an independent reviewer, make a sufficiently strong case for the 150-µg dose. Given the concerns about toxicity with long-term use, the FDA assessed the overall risk–benefit ratio and approved the 75-µg dose of indacaterol. This example illustrates the challenge of accelerating drug development. The prespecified efficacy criteria and adaptive design focused on rapid identification of doses with an encouraging efficacy signal. In the absence of a sufficient amount of patient exposure, safety may not have been adequately evaluated (Chowdhury, Seymour, et al. 2011; FDA CDER et al. 2011).

Adapting a clinical trial to evolving data has also been applied explicitly during the confirmatory phase of therapeutic development (Dragalin 2006; Chow and Chang 2008; Bretz, Koenig, et al. 2009; Mehta, Gao, et al. 2009; FDA CDER et al. 2010a; Mehta and Pocock 2011; Tournoux-Facon, De Rycke, et al. 2011). Adaptations to confirmatory trials present challenges to both investigators and regulatory authorities because of the need to protect the studywide type I (alpha) error and prevent operational biases that could jeopardize the integrity or interpretation of the study (Gallo 2006a, b; Hung, O'Neill et al. 2006; European Medicines Agency and Committee for Medicinal Products for Human Use 2007; Chow and Chang 2008; Chow and Corey 2011; FDA CDER et al. 2011; Wang, Hung, et al. 2011).

The issue of protection of the studywide alpha error bears further discussion. In broad terms, from a regulatory perspective, there is a need to minimize the rate of false-positive inferences so that authorities (and the clinical community) can draw conclusions about specific individual hypotheses without concerns about inflation of the error rate (Dmitrienko, D'Agostino, et al. 2013). In a confirmatory trial, there may be multiple points at which multiplicity concerns arise, such as multiple endpoints (single or composite) and the sequence in which they are being tested, different doses of regimens being tested, and different subgroups of the trial population being examined for any differences in treatment effect. Adaptations to clinical trials add an additional layer or layers of complexity (FDA CDER et al. 2010a). The many choices available to investigators for adapting a confirmatory trial increase the chance that a null hypothesis was rejected inappropriately because of an inflated type I error (FDA CDER et al. 2010a). In the preclinical setting, the rate at which this occurs is referred to as the false discovery rate; in confirmatory clinical trials, this is referred to as the familywise error rate (FWER) (Dmitrienko, D'Agostino, et al. 2013).

When testing m hypotheses, two types of logical relationships can exist: (1) prespecified hypothesis ordering (usually arranged in order of clinical importance), and (2) data-driven hypothesis ordering (no predetermined order and the sequence of testing determined by the significance of the hypothesis test statistics) (Dmitrienko, D'Agostino, et al. 2013). Depending on the distribution of the relationships in the data, investigators will need to use nonparametric, semiparametric, or parametric procedures. Finally, consideration must be given as to whether the multiplicity problem involves a single family or multiple families of hypotheses. Given the array of possible options for adaptation and the necessary procedures for adjustment for multiple testing (e.g., sequence of tests, gatekeeping procedures), investigators are strongly encouraged to seek consultation with regulatory authorities at the planning stage of the trial and prespecify as much of the planned adaptations and testing procedures as possible (European Medicines Agency and Committee for Medicinal Products for Human Use 2007; FDA CDER et al. 2010a; Dmitrienko, D'Agostino, et al. 2013).

In addition to the principles of multiplicity adjustment noted above, there are three statistical penalties that occur during the process of adaptation (Cook and

DeMets 2010). This follows from the difference between a scientific goal and an adaptation goal. For example, the scientific goal may be to compare various doses of a new drug with a standard treatment. Each subject in the trial contributes a fixed amount of information (constrained by the specifics of the protocol, such as the assessment schedule). Adaptations do not increase the information content contributed by an individual subject; however, they allow a more efficient use of the information to answer a specific scientific question. With that perspective, investigators should be aware of the following statistical penalties:

1. Efforts to optimize the likelihood of a successful result may limit the amount of information on other endpoints or research questions. The scope of information that could be used to inform the clinical community may, thus, be limited.
2. Control of the overall type I error is less efficient with respect to the use of information compared with a fixed design trial.
3. Inferential challenges for interpretation of the trial findings may arise, since adaptations to the trial can alter the sampling distributions used in the summary statistics.

Investigators also face logistical issues when designing adaptations to a confirmatory trial: (1) The information on which to base an adaptation must be available in a reasonable timeframe so that it is practical to expect the adaptation to have an impact on the trial (i.e., adaptive design may not be practical in long-term studies). (2) Uncertainty exists about how to project supplies of study drug kits at the start of the trial and the need for flexibility in dosing arms should an adaptation be made (Bretz, Branson, et al. 2009). (3) Blinding of trial personnel must be maintained to avoid operational bias that might arise if the information from an adaptation was used to infer an estimate of the therapeutic response to one or more arms in the study (Gallo 2006a, b; Hung, O'Neill, et al. 2006; European Medicines Agency and Committee for Medicinal Products for Human Use 2007; FDA CDER, et al. 2011; Wang, Hung, et al. 2011). (4) Cook and DeMets (2010) observe that the decision to implement an adaptation is a difficult one for a data monitoring committee (DMC) once it has seen unblinded interim outcome data. Consider an event-driven trial with three arms: a control arm and a high- and a low-dose arm of the experimental therapy (Ruff, Giugliano, et al. 2010). Since both of the experimental arms are to be compared with the control arm, a recommendation by the DMC to discontinue one of the experimental arms while allowing the other to continue could unblind the investigators. By noting the aggregate number of events, the investigators could make an inference about the treatment effect in the arm that is stopped compared with the one that is continued. Therefore, both the low-dose and high-dose arms would need to be continued until the requisite total number of events had been acquired. The operational challenges of decision making for an adaptive design extend to the DMC (or group that has seen unblinded data), causing some authors to propose that adaptations to confirmatory trials be made by an independent group, distinct from the investigators and the DMC (Gallo 2006a, b; Chow, Corey, et al. 2012). Some statisticians have argued that this independent group might also benefit from a sponsor representative who is not directly involved in the trial to understand the drug-development implications of a proposed adaptation (Gallo 2006a, b).

Some adaptations to confirmatory trials are well understood by regulatory authorities. The general principles are that the adaptations discussed below do not involve using unblinded data or involve a well-established group sequential method that minimized that impact on the type I error (FDA CDER et al. 2011).

1. Adaptations to Enrollment Criteria and Sample Size (see Figure 15–4D)
At the design stage, investigators specify what they believe is a patient population that will optimally demonstrate a treatment effect because they are believed to benefit from the mechanism of action of the drug. If during the course of the trial, the population being enrolled does exhibit the anticipated baseline characteristics, an enrichment strategy may be used that involves modifying the enrollment criteria so that patients enrolled subsequently have the desired characteristics. Statistical concerns in this situation are minimal provided the treatment allocation remains blinded. However, if there is an important difference in the treatment effect in the trial population enrolled before and after the adaptation, the regulatory community may have difficulty interpreting the study results and structuring an indication that will be useful to the clinical community (FDA CDER et al. 2011).

The sample size for the trial may be recalculated from blinded aggregate data to protect the power of the study. In the setting of a low-blinded aggregate event rate, investigators cannot distinguish between a lower event rate in the control group and a larger treatment effect than anticipated. For example, at the planning stage of a study, it may be hypothesized that the rate of the primary endpoint in the control arm is 15%, with a 17% relative risk reduction in the investigational arm. With a two-sided alpha of 0.05 and power of 90%, the sample size is estimated to be 8000 subjects and the total number of events 1100. At an interim analysis after 4000 subjects have been enrolled, the aggregate number of events is inspected in a blinded fashion. For m total events in n patients, the revised sample size is calculated as $1100 \times (n/m)$. If 480 events are observed in 4000 patients, the revised sample size to maintain the power of the final is calculated as $1100 \times (4000/480) = 9167$ subjects.

2. Adaptations to Treatments, Allocation Ratio, and Data Collection Schedule (see Figure 15–6D)

Prespecification of the number and timing of interim analyses by the DMC is an adaptive technique that is familiar to investigators and regulatory authorities (European Medicines Agency and Committee for Medicinal Products for Human Use 2007; FDA CDER et al. 2011). Such group sequential designs prespecify stopping boundaries that protect the type I error rate by controlling the spending of alpha at each interim assessment of the accumulating data. Stopping boundaries describe rejection regions by plotting the standardized normal statistic (Z_i) for i number of interim looks. Such stopping boundaries may use a fixed Z value (e.g., 2.6 or 3.0) at each of the i looks or may compare Z_i with $Z^* \sqrt{N/t}$, where Z^* is determined so as to achieve the desired significance level and N is the maximum number of interim looks (Friedman, Furberg, et al. 1998).

Potential decisions that may be made at an interim assessment include termination of the trial because of futility or overwhelming evidence of efficacy or safety concerns; dropping an ineffective dose in a multidose trial while other arms are continued (The PURSUIT Trial Investigators 1998). Response-driven adaptive randomization that alters the allocation ratio such as in the I-SPY2 trial is useful in the exploratory phase of development, but regulatory authorities have expressed concern about the validity, integrity, and interpretability of such "play the winner" approaches in a confirmation trial (FDA CDER et al. 2011).

3. Adaptations to Primary Endpoint, Analytic Methods, or the Trial Hypothesis. (see Figure 15–6D)

External data or a lower-than-anticipated event rate may lead investigators to modify the primary endpoint by adding or removing elements of a composite endpoint (Dargie 2001; Braunwald, Domanski, et al. 2004; European Medicines Agency and Committee for Medicinal Products for Human Use 2007; FDA CDER et al. 2011). In order to protect the validity of the trial, such maneuvers by investigators should be done in a blinded fashion and before database lock. Other adaptations that may be made (and arguably may occur more commonly as our understanding of network medicine expands) include changes to the statistical analysis plan by adding covariates, modifying a regression model, or shifting from parametric to nonparametric techniques if the data do not appear to be normally distributed (FDA CDER et al. 2011). With the increasing number of effective therapies now in clinical use, noninferiority trials are more common when investigational treatments are likely to be roughly therapeutically interchangeable with the standard one but offer clinical advantages (e.g., ease of use, fewer drug interactions, less monitoring required). Investigators may originally hypothesize that they will observe superiority of the new treatment and later adapt the plan to test for noninferiority. Several important principles should be kept in mind. The noninferiority margin should be prespecified (based on historical data) before inspecting any unblinded data (European Medicines Agency and Committee for Medicinal Products for Human Use 2007; FDA CDER et al. 2010b). Since superiority is a special case of noninferiority (where the upper bound of the 95% confidence interval of the treatment effect is not only below the noninferiority margin but is also to the left of the line of unity), a closed testing procedure can be used to test for superiority conditional on first having shown noninferiority (European Medicines Agency and Committee for Medicinal Products for Human Use 2007; Dmitrienko, D'Agostino, et al. 2013). Before embarking on a noninferiority test of the data, investigators should evaluate whether the trial population and protocol for using the standard therapy are similar to the historical precedent that forms the basis for the noninferiority margin. Failure to do so may risk questions about violation of the constancy assumption when the data are reviewed by regulatory authorities.

Regulatory and Ethical Perspectives on Adaptive Designs

Despite the interest in adaptive clinical trials for accelerating drug development and the creativity of biostatisticians in helping design them, (Mehta and Jemiai 2006; Mehta, Gao, et al. 2009; Mehta and Pocock 2011) regulatory authorities are cautious about adaptive designs in confirmatory trials (FDA CDER et al. 2011). A particular concern centers on operational bias occurring after treatment differences are evaluated by analysis of unblinded data. This is considered a serious threat to the integrity of the study and has led regulatory authorities to stress the importance of prestudy consultation, prespecification in writing of operating procedures, identification of the personnel who will perform any interim analyses, measures to control access to unblinded data, and precisely what information will be passed from the DSMB to the investigators and sponsors (FDA CDER, et al. 2011). This caution has led some individuals to conclude that adaptive designs have their greatest utility in the exploratory phase of therapeutic development—a realm in which systems biology and systems pharmacology may have its most significant impact (Editorial 2006).

Clinical research is considered ethical when seven core requirements are fulfilled (Emanuel, Wendler, et al. 2000): value, scientific validity, fair subject selection, favorable risk–benefit ratio, independent review, respect for enrolled subjects, and informed consent. Before approaching a potential research subject for participation, a state of equipoise must exist in which there is a reasonable degree of uncertainty in the clinical community and the enrolling investigator as to which treatment arm is preferable (Freedman 1987). Another important issue in the ethics of clinical trials is therapeutic misconception, which occurs when research subjects believe that the purpose for participating in a clinical trial is to receive "treatment" for their disease—failing to appreciate the distinction between the imperative of clinical research for gaining new knowledge versus the process of ordinary clinical treatment (Appelbaum, Anatchkova, et al. 2012).

Consider the impact of adaptive design of clinical trials on the complex interplay of the ethics of clinical research, equipoise, and therapeutic misconception. The research subjects enrolled early in a clinical trial, before any adaptations occur, face a greater degree of uncertainty than those who enroll later, after an adaptation has been introduced to optimize the response to a given treatment in subjects enrolled after the adaptation. Also, investigators who are aware of the adaptation are in a different position relative to the equipoise they had before the adaptation occurred. Some have argued that response-adaptive randomization is desirable, since it is a "partial remedy" for therapeutic misconception (Meurer, Lewis, et al. 2012). Others have pointed out that adaptive designs may: (1) provide less social and scientific value (since they may make it impossible to test more than the primary objective), (2) challenge scientific validity (potential loss of equipoise, uncertainty about generalizability and reproducibility), and (3) complicate informed consent (Can subjects enrolled truly be considered to have consented to what may or may not take place later in the trial?) (van der Graaf, Roes, et al. 2012). Lipsky and Lewis (2013) developed Bayesian, decision-theoretic, trial designs with response-adaptive randomization. They explored the impact of adaptive designs to improve the efficiency of trial conduct (while protecting type I and II errors) as well as investigated the impact on efficient care of patients by a loss function that includes terms for the per-subject cost of enrollment, a failure cost (for each subject who experiences an inferior outcome), and an error term to account for making an error in the final decision regarding the treatment effect. In their modeling, gains in efficiency of trial conduct did not always translate into large reductions in failed outcomes. While modeling such as that which includes loss functions noted above increases the transparency of the trial, there are additional layers that need to be included. The authors note that the next step will be to incorporate terms that reflect a broader patient horizon—balancing the needs of enrolled subjects against those of future untreated subjects not yet enrolled in the trial.

Conclusion

Advances in the understanding of the molecular aspects of human diseases and improvements in high-throughput screening of candidate compounds coupled with a greater use of computational biology portend a greater use of a systems approach to clinical trials in the future. Notable contemporary examples from the oncology literature underscore these points. Preventive therapy with selective estrogen-receptor modulators (SERMs) can reduce the occurrence of breast cancer in 50% of women. However, SERMs are not widely prescribed because about 51 women need to be treated for 5 years to prevent a single case of breast cancer, and there are concerns about SERM-related side effects such as deep-vein thrombosis, pulmonary embolism, and endometrial carcinoma (Santen, Boyd, et al. 2007). Ingle, Liu, and colleagues (2013) used DNA collected from the National Surgical Adjuvant Breast and Bowel Project (NSABP) trials to perform a nested discovery case–control genome-wide association study to screen for single-nucleotide polymorphisms (SNPs) associated with the occurrence of breast cancer in women treated with SERMs. They analyzed 592 cases and 1171 matched controls from the NSABP trials. SNPs in or near the ZNF423 (chromosome 16) and CTS0 (chromosome 4) genes were associated with breast cancer risk during SERM treatment. Based on the known functions of these genes, the associations could relate to estrogen-dependent induction of *BRCA1* expression. The presence of both risk alleles for ZNF423 and CTS0 was associated with an odds ratio for breast cancer of 5.71. By identifying the SNPs associated with breast cancer risk during SERM therapy, these findings offer the possibility for a future pharmacogenomically individualized program of breast cancer prevention with SERMs in high-risk women.

Evidence has begun to accumulate that biomarkers may be useful for identifying subjects who are more likely to benefit from preventive measures as well as those in whom disease has developed. For example, aspirin users have a lower risk of developing colorectal tumors with an intact *BRAF* gene (Nishihara, Lochhead,et al. 2013). Aspirin use was not associated with a lower risk of *BRAF*-mutated cancers. The biological basis for these findings may be related to upregulation of prostaglandin-endoperoxide synthase 2 by RAF kinases. In addition, individuals with colorectal cancers harboring *PIK3CA* mutations appear to have an improved outcome when treated with aspirin (Pasche 2013). These aspirin findings underscore the tension between guideline-based medical prac-tice and a personalized medicine approach (Goldberger and Buxton 2013). Clin-ical trials have enrollment criteria but also many subgroups of patients who may or may not have features suggesting either a strong benefit or lack of ben-efit from a particular therapy. Once guidelines are written, based on the enroll-ment criteria from a definitive registration-pathway trial, it may be challenging for clinicians to withhold therapy in a subgroup for which the benefit may be limited until additional data in that subpopulation become available.

Recognizing that the standard pathway proceeding from preclinical to clin-ical therapeutic development can take many years, the co-clinical trial concept was introduced (Nardella, Lunardi, et al. 2011). This paradigm calls for the creation of a genetically engineered mouse model of a human cancer, human xenografts of tumors into mouse models, and the simultaneous testing of promising cancer therapeutics in phase 1 and 2 clinical trials and the above animal models. Real-time acquisition of data from the animal models is trans-lated back to clinical studies. The co-clinical project calls for a "mouse hos-pital," a clinical center, and a bioinformatics infrastructure for data mining and analysis. Lunardi et al. used the co-clinical model to study treatments for castration-resistant prostate cancer with androgen deprivation therapy (Lu-nardi, Ala, et al. 2013). The project involved a *Pten*-loss driven mouse model. Castration counteracted tumor progression in the mouse model, but this ben-efit was overcome when there was downregulation of Xaf1 (encoding X-linked inhibitor of apoptosis-protein associated factor 1) and upregulation of *Srd5a1* (encoding 3-oxo-5-α-steroid 4-dehydrogenase 1) and the androgen receptor is relocalized to the nucleus. They hypothesize that patients with prostate cancer characterized by deregulation in Xaf1 and *SRD5A1* should be evaluated in future clinical studies with embelin and dutasteride.

Much of the discussion and many of the examples in this chapter center on therapeutics that are small molecules. Advances in systems biology have spawned the development of cellular and gene therapy (CGT) products, prompting the FDA to issue a draft guidance document on considerations for the design of early-phase clinical trials with those entities (Food and Drug Ad-ministration and Center for Biologics Evaluation and Research (CBER) 2013). The unique features of CGT products that influence the design of early-stage clinical trials include the relative lack of clinical experience with them and the complex nature of living cell products that may be affected by the microenvi-ronment, resulting in differentiation into undesired cell types. These consider-ations may dictate a larger cohort size than the 3+3 scheme used in oncology, not using healthy volunteers for initial studies, and foregoing blinding if it cannot be accomplished safely in a control group.

In addition to a systems approach to clinical trials, the concept of adaptive designs has led to new regulatory approaches to drug approval (Eichler, Oye, et al. 2012). It was proposed that an initial restricted license be granted for a new drug based on clinical trials in an enriched population with the caveat that initial prescribing experience is monitored by registries and electronic medical records. A broader license would be granted when trials in a wider population are submitted, provided the earlier monitoring experience is favorable. The gap between efficacy (ideal results in a clinical trial setting) and effectiveness (assessment of treatment effect in a real-world setting) can be bridged by assembling a database of the biologic sources of variability (e.g., genomics, comorbidities, disease-state factors, drug–drug interaction) and behavioral sources of variability (e.g., prescribing patterns and patient adherence) (Eichler, Abadie, et al. 2011). Systems approaches have been proposed for monitoring adverse drug events through a combination of a top-down approach (mapping clinical reports back down through drug-centric, mechanism-centric, and network-centric levels) and a bottom-up approach (predicting a drug-induced effect by starting with a network-centric approach built on informatics and -omics and then projected upward to anticipated clinical reports) (Lesko, Zheng, et al. 2013).

Finally, medical applications of wireless communications have spawned a bioengineering field of wireless body area networks (WBANs) (Khan and Yuce 2010). This involves a network of sensors located inside or outside of a subject's body. A WBAN system allows a subject to be mobile and is location-independent since it can be connected to a monitoring hub but can also transmit data over WiFi, Bluetooth, and mobile networks. By transmitting real-time physiological data from research subjects, investigators can assess the dynamic response to an intervention and are freed from the extrapolations that must be made from periodic snapshots of a clinical response as might be recorded during a routine clinic visit. The "big data" needs generated by such an approach will require advanced informatics approaches. They offer the exciting potential to view network medicine in a way that was not possible without the advances in semiconductor technology originally predicted by Moore 50 years ago!

References

Allison, M. (2012). Reinventing clinical trials. Nat Biotechnol 30(1): 41–49.

Antman, E., S. Weiss, et al. (2012). Systems pharmacology, pharmacogenetics, and clinical trial design in network medicine. Wiley Interdiscip Rev Syst Biol Med 4(4): 367–83.

Antman, E. M., C. M. Gibson, et al. (2000). Combination reperfusion therapy with abciximab and reduced dose reteplase: results from TIMI 14. The Thrombolysis in Myocardial Infarction (TIMI) 14 Investigators. Eur Heart J 21(23): 1944–53.

Antman, E. M., R. P. Giugliano, et al. (1999). Abciximab facilitates the rate and extent of thrombolysis: results of the thrombolysis in myocardial infarction (TIMI) 14 trial. The TIMI 14 Investigators. Circulation 99(21): 2720–32.

Appelbaum, P. S., M. Anatchkova, et al. (2012). Therapeutic misconception in research subjects: development and validation of a measure. Clin Trials 9(6): 748–61.

Barker, A. D., C. C. Sigman, et al. (2009). I-SPY 2: an adaptive breast cancer trial design in the setting of neoadjuvant chemotherapy. Clin Pharmacol Ther 86(1): 97–100.

Barnes, P. J., S. J. Pocock, et al. (2010). Integrating indacaterol dose selection in a clinical study in COPD using an adaptive seamless design. Pulm Pharmacol Ther 23(3): 165–71.

Berry, D. A., R. S. Herbst, et al. (2012). Reports from the 2010 Clinical and Translational Cancer Research Think Tank meeting: design strategies for personalized therapy trials. Clin Cancer Res 18(3): 638–44.

Braunwald, E., M. J. Domanski, et al. (2004). Angiotensin-converting-enzyme inhibition in stable coronary artery disease. N Engl J Med 351(20): 2058–68.

Bretz, F., M. Branson, et al. (2009). Adaptivity in drug discovery and development. Drug Dev Res 70: 169–90.

Bretz, F., F. Koenig, et al. (2009). Adaptive designs for confirmatory clinical trials. Stat Med 28(8): 1181–217.

Buckman, S., S. M. Huang, et al. (2007). Medical product development and regulatory science for the 21st century: the critical path vision and its impact on health care. Clin Pharmacol Ther 81(2): 141–44.

Chapman, P. B., A. Hauschild, et al. (2011). Improved survival with vemurafenib in melanoma with BRAF V600E mutation. N Engl J Med 364(26): 2507–16.

Chow, S. C., and M. Chang (2008). Adaptive design methods in clinical trials—a review. Orphanet J Rare Dis 3: 11.

Chow, S. C., and R. Corey (2011). Benefits, challenges and obstacles of adaptive clinical trial designs. Orphanet J Rare Dis 6(1): 79.

Chow, S. C., R. Corey, et al. (2012). On the independence of data monitoring committee in adaptive design clinical trials. J Biopharm Stat 22(4): 853–67.

Chowdhury, B. A., S. M. Seymour, et al. (2011). The risks and benefits of indacaterol—the FDA's review. N Engl J Med 365(24): 2247–49.

Cokol, M., H. N. Chua, et al. (2011). Systematic exploration of synergistic drug pairs. Mol Syst Biol 7: 544.

Cook, T., and D. L. DeMets (2010). Review of draft FDA adaptive design guidance. J Biopharm Stat 20(6): 1132–42.

Dargie, H. J. (2001). Effect of carvedilol on outcome after myocardial infarction in patients with left-ventricular dysfunction: the CAPRICORN randomised trial. Lancet 357(9266): 1385–90.

Dmitrienko, A., R. B. D'Agostino, Sr., et al. (2013). Key multiplicity issues in clinical drug development. Stat Med 32(7): 1079–111.

Dragalin, V. (2006). Adaptive designs: terminology and classification. Drug Informat J 40: 425–35.

Editorial (2006). Adapting to circumstances. Nat Rev Drug Discov 5(8): 617.

Eichler, H. G., E. Abadie, et al. (2011). Bridging the efficacy-effectiveness gap: a regulator's perspective on addressing variability of drug response. Nat Rev Drug Discov 10(7): 495–506.

Eichler, H. G., K. Oye, et al. (2012). Adaptive licensing: taking the next step in the evolution of drug approval. Clin Pharmacol Ther 91(3): 426–37.

Emanuel, E. J., D. Wendler, et al. (2000). What makes clinical research ethical? JAMA 283(20): 2701–11.

Esserman, L. J., and J. Woodcock (2011). Accelerating identification and regulatory approval of investigational cancer drugs. JAMA 306(23): 2608–9.

European Medicines Agency and Committee for Medicinal Products for Human Use (2007). Reflection paper on methodological issues in confirmatory clinical trials planned with an adaptive design (http://www.ema.europa.eu/docs/en_GB/document_library/Scientific_guideline/2009/09/WC500003616.pdf).

Flaherty, K. T., I. Puzanov, et al. (2010). Inhibition of mutated, activated BRAF in metastatic melanoma. N Engl J Med 363(9): 809–19.

Fleming, T. R. and D. L. DeMets (1996). Surrogate end points in clinical trials: are we being misled? Ann Intern Med125(7): 605–13.

Food and Drug Administration and Center for Biologics Evaluation and Research (CBER) (2013). Guidance for industry: considerations for the design of early-phase clinical trials of cellular and gene therapy products. Draft guidance (http://www.fda.gov/downloads/BiologicsBloodVaccines/GuidanceComplianceRegulatoryInformation/Guidances/CellularandGeneTherapy/UCM359073.pdf).

Food and Drug Administration, Center for Drug Evaluation and Research (CDER), et al. (2011). Identifying CDER's science and research needs report (http://www.fda.gov/downloads/drugs/scienceresearch/ucm264594.pdf).

Food and Drug Administration, Center for Drug Evaluation and Research (CDER), et al. (2010A) Guidance for industry: adaptive design clinical trials for drugs and biologics (http://www.fda.gov/downloads/Drugs/GuidanceComplianceRegulatoryInformation/Guidances/ucm201790.pdf).

Food and Drug Administration, Center for Drug Evaluation and Research (CDER), et al. (2010B) Guidance for industry: non-inferiority clinical trials (http://www.fda.gov/downloads/drugs/guidancecomplianceregulatoryinformation/guidances/ucm202140.pdf).

Fox, S., S. Farr-Jones, et al. (2006). High-throughput screening: update on practices and success. J Biomol Screen 11(7): 864–69.

Freedman, B. (1987). Equipoise and the ethics of clinical research. N Engl J Med 317(3): 141–45.

Freidlin, B., L. M. McShane, et al. (2010). Randomized clinical trials with biomarkers: design issues. J Natl Cancer Inst 102(3): 152–60.

Friedman, L. M., C. D. Furberg, et al. (1998). Monitoring Response Variables: Fundamentals of Clinical Trials. New York: Springer, pp. 246–83.

Fusaro, V. A., P. Patil, et al. (2013). A systems approach to designing effective clinical trials using simulations. Circulation 127(4): 517–26.

Gallo, P. (2006a). Confidentiality and trial integrity issues for adaptive designs. Drug Inf J 40: 445–50.

Gallo, P. (2006b). Operational challenges in adaptive design implementation. Pharm Stat 5(2): 119–24.

Gallo, P., C. Chuang-Stein, et al. (2006). Adaptive designs in clinical drug development—an Executive Summary of the PhRMA Working Group. J Biopharm Stat 16(3): 275–83; discussion 285–91, 293–98, 311–12.

Goldberger, J. J., and A. E. Buxton (2013). Personalized medicine vs guideline-based medicine. JAMA 309(24): 2559–60.

Hamren, B., E. Bjork, et al. (2008). Models for plasma glucose, HbA1c, and hemoglobin interrelationships in patients with type 2 diabetes following tesaglitazar treatment. Clin Pharmacol Ther 84(2): 228–35.

Huang, S. M., and R. Temple (2008). Is this the drug or dose for you? Impact and consideration of ethnic factors in global drug development, regulatory review, and clinical practice. Clin Pharmacol Ther 84(3): 287–94.

Hung, H. M., R. T. O'Neill, et al. (2006). A regulatory view on adaptive/flexible clinical trial design. Biom J 48(4): 565–73.

Ingle, J. N., M. Liu, et al. (2013). Selective estrogen receptor modulators and pharmacogenomic variation in ZNF423 regulation of BRCA1 expression: individualized breast cancer prevention. Cancer Discov 3(7):812–25.

Institute of Medicine (2010). Evaluation of Biomarkers and Surrogate Endpoints in Chronic Disease. Washington, DC: National Academies Press.

Ishizuka, N., and Y. Ohashi (2001). The continual reassessment method and its applications: a Bayesian methodology for phase I cancer clinical trials. Stat Med 20(17–18): 2661–81.

Ivy, S. P., L. L. Siu, et al. (2010). Approaches to phase 1 clinical trial design focused on safety, efficiency, and selected patient populations: a report from the clinical trial design task force of the national cancer institute investigational drug steering committee. Clin Cancer Res 16(6): 1726–36.

Karlsson, K. E., C. Vong, et al. (2013). Comparisons of analysis methods for proof-of-concept trials. CPT: Pharmac Syst Pharmacol 2: e23.

Khan, J. Y., and M. R. Yuce (2010). Wireless body area network (WBAN) for medical applications. In: D. Campolo, ed., New Developments in Biomedical Engineering. InTech (http://www.intechopen.com/books/new-developments-in-biomedical-engineering/wireless-body-area-network-wban-for-medical-applications).

Lalonde, R. L., K. G. Kowalski, et al. (2007). Model-based drug development. Clin Pharmacol Ther 82(1): 21–32.

Lee, J. A., S. Chu, et al. (2011). Open innovation for phenotypic drug discovery: the PD2 assay panel. J Biomol Screen 16(6): 588–602.

Lee, M. J., A. S. Ye, et al. (2012). Sequential application of anticancer drugs enhances cell death by rewiring apoptotic signaling networks. Cell 149(4): 780–94.

Lehar, J., G. R. Zimmermann, et al. (2007). Chemical combination effects predict connectivity in biological systems. Mol Syst Biol 3: 80.

Lesko, L. J. (2007). Paving the critical path: how can clinical pharmacology help achieve the vision? Clin Pharmacol Ther 81(2): 170–77.

Lesko, L. J., S. Zheng, et al. (2013). Systems approaches in risk assessment. Clin Pharmacol Ther 93(5): 413–24.

Lewis, R. J., J. T. Connor, et al. (2011). Application of adaptive design and decision making to a phase II trial of a phosphodiesterase inhibitor for the treatment of intermittent claudication. Trials 12: 134.

Lindsay, M. A. (2003). Target discovery. Nat Rev Drug Discov 2(10): 831–38.

Lipsky, A. M., and R. J. Lewis (2013). Response-adaptive decision-theoretic trial design: operating characteristics and ethics. Stat Med 32(21):3752–65.

Loscalzo, J., and A. L. Barabási (2011). Systems biology and the future of medicine. Wiley Interdiscip Rev Syst Biol Med 3(6): 619–27.

Lumpkin, M. M., H. G. Eichler, et al. (2012). Advancing the science of medicines regulation: the role of the 21st-century medicines regulator. Clin Pharmacol Ther 92(4): 486–93.

Lunardi, A., U. Ala, et al. (2013). A co-clinical approach identifies mechanisms and potential therapies for androgen deprivation resistance in prostate cancer. doi 10.1038/ng.2650. Nature Genet 45(7):747–55.

Mehta, C. R., and Y. Jemiai (2006). A consultant's perspective on the regulatory hurdles to adaptive trials. Biom J 48(4): 604–8; discussion 613–22.

Mehta, C., P. Gao, et al. (2009). Optimizing trial design: sequential, adaptive, and enrichment strategies. Circulation 119(4): 597–605.

Mehta, C. R., and S. J. Pocock (2011). Adaptive increase in sample size when interim results are promising: A practical guide with examples. Stat Med 30(28): 3267–84.

Meurer, W. J., R. J. Lewis, et al. (2012). Adaptive clinical trials: a partial remedy for the therapeutic misconception? JAMA 307(22): 2377–78.

Miller, R., W. Ewy, et al. (2005). How modeling and simulation have enhanced decision making in new drug development. J Pharmacokinet Pharmacodyn 32(2): 185–97.

Milligan, P. A., M. J. Brown, et al. (2013). Model-based drug development: a rational approach to efficiently accelerate drug development. Clin Pharmacol Ther 93(6): 502–14.

Moore, G. E. (1965). Cramming more components onto integrated circuits. Electronics 38(8): 1–4.

Nardella, C., A. Lunardi, et al. (2011). The APL paradigm and the co-clinical trial project. Cancer Discov 1(2): 108–16.

National Center for Advancing Translational Sciences National Center for Advancing Translational Sciences (NCATS) website (http://www.ncats.nih.gov/index.html).

National Center for Advancing Translational Sciences. Rescuing and Repurposing Drugs (http://www.ncats.nih.gov/research/reengineering/rescue-repurpose/rescue-repurpose.html).

Nishihara, R., P. Lochhead, et al. (2013). Aspirin use and risk of colorectal cancer according to BRAF mutation status. JAMA **309**(24): 2563–71.

Orloff, J., F. Douglas, et al. (2009). The future of drug development: advancing clinical trial design. Nat Rev Drug Discov. **8**(12): 949–57.

Pasche, B. (2013). Differential effects of aspirin before and after diagnosis of colorectal cancer. JAMA **309**(24): 2598–99.

Peck, C. C. (2010). Quantitative clinical pharmacology is transforming drug regulation. J Pharmacokinet Pharmacodyn **37**(6): 617–28.

Rawlins, M. D. (2004). Cutting the cost of drug development? Nat Rev Drug Discov **3**(4): 360–64.

Ruff, C. T., R. P. Giugliano, et al. (2010). Evaluation of the novel factor Xa inhibitor edoxaban compared with warfarin in patients with atrial fibrillation: design and rationale for the Effective aNticoaGulation with factor xA next GEneration in Atrial Fibrillation-Thrombolysis In Myocardial Infarction study 48 (ENGAGE AF-TIMI 48). Am Heart J **160**(4): 635–41.

Salazar, D. E., J. Mendell, et al. (2012). Modelling and simulation of edoxaban exposure and response relationships in patients with atrial fibrillation. Thromb Haemost **107**(5): 925–36.

Santen, R. J., N. F. Boyd, et al. (2007). Critical assessment of new risk factors for breast cancer: considerations for development of an improved risk prediction model. Endocr Relat Cancer **14**(2): 169–87.

Scannell, J.W., A. Blanckley, et al. (2012) Diagnosing the decline in pharmaceutical R&D efficiency. Nat Rev Drug Disc **11**(3): 191–200.

Sheiner, L.B. (1997). Learning versus confirming in clinical drug development. Clin Pharmacol Ther **61**(3): 275–91

Sheiner, L. B., S. L. Beal, et al. (1989). Study designs for dose-ranging. Clin Pharmacol Ther **46**(1): 63–77.

Simon, R., B. Freidlin, et al. (1997). Accelerated titration designs for phase I clinical trials in oncology. J Natl Cancer Inst **89**(15): 1138–47.

Tallarida, R. J. (2006). An overview of drug combination analysis with isobolograms. J Pharmacol Exp Ther **319**(1): 1–7.

The PURSUIT Trial Investigators (1998). Inhibition of platelet glycoprotein IIb/IIIa with eptifibatide in patients with acute coronary syndromes. N Engl J Med **339**(7): 436–43.

Topol, E. J. (2001). Reperfusion therapy for acute myocardial infarction with fibrinolytic therapy or combination reduced fibrinolytic therapy and platelet glycoprotein IIb/IIIa inhibition: the GUSTO V randomised trial. Lancet **357**(9272): 1905–14.

Tournoux-Facon, C., Y. De Rycke, et al. (2011). Targeting population entering phase III trials: a new stratified adaptive phase II design. Stat Med **30**(8): 801–11.

van der Graaf, P. H. (2012). CPT: pharmacometrics and systems pharmacology. CPT: Pharmacometrics Syst Pharmacol **1**: e8.

van der Graaf, R., K. C. Roes, et al. (2012). Adaptive trials in clinical research: scientific and ethical issues to consider. JAMA **307**(22): 2379–80.

Wang, S. J., H. M. Hung, et al. (2011). Regulatory perspectives on multiplicity in adaptive design clinical trials throughout a drug development program. J Biopharm Stat **21**(4): 846–59.

Yeh, P., and R. Kishony (2007). Networks from drug-drug surfaces. Mol Syst Biol **3**: 85.

Zineh, I., and J. Woodcock (2013). Clinical pharmacology and the catalysis of regulatory science: opportunities for the advancement of drug development and evaluation. Clin Pharmacol Ther **93**(6): 515–25.

16

Microbiomics in Network Medicine

Joanne E. Sordillo, George M. Weinstock,
and Augusto A. Litonjua

Introduction

While it has been classically thought that microbes are pathogenic, it is becoming clear that human evolution was dependent to some degree on symbiosis with certain microbial organisms in the gut, which allowed early humans to acquire new foods and expand their diet (Ley, Hamady, et al. 2008; Ley, Lozupone, et al. 2008; Fraune and Bosch 2010). For example, the early hominid diet consisted of plant roots, bulbs, and tubers; then a shift occurred to a diet consisting of more meat, until the adoption of agricultural practices and domestication of animals again caused another shift in diet, incorporating dairy in addition to meat and plants. The gut microbiome was critical in these shifts in diet, enabling early humans to access nutrients fully. This is reflected in the findings that the lower-gut microbiomes of herbivores, carnivores, and omnivores are different (Ley, Hamady, et al. 2008).

Dating back to the mid-to-late twentieth century, there has been interest in studying the role of the gut microbiota in human health (Luckey 1970). Early studies used culture methods to identify bacteria and were limited to those that were potentially pathogenic. Clearly, these culture-based techniques were limited, as the vast majority of microorganisms in the human gut were either difficult or impossible to grow. With the advent of modern sequencing methods, the study of the microbiome has exploded in the past decade. Being culture-independent, these methods allow for a deeper and more expansive view of the community of microorganisms that reside in the human gut. The human microbiota was defined originally as "the ecological community of . . . microorganisms that literally share our body space" (Lederberg and McCray 2001). This collection of communities of microorganisms inhabiting different anatomical locations in humans is also a collection of genomes, defined as the metagenome (Handelsman, Rondon, et al. 1998). Metagenomics is the study of these genomes and their genes. Using culture methods, it has been estimated that there are over 100-fold more bacteria than human cells in the colon (Luckey 1970), and this figure has been upheld by sequencing methods (Qin,

Li, et al. 2010). This number may even be an underestimate, as these studies have not included viruses and other types of nonbacterial microorganisms. It is interesting to note that microorganisms are commonly found in complex communities in which different organisms share a similar ecological niche (Tyler, Smith, et al. 2014). Commonly, these organisms are dependent on other organisms or the whole community of organisms, requiring metabolic support for survival (Lozupone, Faust, et al. 2012). In addition, these communities of organisms need to maintain a delicate and mutually beneficial balance with the human host in order to ensure that both symbionts survive and prosper (Xu, Mahowald, et al. 2007). The complex nature of these microbe–microbe, microbe–community, microbe–host interactions, and various iterations of these interactions is only beginning to be understood. Network approaches will be necessary to better understand these complex relationships and how they affect human health.

This chapter will first review the important effects of the microbiome on human health. Next, the contributions of the human microbiome consortiums will be reviewed, as they have jump-started research into the microbiome with their basic data and tools. A basic workflow of microbiome research follows. Because the microbiome contains at least thousands of bacteria, viruses, fungi, and other microorganisms that interact with each other, network approaches will be necessary to understand fully the functions of these communities of organisms. We present a brief review of the emerging methods available that will enable researchers to begin to ask the important questions of how these interactions occur. While most of the discussion and the examples presented here relate to the gut microbiome, these methods are applicable to the study of any microbiome niche.

Examples of Function of the Gut Microbiome in Human Health

Harvest of otherwise inaccessible nutrients and/or sources of energy in the diet.
The composition of the gut microbiota of people with very dissimilar diets differ from each other, presumably to maximize the extraction of nutrients from these diets. For example, children from a rural African village who eat a diet rich in fiber have a gut microbiome that shows enrichment for bacteria from the phylum Bacteroidetes but depletion of Firmicutes. Specifically, their microbiome has a unique abundance of bacteria from the *Prevotella* and *Xylanibacter* genera, which are known to contain genes for

cellulose and xylan hydrolysis; these are completely lacking in age-matched European children (De Filippo, Cavalieri, et al. 2011). This is consistent with other studies that have shown that microbiomes of carnivores are enriched with bacterial genes that degrade protein while those of herbivores are enriched with bacterial genes that synthesize amino acid building blocks (Ley, Hamady, et al. 2008; Muegge, Kuczynski, et al. 2011). Thus, it is clear that the gut microbiome allows adaptation to the environment (diet) of the human host.

However, it is also apparent that the gut microbiome can confer disease risk given the right environment, and it has recently been suggested that the gut microbiome is the driving force for obesity (Kovatcheva-Datchary and Arora 2013). In murine models, obesity has been associated with a decreased abundance in Bacteroidetes and a proportional increase in Firmicutes (Ley, Backhed, et al. 2005; Turnbaugh, Backhed, et al. 2008). However, the picture is not as clear in humans. While several studies have shown an increase in the ratio of Firmicutes to Bacteroidetes (Ley, Turnbaugh, et al. 2006; Santacruz, Collado, et al. 2010), which is in line with the murine data, other studies have not shown this pattern (Duncan, Lobley, et al. 2008; Zhang, DiBaise, et al. 2009). Rather than the composition of the microbiome, it appears that an altered functionality of the microbiome is associated with obesity. Turnbaugh and colleagues have shown that despite differences in microbiome composition between individuals, there appears to be a wide array of shared microbial genes that likely comprises the functional core microbiome (Turnbaugh and Gordon 2009; Turnbaugh, Hamady, et al. 2009). Deviations from this core with respect to genes and pathways involved in energy harvest are associated with obesity. Furthermore, in a systems-level analysis of metabolic networks, microbial genes associated with obesity are located at the periphery of the metabolic networks, suggesting that lean and obese microbiomes differ in their interface with the human host and in the way they interact with host metabolism (Greenblum, Turnbaugh, et al. 2012).

Synthesis of vitamins. Humans are incapable of synthesizing most vitamins, which are essential micronutrients usually found as cofactors of various enzymes involved in biochemical reactions in cells. Aside from exogenous sources, the gut microbiome is capable of producing these vitamins, such as vitamin K (Suttie 1995). Gut bacteria also produce several B vitamins. Several strains of bacteria from the genus *Bifidobacteria* have been shown to produce folate both in vitro (D'Aimmo, Mattarelli, et al. 2012) and in vivo (Strozzi and Mogna 2008), leading to the identification of high-level (e.g., *Bifidobacterium bifidum* and *B. longum* subsp. *infantis*) and low-level folate-producing species (e.g., *B. breve, B. longum* subsp. *longum* and *B. adolescentis*) (Pompei, Cordisco, et al. 2007). Bacteria from the genus *Lactobacillus* generally need folate for growth, but one strain, *L. plantarum,* has been shown to be a folate producer (Rossi, Amaretti, et al. 2012). Other B vitamins, such as riboflavin and B_{12}, may also be produced by gut microbiota (LeBlanc, Milani, et al. 2013).

Metabolism of xenobiotics. Xenobiotics include any compound that is found in an organism but that is foreign to humans in that it is not normally produced or consumed by them. Humans are exposed to therapeutic and diet-derived xenobiotics on a daily basis, and the role of the microbiome in the metabolism of these compounds will be an important focus of investigation. Known involvement of the gut microbiome in xenobiotic metabolism occurs through several direct mechanisms: (1) production of active compounds, (2) detoxification, and (3) direct binding to bacterial cells (Carmody and Turnbaugh 2014). Indirect mechanisms may also be involved and occur via microbial manipulation of host physiology; they include such pathways as microbial participation in enterohepatic cycling and microbial production of metabolic pathway intermediates (Carmody and Turnbaugh 2014). Two studies have highlighted the importance of this role of the microbiome in human health. The first involved a series of experiments using untargeted metabolomic analyses of plasma samples, in which three metabolites linked with ingestion of phosphatidylcholine—choline, betaine, and trimethylamine-N-oxide (TMAO)—were reproducibly correlated with cardiovascular risk (Wang, Klipfell, et al. 2011). TMAO, the metabolite most strongly correlated with cardiovascular disease risk, arises from bacterial metabolism of choline via an intermediate, trimethylamine, which is not produced by humans (Barrett and Kwan 1985; Zhang, Mitchell et al. 1999; Tang, Wang, et al. 2013). The second study investigated the relationship of artificial sweeteners and the development of glucose intolerance (Suez, Korem, et al. 2014). Because of the contradictory epidemiological evidence for improvement in glycemic response, weight gain, and risk of type 2 diabetes, and because these artificial sweeteners pass through the gastrointestinal (GI) tract undigested, the authors speculated that the gut microbiome may have a role in the effects of these artificial sweeteners. Suez, Korem, and colleagues (2014) showed that mice fed saccharin, sucralose, or aspartame developed glucose intolerance; that this effect could be blocked by the co-administration of antibiotics; and that this glucose-intolerant phenotype could be transferred to germ-free mice by transplanting fecal material from saccharin-fed mice. Metagenomic sequencing analysis confirmed that saccharin consumption induced changes in both the composition and the function of the gut microbiome, resulting in expansion of genes for glycan degradation and leading to increases in short-chain fatty acid levels in the stool. This is characteristic of increased energy harvest by the microbiota. The authors extended these findings to human subjects. First, they categorized a cohort of subjects according to their consumption of artificial sweeteners (based on responses to a food frequency questionnaire) and found that high consumers had higher glycated hemoglobin (HbA_{1c}) levels than low consumers. Next, they studied seven healthy volunteers and fed them the equivalent of 5 g/day of saccharin and performed glucose-tolerance tests and collected stool samples for 7 days. Four of the seven began to develop impaired glucose responses after 4 days of consuming saccharin. They then transplanted stool from two human subjects who developed impaired glucose responses and two who did not into germ-free mice. They showed that the impaired glucose-tolerance phenotype could be transferred by stool transplants, thus implicating the distal gut microbiome in conferring impaired glucose tolerance in the face of saccharin ingestion.

Development and activity of the immune system. The gut microbiome is, quantitatively, the most important postnatal source of microbial stimulation of the immune system (Salminen, Bouley, et al. 1998; Guarner and Malagelada 2003) and has a role in its development and programming (Bengmark 2012; Weng and Walker 2013). Both innate (Hooper, Stappenbeck, et al. 2003) and adaptive (Mazmanian, Liu, et al. 2005; Lee and Mazmanian 2010) immune responses are modulated by gut bacteria, and changes in the composition and function of the gut microbiome have been postulated to be a cause of the rise in prevalence of autoimmune and allergic disorders (Weng and Walker 2013). Emerging evidence also points to the important role of gut microbiota in shaping the anticancer immune response to chemotherapeutic agents (Iida, Dzutsev, et al. 2013; Viaud, Saccheri, et al. 2013).

Other effects. Gut microbiota have also been implicated in gut epithelial cell renewal (Pull, Doherty, et al. 2005) and function (Backhed, Manchester, et al. 2007). No doubt other effects will be related to the gut microbiome. Animal models are being used to investigate the relationship between the gut microbiome and brain development and nervous system disorders (Diaz Heijtz, Wang, et al. 2011; Clarke, Grenham, et al. 2013) and research is ongoing to define a lung microbiome (Beck, Young, et al. 2012; Lynch and Bruce 2013; Dickson, Martinez, et al. 2014). The concept of a tissue and blood microbiome has also been proposed, and initial prospective relationships between sequenced circulating bacterial DNA and the onset of diabetes and cardiovascular disease has been described (Amar, Serino, et al. 2011; Amar, Lange, et al. 2013). The advent of modern methods ushered in by large consortiums, such as the Human Microbiome Project (HMP) and the European Commission Metagenomics of the Human Intestinal Tract (MetaHIT) Project, has already facilitated research into the role of the various microbiomes in human health. Because there are complex relationships between microbes and their local communities, between communities of microbes in various niches, and between microbes and the human host, network approaches will be necessary to elucidate these relationships fully.

Human Microbiome Projects

To better to understand the role of these microorganisms in human health, it is first necessary to describe the various niches of microorganisms in the human body. To begin to accomplish this task, two consortiums were established—the U.S. National Institutes of Health–funded HMP and the European Commission's MetaHIT. The first phase of the HMP was launched in 2007. This first phase (2007–2013) aimed to characterize the composition and diversity of microbial communities that inhabit major mucosal surfaces of the human body, including nasal passages, oral cavities, skin, and gastrointestinal and urogenital tracts, and to evaluate the genetic metabolic potential of these communities, (HMP Consortium, 2014) and was tasked with six initiatives:

- Develop a reference set of microbial genomic sequences and give a preliminary characterization of the human microbiome.
- Elucidate the relationship between disease and changes in the human microbiome.
- Develop new technologies for computational analysis.
- Develop new tools for computational analysis.
- Establish a data analysis and coordinating center (DACC).
- Establish research repositories.

Because new methods are expected to give rise to new and unexplored concerns, an Ethical, Legal and Societal Implications (ELSI) program was also created to address the issues that will arise from human microbiome research.

The HMP recruited 300 healthy adults, 18 to 40 years of age, who were carefully screened and phenotyped (HMP Consortium 2012a). These subjects then underwent sampling one to three times from 15 male or 18 female body sites. Each body habitat was characterized by distinct microbial communities, with the oral and stool communities being most diverse while vaginal sites harbored particularly simple communities (HMP Consortium 2012b). A particularly important finding was that within-subject variation over time was consistently lower than between-subject variation, both in the organisms present and in the metabolic functions represented by the microbes. This finding suggests that a feature of the microbiome in healthy individuals is stability over time and that deviations from this could be associated with diseases. While no taxa were universally present among all body habitats and individuals, several metabolic pathways were present in all habitats and in all individuals (Figure 16–1). The most abundant of these core metabolic pathways include the ribosome and translational machinery, nucleotide charging and ATP synthesis, and glycolysis (HMP Consortium 2012b).

The MetaHIT project ran from 2008 to 2012. Its central objective was to establish associations between the microbiome and human health and disease. Unlike the HMP, the MetaHIT concentrated only on the gut microbiome. MetaHIT undertook several activities. First, it established an extensive reference catalog of microbial genes present in the human intestine. Second, it developed bioinformatics tools to store, organize, and interpret the sequence information. Third, it developed tools to determine which genes of the reference catalog were present in different individuals and at what frequency. Fourth, it gathered cohorts of individuals; focused on healthy subjects, subjects with

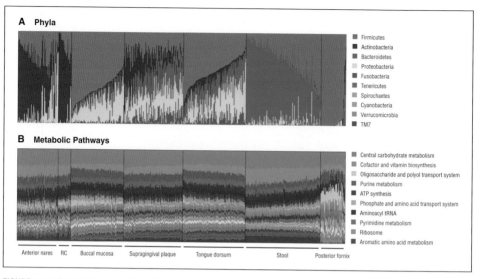

FIGURE 16–1. Taxonomic composition of the microbiome (top) varies while metabolic pathways (bottom) are relatively conserved in healthy subjects. RC, retroauricular crease; tRNA, transfer RNA. (Adapted with permission from HMP Consortium (2012b). Structure, function, and diversity of the healthy human microbiome. *Nature* **486**(7402): 207–14.)

inflammatory bowel disease, and obese subjects; and determined for most which microbial genes they carry. Fifth, it developed methods to study the function of bacterial genes associated with disease, with the aim of understanding the underlying mechanisms and host–microbe interactions.

MetaHIT collected stool samples from 124 healthy, overweight, and obese subjects, as well as from patients with inflammatory bowel disease. The initial results from MetaHIT cataloged 3.3 million nonredundant microbial genes, approximately 150 times more than the human gene complement (Qin, Li, et al. 2010). MetaHIT also identified three discrete enterotypes in the human gut microbiome (Figure 16–2) (Arumugam, Raes, et al. 2011). Based on species composition, enterotype 1 is dominated by *Bacteroides,* enterotype 2 by *Prevotella,* and enterotype 3 (the most frequent) by *Ruminococcus.* However, other researchers have not found the same discrete enterotypes and instead suggest a continuum or gradient of species and functionality (Wu, Chen, et al. 2011) and that individuals cross over from one putative cluster to another over time (Caporaso, Lauber, et al. 2011). Thus, it is likely that the members of the communities change over time, but that the stability of the core functionality of the gut microbiome is important for health.

Both the HMP and MetaHIT have helped to expand our knowledge of the human microbiome, and they have stimulated more research on this topic. Aside from the initial catalog of microbial genes and identification of members

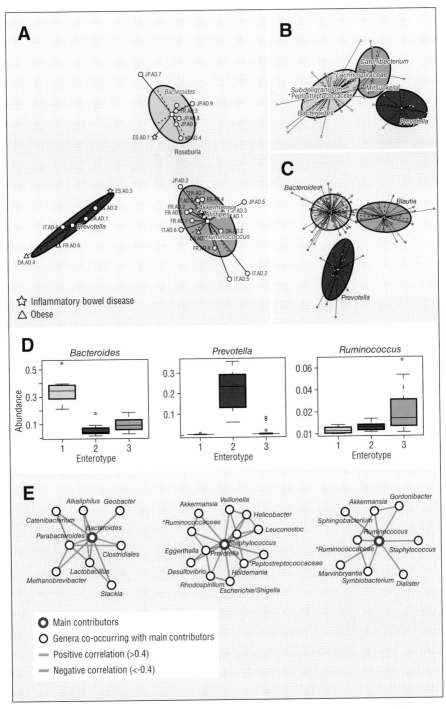

FIGURE 16–2. Enterotypes in the human gut microbiome. Panels A to C show enterotype clusters. A, Genus compositions of 33 Sanger metagenomes; B, a subset containing 85 metagenomes from an Illumina data set; and C, 154 pyrosequencing-based 16S sequences. D, Abundance of taxa that are the main contributors to enterotypes. E, Analysis of co-occurrence networks for the three enterotypes. (Adapted with permission from Arumugam, M., J. Raes, et al. (2011). Enterotypes of the human gut microbiome. Nature 473(7346): 174–80.)

of each microbiome niche, an important contribution is the development of methods for both sequencing and analysis. The HMP has made their protocols and tools available to the general research community through their Data Analysis and Coordination Center website (http://www.hmpdacc.org). With initial answers to the question of what organisms are present in a particular region of the body, the HMP and MetaHIT have only scratched the surface of microbiome research. A second phase of the HMP has just been launched to answer questions regarding the interactions between these organisms, how these organisms and their interactions affect the human host, and how the human host responds to these organisms. The Integrative Human Microbiome Project (iHMP, http://hmp2.org) will study these interactions by analyzing microbiome and host responses in disease-specific cohorts with longitudinal data and by creating integrated multi-omic datasets of microbiome and host characteristics and responses to perturbations (Integrative Human Microbiome Project Consortium 2014).

Workflow for Microbiome Analysis

Detailed workflows for microbiome analyses, which encompass sample collection through sequencing and bioinformatic analysis of sequence data, have been published (Morgan and Huttenhower 2012; Weinstock 2012; Tyler, Smith, et al. 2014). A summary of the workflow is presented in Figure 16–3.

> *Sample collection and storage.* Before embarking on a microbiome project, the appropriate study design needs to be decided (e.g., case–control, diseased only, cohort, etc.) and then sample collection can proceed. Once the sample is collected, consideration must be given to whether immediate extraction should be performed or whether the sample should be frozen at −80°C, as this can have effects on measurements (Bahl, Bergstrom, et al. 2012). Once a decision is made, then all samples collected for the particular study should use the same method.
>
> *DNA extraction.* The next step in the process of analyzing the microbiome is extracting total DNA. The choice of extraction method can affect apparent community composition (Carrigg, Rice, et al. 2007; Kaser, Ruf, et al. 2009; Salonen, Nikkila, et al. 2010) because samples are heterogeneous with regard to the organisms present, with differences in the structures of their cell walls. Currently, no method allows a truly unbiased view of the bacterial community

structure in any sample, (Ó Cuív, Aguirre de Carcer, et al. 2011; Yuan, Cohen, et al. 2012), and this needs to be taken into account in any microbiome study.

16S rRNA and shotgun sequencing. Bacterial ribosomal RNA (rRNA) genes are transcribed from the ribosomal operon as 30S rRNA, then cleaved into 16S, 23S, and 5S rRNA units. Of these units, 16S is the most conserved and has been the mainstay for characterizing microbial community structure for many decades (Tringe and Hugenholtz 2008). Modern methods have made sequencing this gene easier, and microbiome studies rely on this method for identifying the bacteria that are present and determining the taxonomic diversity in the sample. Once sequencing is completed, filtering is employed to ensure that the data are of good quality. This entails addressing such issues as read quality, chimerism (a read formed from different 16S rRNA genes), and read length (Weinstock 2012). Next, tables of taxa and abundance are produced by comparisons of the generated sequences with 16S rRNA sequence databases such as GreenGenes (DeSantis, Hugenholtz, et al. 2006), the Ribosomal Database Project (Cole, Wang, et al. 2009), and SILVA (Pruesse, Quast, et al. 2007) to assign the sequences to specific taxa (i.e., phylotyping). Alternatively, bioinformatic software packages can also cluster the reads into operational taxonomic units, or OTUs (Schloss, Westcott, et al. 2009; Lozupone, Lladser, et al. 2011). OTUs are sequences that are grouped together based on similarity; generally, sequences that are 97% similar are binned into one OTU (Schloss 2010). Analyses can then proceed, and ecological metrics are computed. With the OTU information, networks of bacterial communities can be constructed based on what bacteria are present, as shown in Figure 16–2.

While 16S rRNA sequencing allows us to determine what organisms are present and their relative abundance, shotgun sequencing complements this by allowing us to know what genes are present and to infer the functional pathways that are encoded. Shotgun sequencing is followed by assembly of the entire microbiome to allow reconstruction of microbial genomes and pathways within a given habitat. As highlighted earlier, metagenomic sequencing of a relatively large number of healthy individuals performed by the HMP and MetaHIT consortiums revealed similarities in gene profiles between these individuals despite the large variation in taxonomic configuration (Arumugam, Raes et al. 2011; HMP Consortium 2012b).

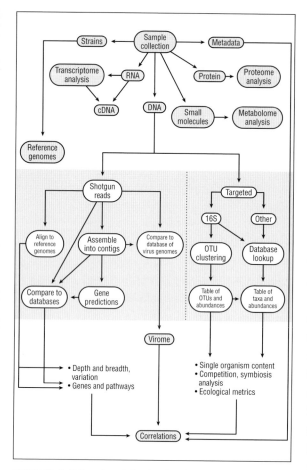

By comparing the sequences from shotgun reads with gene databases, such as GenBank or Kyoto Encyclopedia of Genes and Genomes (KEGG), using the Basic Local Alignment Search Tool (BLAST), lists of genes can be produced (HMP Consortium 2012,b; Abubucker, Segata, et al. 2012), which can then be used to build metabolic and biochemical pathways for reconstruction of community function (Abubucker, Segata, et al. 2012).

Both results from 16S rRNA sequencing analyses and shotgun sequencing analyses can then be correlated with human phenotypes, exposures (e.g., diet), and disease. This is the basic workflow for human microbiome analyses. However, as technology improves and throughput becomes higher at a reasonable cost, multi-omic studies will be needed to better understand the relationship humans have with their microbiome. Studies such as metatranscriptomics, metabolomics, and metaproteomics all hold promise for expanding microbiome studies. Network approaches will then be needed to integrate and understand all these -omics datasets.

FIGURE 16–3. Data and work flow in microbiome analysis. cDNA, complementary DNA; contig= a stretch of contiguous sequence in a genome assembly; OTU, operational taxonomic unit. (Adapted with permission from Weinstock, G. M. (2012). Genomic approaches to studying the human microbiota. Nature **489**(7415): 250–6.)

Community Analyses and Network Approaches to the Study of the Microbiome

Characterization of the human microbiome in recent years has led to tremendous gains in our understanding of the microbial taxa that live on and within us, and the functions they may serve as inhabitants of various body sites. Sequencing of the human microbiome provides more than just the opportunity for compiling data on the taxonomic composition or functional genetic potential of a biological sample. Relative abundance profiles of microbial communities may be used in: (1) statistical analyses to compare the microbiome by a given phenotype or group characteristic; and (2) network analyses to determine: (a) connections within the microbial ecosystem and the effect of perturbations, and (b) the relationship between the microbiome and other -omics data. These computational tools and techniques go beyond basic descriptive analyses. They will allow us to account for the multidimensional features of the microbiome, to consider the complex microbial community itself as an outcome, and to explore dynamics of microbial ecology.

Community comparisons. Statistical analysis of the microbiome in relation to environmental perturbations, human physiological states, and/or disease phenotypes is challenging because of the somewhat constrained nature of relative abundance data, as well as its high dimensionality. A number of statistical tools have been developed to account for the compositional distribution and complexity of microbiome data. One of the most commonly used techniques for dimensionality reduction and visualization of overall taxonomic composition is the UniFrac method (Lozupone and Knight 2005; Lozupone, Hamady, et al. 2006; Lozupone, Lladser, et al. 2011). UniFrac may be summarized as a phylogenetic analysis technique that measures the distance between two community samples in terms of the amount of sequence divergence on a phylogenetic tree that is unique to each of the samples (Ley, Hamady, et al. 2008). In this method, all of the biological samples in a given study are used to construct a master or central phylogenetic tree. For each pair of samples (communities), a value known as the UniFrac metric is calculated to determine how similar they are based on the degree of branch length that they share on the master phylogenetic tree (Figure 16–4) (Boon, Meehan, et al. 2014). Principal coordinates analysis (PCoA) can be applied to the unweighted UniFrac distances to show which samples contain similar taxonomic composition (these will cluster together on the PCoA plot) and which samples have markedly different compositions (these will appear far apart on the PCoA plot). Furthermore, the UniFrac tool allows statistical pairwise comparisons between different types of community samples (i.e., microbial communities from different body sites or from sub-

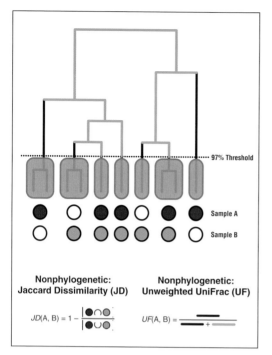

FIGURE 16–4. Community comparisons by Jaccard Dissimilarity Index and UniFrac Distance. Nonphylogenetic (Jaccard dissimilarity index) and phylogenetic diversity (UniFrac) in two hypothetical microbiome samples. Red circles indicate OTUs present in sample A; blue circles indicate OTUs present in sample B; white circles show the absence of an OTU from a sample. Green edges of the tree show overlap between the two samples, black edges in the tree have branches from one, but not both samples.

jects with different phenotypes) in order to determine which communities are significantly different after adjusting for multiple comparisons (Lozupone, Hamady, et al. 2006). For instance, in a study of host diet and bacterial phylogeny, UniFrac-based principal coordinates of gut microbiome data from humans demonstrated significantly different clusters for carnivores, herbivores, and omnivores ($p<0.005$) (Ley, Hamandy 2008). Use of the UniFrac method in a study of the biogeography of the human microbiome showed that body habitat was the most important determinant of community composition and that for a given body site, the most abundant taxa were relatively stable across individuals and over time (Costello, Lauber, et al. 2009).

The Jaccard dissimilarity index provides an alternative to the unweighted UniFrac distance for assessing overall differences in community composition between samples. The Jaccard dissimilarity index is computed using data on the presence and/or absence of taxa, but does not incorporate information on the phylogenetic overlap between samples (see Figure 16–4) (Boon, Meehan, et al. 2014).

Another community comparison approach, developed by La Rosa, Brooks, and colleagues (2012), utilizes a parametric model (assuming a Dirichlet multinomial [DM] distribution) to perform multivariate statistical hypothesis testing for differences in bacterial taxa composition between groups of metagenomic samples. Unlike many nonparametric methods that rely on permutation testing, this parametric model is computationally efficient, can quantify the difference between community compositions, and is unlikely to have an inflated type I error rate. This method also preserves more of the unique information in the micro-

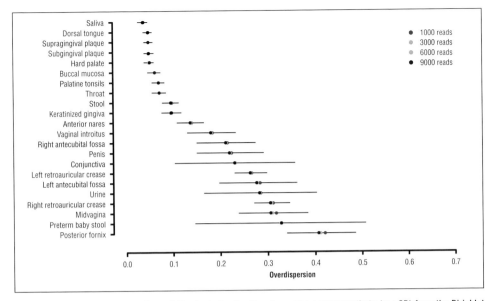

FIGURE 16–5. Bacterial community variation by body site. Overdispersion parameter theta ($m \pm$ SD) from the Dirichlet multinomial model was used to evaluate microbial community variation. Samples with higher theta values had greater variation. Variation within a bacterial community was consistent across different read depths (1000, 3000, 6000, and 9000 read depths).

biome, since no initial data-reduction step is required prior to analysis (as in Uni-Frac). Theta, the overdispersion parameter in the DM model ranging from 0 to 1, reflects the variance of each taxon and covariance across taxa (higher theta values denote higher variation). An HMP analysis of microbiome biogeography by body habitat using this DM model for community comparison showed the greatest community variation (theta) for vaginal (posterior fornix) samples, but the lowest for oral and stool microbiomes (Figure 16–5) (Zhou, Gao, et al. 2013). Even though there was little variability within specific oral sites, taxonomic composition data analysis using this model showed significant differences between oral sites (subgingival plaque, supragingival plaque, and saliva) revealing that these bacterial communities are distinct from one another, despite the close proximity of sampling locations (subgingival vs. supragingival plaque comparison shown in Figure 16–6) (La Rosa, Brooks, et al. 2012). A third type of computational analysis for community-level microbiome data compares taxonomic trees built using sequence data from the bacterial 16S rRNA gene. This statistical method takes into account the entire branched, hierarchical structure of the bacterial taxonomy in a given sample (rather than analyzing the data at only one specific taxonomic level) and uses a form of object-oriented data analysis (OODA) to construct individual weighted tree structures for each biological sample (La Rosa, Shands, et al. 2012). Maximum likelihood estimation is used to derive a group-level tree for each

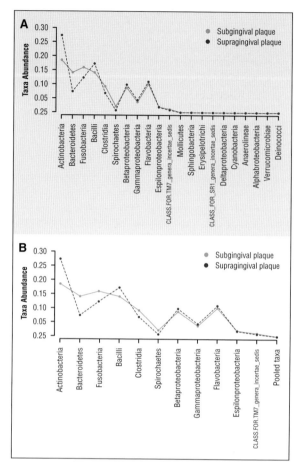

FIGURE 16–6. Comparison of two metagenomic groups using a taxa composition data analysis approach. Taxon abundance curves (frequency means) are plotted for subgingival plaque samples (blue) and supragingival plaque samples (red). A, Taxa frequency means for each group. For the plot in B, rare taxa (with abundance less than 1%) are pooled into an additional taxon labeled as "Pooled taxa."

sample type, as well as an overall central tree across all samples (i.e., assuming no difference in the microbiome by sample grouping). Using the OODA model, likelihood-ratio test statistics are computed to compare the taxonomic tree distributions of the two metagenomic populations. This method was used to demonstrate differences in hierarchical taxonomy in the core microbiomes of saliva and stool samples in 24 human subjects sequenced as part of the HMP (Figure 16–7).

Feature selection. While statistical analysis of overall community differences between sample types often yields meaningful insights, it may be difficult to determine which features of the community are driving these effects. LEfSe (linear discriminant analysis with effect size) is a bioinformatics tool that utilizes all forms of community-level microbiome data (taxonomic composition, functional gene abundances, gene expression and/or metabolomics) to identify features that distinguish between different biological classes (phenotypes, biological sample type, or environmental source) (Segata, Izard, et al. 2011). In the initial step of the algorithm, a nonparametric Kruskal–Wallis test is performed to determine whether there are any discriminating features between two classes (groups), then pairwise Wilcoxon tests are performed on the subclasses to ensure that they also follow the class-level trend. Finally, a linear discriminant analysis model is built and used to rank features that have the greatest discriminatory power. For instance, an LEfSe analysis of HMP data comparing mucosal and nonmucosal body sites determined that Actinobacteria enrichment was a discriminating feature of mucosal microbiomes (Figure 16–8) (Segata, Izard, et al. 2011). In another LEfSe analysis of HMP data, functional genetic profiles of digestive-tract samples varied markedly by sampling location (buccal mucosa, dorsal tongue, supragingival plaque, and stool). For example, phosphotransferase system (PTS) transporters for monosaccharides were more abundant in the oral sampling sites, while the stool microbiome demonstrated enrichment for polysaccharide transport pathways (Segata, Haake, et al. 2012). LEfSe has also been used to identify several *Lactobacillus* OTUs of the vaginal microbiome that show relatively greater abundance during pregnancy (Figure 16–9) (Aagaard, Riehle, et al. 2012).

MetaStats (White, Nagarajan, et al. 2009) and STAMP (Parks and Beiko 2010) are two additional tools that can be used to identify differentially abundant features when comparing microbiomes. The MetaStats method compares features using a nonparametric *t*-test with correction for multiple comparisons and performs a separate analysis (Fisher exact test) for features with sparse count data. Using MetaStats for a reanalysis of gut microbiome data revealed differences in the microbial communities in lean versus obese individuals that were not observed in the original analysis (a higher abundance of Actinobacteria was shown in obese vs. lean subjects). STAMP is a software package with a wide variety of statistical analyses available for comparison of taxonomic and functional profiles in metagenomic samples. Some of the statistical tests in STAMP include the Fisher exact test for metagenomic data, a nonparametric bootstrapping method, and an implementation of the Barnard test.

Network methods and meta-omics analysis. Although community-level statistical models consider the microbiome as an outcome, or as a potential source of discriminatory biomarkers, network analyses focus more on the connections between the microbial community members, their relationship to other types of data, and their response to external perturbations. Networks based on microbiome data are similar to many other types of biological networks in that they are scale-free. As detailed in Chapters 1 and 2, scale-free networks have few highly connected nodes

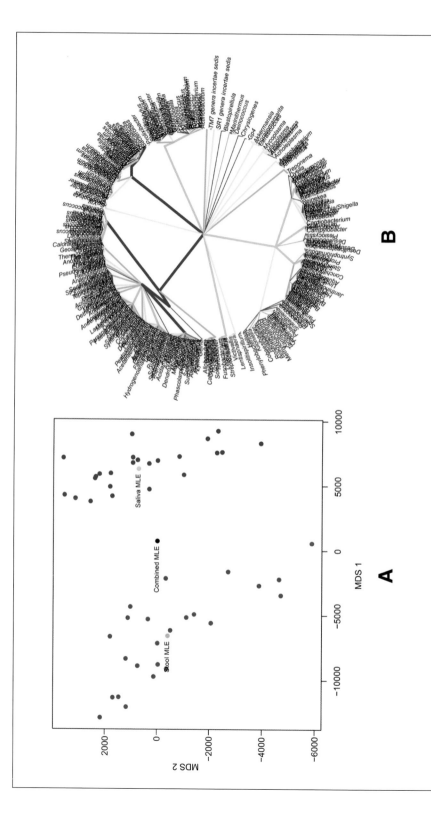

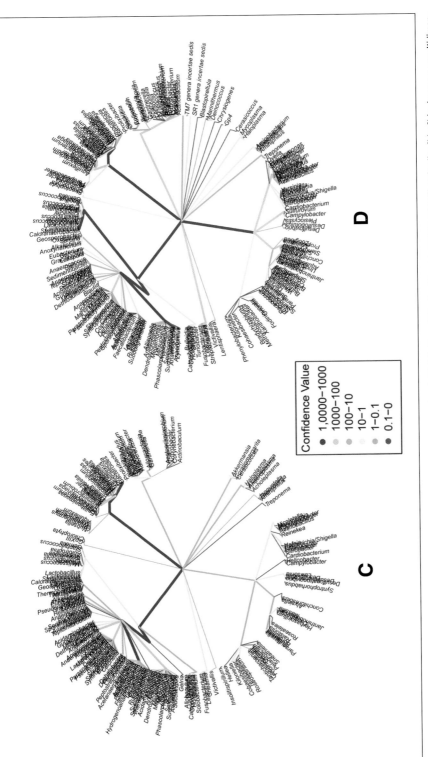

FIGURE 16–7. Hierarchical taxonomy in the core microbiomes of saliva vs. stool in HMP samples. A, Distribution of 48 microbiome trees (stool [red]) and saliva [blue]) is shown on a multidimensional scaling plot, showing distinct differences by sample type. B, Combined (stool + saliva) Maximum Likelihood Estimated (MLE) tree. C and D, MLE trees from stool and saliva samples, respectively.

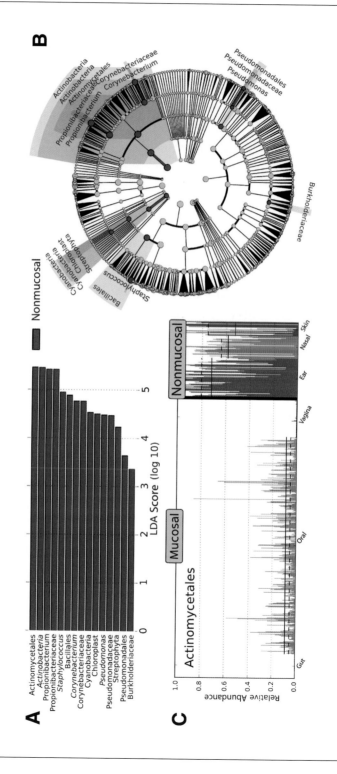

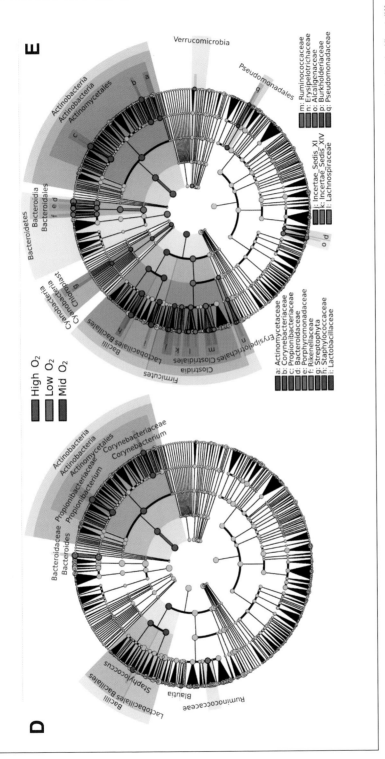

FIGURE 16–8. LEfSe results on the human microbiome. A, LEfSe Linear Discriminant Analysis Effective Size (LDA) scores for taxa demonstrating biologically and statistically significant differences between mucosal and nonmucosal sites. B, Taxonomic representation of statistically and biologically consistent differences between mucosal and nonmucosal body sites (red indicating nonmucosal, yellow nonsignificant; circle diameter proportional to abundance). C, Actinomycetales abundances in mucosal versus nonmucosal body sites. D and E, Differential features by high, mid, and low O_2 body sites (D reflects the most strict version of LEfSe [all O_2 classifications differential] while the results shown in E are from less strict LEfSe analysis [at least one O_2 class is differential]).

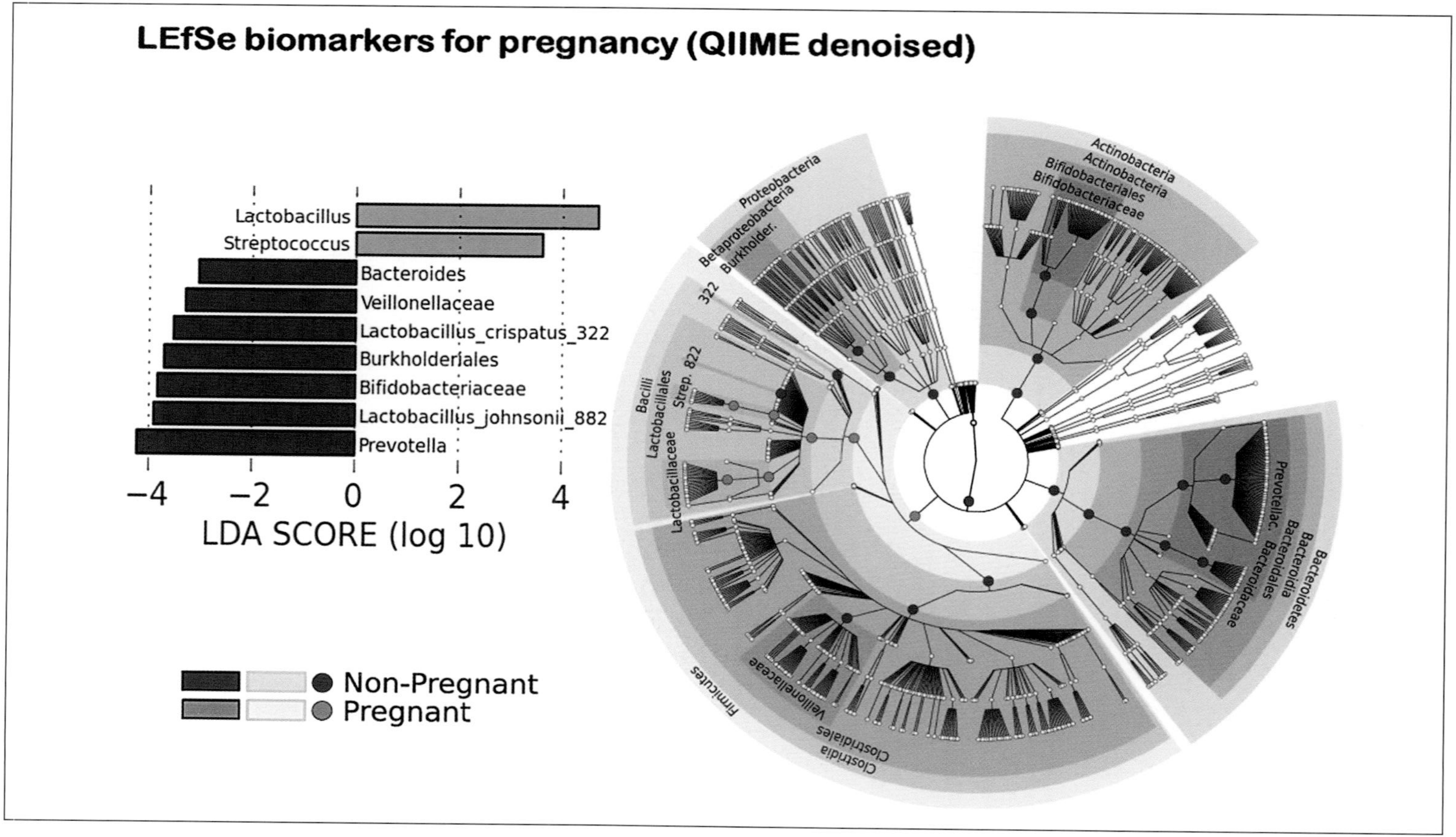

FIGURE 16—9. Taxonomic features of the vaginal microbiome vary by pregnancy status.

(hubs) and many nodes with few connections (Arita 2005). As is described in the comprehensive review by Faust and Raes (2012), there are two general types of networks in microbiome analyses: similarity-based networks, and regression- or rule-based networks of complex relationships. The similarity-based network approach shows the pattern of pairwise connections between bacterial taxa, using a measure that quantifies the co-occurrence of each pair of species. Commonly used similarity-based measures are correlations (Pearson or Spearman) and the Jaccard index. Edges are drawn between nodes if the p value or False Discovery Rate (FDR) for the correlation coefficient meets some minimum value and if the correlation coefficient is above some predetermined threshold. Owing to the nature of relative abundance data, care should be taken when assessing the statistical significance of correlation coefficients (correlations may be distorted as a result of compositionality bias, resulting in the apparent association between two rare taxa in the presence of highly abundant community members). Computational packages such as CCREPE (Faust, Sathirapongsasuti, et al. 2012) and SparCC (Friedman and Alm 2012) are available for the calculation of correlation coefficients and associated p values in compositional data. Although similarity-based networks may capture relevant pairwise associations between bacterial taxa, they miss complex interactions between members of the microbial community (how groups of taxa, rather than just a single species, influence the abundance of a particular microbe).

In network models of complex relationships between microbes, connections are identified using either multiple-regression techniques or association-rule mining (Agrawal, Imielinski, and Swami 1993) (a technique that derives logical rules about the presence or absence of taxa in microbiome data; i.e., "taxon A is always absent if taxon B is present"). In addition to modeling relationships between microbiome community members, networks can take into account the influence of environmental perturbations, phenotypes, or subject characteristics thought to influence the microbiome in a biological sample. Furthermore, new network methods are being developed to uncover the dynamic changes in these connections over time (as opposed to modeling the relationships as static). Classical Lotka–Volterra (LV) modeling of predator-prey relationships, based on a system of differential equations (Das and Gupta 2011) was extended in generalized LV predictive networks to capture dynamic

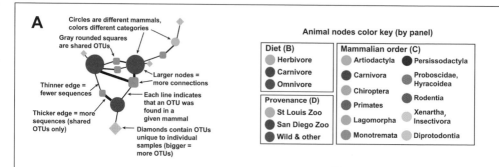

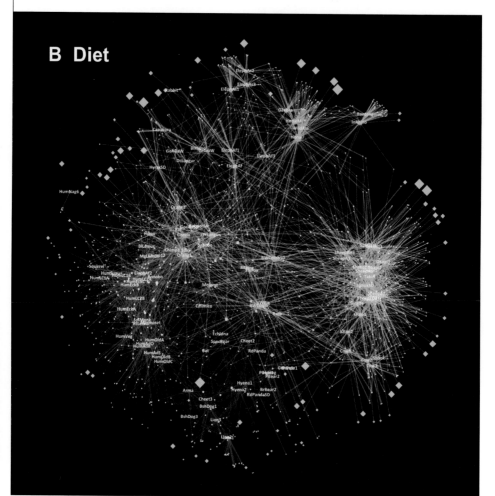

FIGURE 16–10. Network-based analysis of gut microbiome in 60 mammalian species. (A) Schematic of a host-gut microbe network. Color-coded networks are shown for (B) diet, (C) animal taxonomy, (D) animal provenance, or represent randomized assignments of OTUs to animal nodes (E). (Reprinted with permission from AAAS from Ley, R.E., et al. (2008). Evolution of mammals and their gut microbes. Science **320**(5883): 1641–51.)

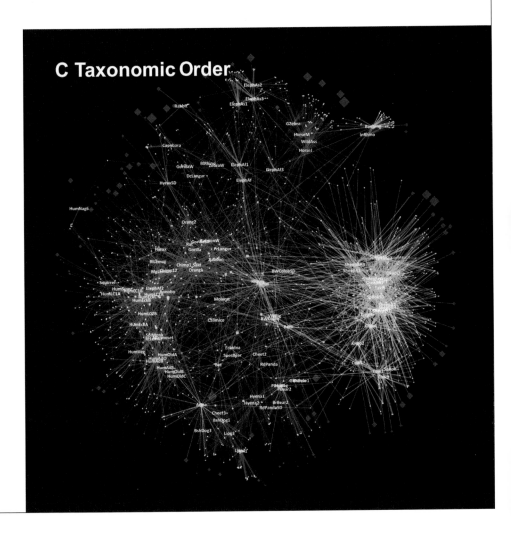

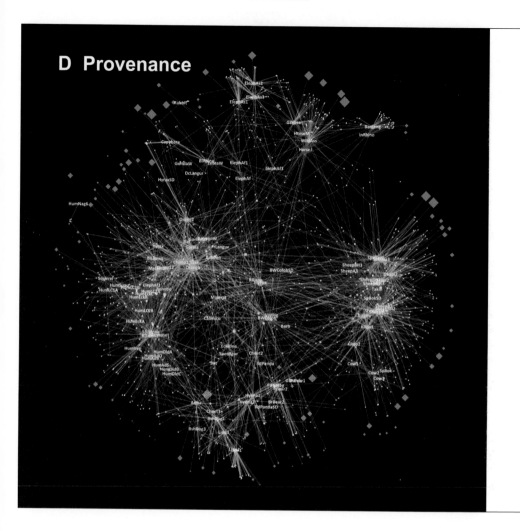

changes in interactions between microbial species, as well as responses to time-varying external perturbations (Munoz-Tamayo, Laroche, et al. 2010; Bucci and Xavier 2014). It is important to note that although network methods are capable of identifying connections between microbial community members, these network connections are not necessarily causal associations. The incorporation of other types of -omics data into network analysis of the microbiome (metatranscriptomics, metaproteomics, metabolomics) may lend additional evidence for biological plausibility for the associations identified between nodes.

Although network analysis of microbiome data is still relatively new, a number of studies have implemented the approaches described above. The majority of published microbiome network analyses employ similarity-based net-

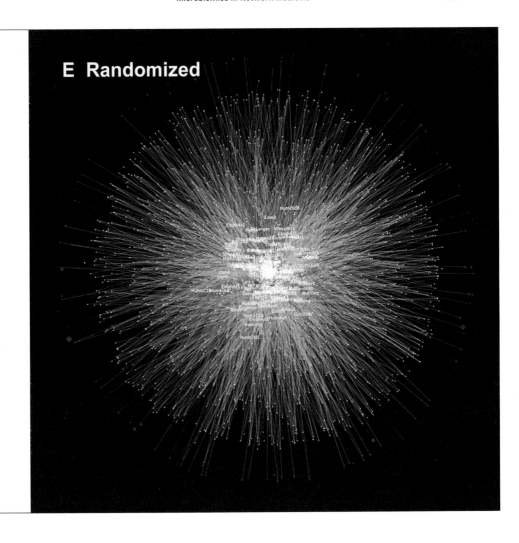

works. In a 2008 publication in *Science* on the evolution of mammals and their gut microbes, Ley, Hamady, and colleagues (2008) used a similarity-based bipartite network to map connections between gut microbial community members and then color-coded the connections observed for particular groupings by mammalian taxonomic order and diet. The resulting network visualizations showed clear clusters by diet (herbivore, carnivore, or omnivore) as well as by mammalian order (Figure 16–10). A correlation network approach (based on the Kendall tau rank-correlation coefficient) to study the effects of a short-term high-fat diet in healthy adult men revealed a negative correlation between members of the Bacteriodetes phylum and carbohydrate oxidation and a positive correlation between abundance of the Firmicute genus Clostridium and order Clostridialesand short-chain fatty acid oxidation (Kelder,

Stroeve, et al. 2014). A report on co-occurrence networks of gut microbiota in apparently healthy, borderline and severely malnourished children demonstrated differences in species connections and a visible hub for potentially pathogenic bacteria in the microbiome network for the malnourished group (but not for borderline malnourished or apparently healthy groups) (Ghosh, Gupta, et al. 2014). Co-occurrence networks in this study were based on Spearman correlation coefficients (with p values calculated using the ReBoot Method [Faust, Sathirapongsasuti, et al. 2012]). In a case–control study of anti–islet-cell immunity, children who tested positive for islet-cell autoantibodies showed substantially different interaction networks for gut microbiota in early life. The authors built separate networks for autoantibody-positive and autoantibody-negative children, using Spearman correlations for all possible pairs of genera (with permutation testing to compute p values for correlation coefficients) (Endesfelder, zu Castell, et al. 2014). In another study, a similarity-based network-building approach of 16S rRNA gene sequence data was combined with generalized boosted linear regression to build a global network of microbial taxa across all body sites. Results of this network showed highly specialized niches of microbial interactions within body sites (with few connections between body sites) (Faust, Sathirapongsasuti, et al. 2012). Hub microbes that may drive overall microbiome composition were observed in networks for specific body sites, including *Streptococcus* for the oral cavity and *Bacteroides* for the gut.

Network studies that go beyond similarity-based methods, and also incorporate dynamic changes in the microbiome over time, have now begun to emerge. In an example of a dynamic network analysis of microbe–microbe interactions, a generalized LV modeling system was used to study temporal changes of the gut microbiota in a mouse model of antibiotic-mediated *Clostridium difficile* infection (Stein, Bucci, et al. 2013). The LV network method developed by these authors enabled the quantification of growth rates of microbial species, species–species interactions, and susceptibilities of microbial groups to time-variable external perturbations. Dynamic network analyses of the 16S sequence data from this mouse model revealed intrinsic stability of the gut microbiome composition following antibiotic perturbation or *C. difficile* infection (implying that external perturbations can have lasting impact on gut microbial communities), and highlighted a potential subnetwork in the protection against *C. difficile* infection. In a human gut microbiome study, LV modeling also formed the basis for a dynamic network modeling approach, called LIMITS (learning interactions from microbial time series), that uses sparse linear regression with bootstrap aggregation (Fisher and Mehta 2014). A LIMITS analysis of dynamic changes in the gut microbiome of two human subjects showed unique microbial interaction networks for each individual (Figure 16–11). Within the inter-

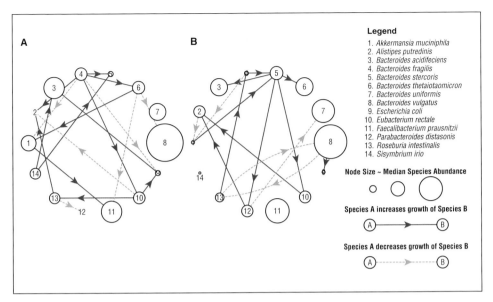

FIGURE 16–11. Interaction topologies of abundant species in the guts of two human subjects. Solid red arrows denote beneficial interactions, dashed blue arrows denote competitive interactions, and node size indicates median relative species abundance. In individual A, *Bacteroides fragilis* (species 4) acts as a keystone species. In individual B, *Bacteroides stercoris* (species 5) acts as a keystone species. The top 10 most abundant species in individuals A and B were used to create this model (14 species in total represent the union of the top 10 taxa in these two individuals).

action networks, keystone species or bacterial taxa with a disproportionately high influence on other community members were identified for each of the individuals. LV analyses in large cohorts of human subjects may help determine whether keystone species of the microbiome are similar across populations and the extent to which they are influenced by disease phenotypes and/or environmental perturbations.

An important future direction in network analysis will be to unite meta-omics data of the microbiome (including shotgun metagenomics, 16S rRNA gene sequencing, metatranscriptomics, metametabolomics. and metaproteomics), in conjunction with host factors, disease states, and environmental perturbations, to construct global networks of the microbial ecosystem (Figure 16–12) (Segata, Boernigen, et al. 2013). A review by Morgan and Huttenhower (2014) describes the currently available tools for various meta-omics platforms. The majority of microbiome studies implement metagenomics, with some emerging work on metatranscriptomics and metabolomics. The most underderdeveloped area is metaproteomics, which, in conjunction with metabolomic data, could provide valuable insight into microbial metabolic pathways (Hettich, Pan, et al. 2013). Although true network analyses for combining different types of meta-omic data are still under development, Morgan, Tickle, and colleagues

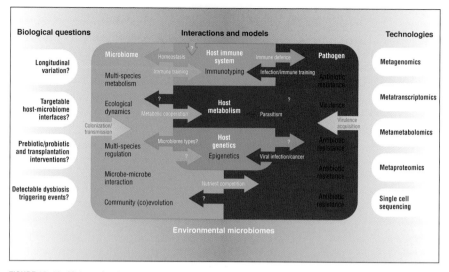

FIGURE 16–12. Meta-omics data may help answer open biological questions in microbiome studies. Microbial communities interact with the environment, host organisms, and transient microbes. Future studies integrating meta-omics data may provide important insights into factors that influence the complex microbial ecosystem.

(2012) used a novel multivariate technique to assess both taxonomic and functional features of the gut microbiome in healthy subjects versus those with inflammatory bowel disease. Interestingly, the authors discovered a greater perturbation of pathways (12% were different in subjects with inflammatory bowel disease [IBD] vs. controls) as compared to taxonomy (only a 2% difference in genera of the intestinal microbiome by disease status). Notable changes included shifts in oxidative stress pathways, and altered carbohydrate and amino acid biosynthesis of microbiota (nutrient transport and uptake were decreased in patients with IBD) (Figure 16–13).

Conclusion

The distinct microbiomes in different parts of the body are important for human health. The HMP and MetaHIT are important consortiums that provided answers regarding what organisms are present in different regions of the body and provided a first view of the function of these organisms. In addition, these consortiums provided researchers with basic tools to begin to dissect the different microbiomes. The second phase of the HMP (iHMP) aims to collect integrated multi-omic datasets that should enable multi-omic and network analyses. Statistical analysis tools for microbial communities and network modeling strategies for microbiome data are evolving at a rapid pace. These methods will

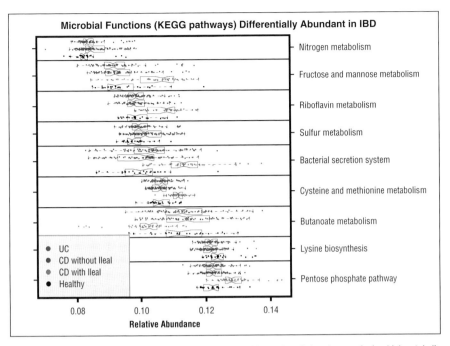

FIGURE 16–13. Patients with inflammatory bowel disease (IBD) have altered abundances of microbial metabolic pathways. KEGG metabolic pathways abundance is color-coded by disease state (and by ileal involvement in the subjects within the IBD group). CD, Crohn disease; UC, ulcerative colitis.

become essential to our understanding of interactions between the microbes that inhabit us, the factors that determine human microbial ecology, perturbations that destabilize our microbiota, and the influence of the microbiome on physiological processes that either promote health or induce disease.

References

Aagaard, K., K. Riehle, et al. (2012). A metagenomic approach to characterization of the vaginal microbiome signature in pregnancy. PLoS One 7(6): e36466.

Abubucker, S., N. Segata, et al. (2012). Metabolic reconstruction for metagenomic data and its application to the human microbiome. PLoS Comput Biol 8(6): e1002358.

Agrawal, R, T. Imielinski, A. Swami (1993). Mining association rules between sets of items in large databases. Proceedings of the 1993 ACM SIGMOID Conference, Washington, D.C., May 1993. AMC SIGMOID Record 22: 207–216.

Amar, J., C. Lange, et al. (2013). Blood microbiota dysbiosis is associated with the onset of cardiovascular events in a large general population: the D.E.S.I.R. study. PLoS One 8(1): e54461.

Amar, J., M. Serino, et al. (2011). Involvement of tissue bacteria in the onset of diabetes in humans: evidence for a concept. Diabetologia 54(12): 3055–61.

Arita, M. (2005). Scale-free networks in cell biology. J Cell Sci (2005) 118: 4947–57.

Arumugam, M., J. Raes, et al. (2011). Enterotypes of the human gut microbiome. Nature 473(7346): 174–80.

Backhed, F., J. K. Manchester, et al. (2007). Mechanisms underlying the resistance to diet-induced obesity in germ-free mice. Proc Natl Acad Sci U S A **104**(3): 979–84.

Bahl, M. I., A. Bergstrom, et al. (2012). Freezing fecal samples prior to DNA extraction affects the Firmicutes to Bacteroidetes ratio determined by downstream quantitative PCR analysis. FEMS Microbiol Lett **329**(2): 193–97.

Barrett, E. L., and H. S. Kwan (1985). Bacterial reduction of trimethylamine oxide. Annu Rev Microbiol **39**: 131–49.

Beck, J. M., V. B. Young, et al. (2012). The microbiome of the lung. Transl Res **160**(4): 258–66.

Bengmark, S. (2012). Gut microbiota, immune development and function. Pharmacol Res **69**(1): 87–113.

Boon, E., C. J. Meehan, et al. (2014). Interactions in the microbiome: communities of organisms and communities of genes. FEMS Microbiol Rev **38**(1): 90–118.

Bucci, V., and J. B. Xavier (2014). Towards predictive models of the human gut microbiome. J Mol Biol **426**(23): 3907–16.

Caporaso, J. G., C. L. Lauber, et al. (2011). Moving pictures of the human microbiome. Genome Biol **12**(5): R50.

Carmody, R. N., and P. J. Turnbaugh (2014). Host-microbial interactions in the metabolism of therapeutic and diet-derived xenobiotics. J Clin Invest **124**(10): 4173–81.

Carrigg, C., O. Rice, et al. (2007). DNA extraction method affects microbial community profiles from soils and sediment. Appl Microbiol Biotechnol **77**(4): 955–64.

Clarke, G., S. Grenham, et al. (2013). The microbiome-gut-brain axis during early life regulates the hippocampal serotonergic system in a sex-dependent manner. Mol Psychiatry **18**(6): 666–73.

Cole, J. R., Q. Wang, et al. (2009). The Ribosomal Database Project: improved alignments and new tools for rRNA analysis. Nucleic Acids Res **37**(Database issue): D141–45.

Costello, E. K., C. L. Lauber, et al. (2009). Bacterial community variation in human body habitats across space and time. Science **326**(5960): 1694–97.

D'Aimmo, M. R., P. Mattarelli, et al. (2012). The potential of bifidobacteria as a source of natural folate. J Appl Microbiol **112**(5): 975–84.

Das, S., and P. K. Gupta (2011). A mathematical model on fractional Lotka-Volterra equations. J Theor Biol **277**(1): 1–6.

De Filippo, C., D. Cavalieri, et al. (2011). Impact of diet in shaping gut microbiota revealed by a comparative study in children from Europe and rural Africa. Proc Natl Acad Sci U S A **107**(33): 14691–96.

DeSantis, T. Z., P. Hugenholtz, et al. (2006). Greengenes, a chimera-checked 16S rRNA gene database and workbench compatible with ARB. Appl Environ Microbiol **72**(7): 5069–72.

Diaz Heijtz, R., S. Wang, et al. (2011). Normal gut microbiota modulates brain development and behavior. Proc Natl Acad Sci U S A **108**(7): 3047–52.

Dickson, R. P., F. J. Martinez, et al. (2014). The role of the microbiome in exacerbations of chronic lung diseases. Lancet **384**(9944): 691–702.

Duncan, S. H., G. E. Lobley, et al. (2008). Human colonic microbiota associated with diet, obesity and weight loss. Int J Obes (Lond) **32**(11): 1720–24.

Endesfelder, D., W. zu Castell, et al. (2014). Compromised gut microbiota networks in children with anti-islet cell autoimmunity. Diabetes **63**(6): 2006–14.

Faust, K., and J. Raes (2012). Microbial interactions: from networks to models. Nat Rev Microbiol **10**(8): 538–50.

Faust, K., J. F. Sathirapongsasuti, et al. (2012). Microbial co-occurrence relationships in the human microbiome. PLoS Comput Biol **8**(7): e1002606.

Fisher, C. K., and P. Mehta (2014). Identifying keystone species in the human gut microbiome from metagenomic timeseries using sparse linear regression. PLoS One **9**(7): e102451.

Fraune, S., and T. C. Bosch (2010). Why bacteria matter in animal development and evolution. Bioessays **32**(7): 571–80.

Friedman, J., and E. J. Alm (2012). Inferring correlation networks from genomic survey data. PLoS Comput Biol **8**(9): e1002687.

Ghosh, T. S., S. S. Gupta, et al. (2014). Gut microbiomes of Indian children of varying nutritional status. PLoS One **9**(4): e95547.

Greenblum, S., P. J. Turnbaugh, et al. (2012). Metagenomic systems biology of the human gut microbiome reveals topological shifts associated with obesity and inflammatory bowel disease. Proc Natl Acad Sci U S A **109**(2): 594–99.

Guarner, F., and J. R. Malagelada (2003). Gut flora in health and disease. Lancet **361**(9356): 512–19.

Handelsman, J., M. R. Rondon, et al. (1998). Molecular biological access to the chemistry of unknown soil microbes: a new frontier for natural products. Chem Biol **5**(10): R245–49.

Hettich, R. L., C. Pan, et al. (2013). Metaproteomics: harnessing the power of high performance mass spectrometry to identify the suite of proteins that control metabolic activities in microbial communities. Anal Chem **85**(9): 4203–14.

HMP Consortium (2012a). A framework for human microbiome research. Nature **486**(7402): 215–21.

HMP Consortium (2012b). Structure, function, and diversity of the healthy human microbiome. Nature **486**(7402): 207–14.

HMP Consortium (2014). Human Microbiome Project (http://commonfund.nih.gov/hmp /index).

Hooper, L. V., T. S. Stappenbeck, et al. (2003). Angiogenins: a new class of microbicidal proteins involved in innate immunity. Nat Immunol **4**(3): 269–73.

Iida, N., A. Dzutsev, et al. (2013). Commensal bacteria control cancer response to therapy by modulating the tumor microenvironment. Science **342**(6161): 967–70.

Integrative Human Microbiome Project Consortium (2014). Dynamic analysis of microbiome-host omics profiles during periods of human health and disease. Cell Host Microbe **16**(3): 276–89.

Kaser, M., M. T. Ruf, et al. (2009). Optimized method for preparation of DNA from pathogenic and environmental mycobacteria. Appl Environ Microbiol **75**(2): 414–18.

Kelder, T., J. H. Stroeve, et al. (2014). Correlation network analysis reveals relationships between diet-induced changes in human gut microbiota and metabolic health. Nutr Diabetes **4**: e122.

Kovatcheva-Datchary, P., and T. Arora (2013). Nutrition, the gut microbiome and the metabolic syndrome. Best Pract Res Clin Gastroenterol **27**(1): 59–72.

La Rosa, P. S., J. P. Brooks, et al. (2012). Hypothesis testing and power calculations for taxonomic-based human microbiome data. PLoS One **7**(12): e52078.

La Rosa, P. S., B. Shands, et al. (2012). Statistical object data analysis of taxonomic trees from human microbiome data. PLoS One **7**(11): e48996.

LeBlanc, J. G., C. Milani, et al. (2013). Bacteria as vitamin suppliers to their host: a gut microbiota perspective. Curr Opin Biotechnol **24**(2): 160–68.

Lederberg, J., and A. T. McCray (2001). 'Ome sweet 'omics—a genealogical treasury of words. Scientist **15**(7): 8 (Abstract).

Lee, Y. K., and S. K. Mazmanian (2010). Has the microbiota played a critical role in the evolution of the adaptive immune system? Science **330**(6012): 1768–73.

Ley, R. E., F. Backhed, et al. (2005). Obesity alters gut microbial ecology. Proc Natl Acad Sci U S A **102**(31): 11070–75.

Ley, R. E., M. Hamady, et al. (2008). Evolution of mammals and their gut microbes. Science **320**(5883): 1647–51.

Ley, R. E., C. A. Lozupone, et al. (2008). Worlds within worlds: evolution of the vertebrate gut microbiota. Nat Rev Microbiol **6**(10): 776–88.

Ley, R. E., P. J. Turnbaugh, et al. (2006). Microbial ecology: human gut microbes associated with obesity. Nature **444**(7122): 1022–23.

Lozupone, C., K. Faust, et al. (2012). Identifying genomic and metabolic features that can underlie early successional and opportunistic lifestyles of human gut symbionts. Genome Res **22**(10): 1974–84.

Lozupone, C., M. Hamady, et al. (2006). UniFrac—an online tool for comparing microbial community diversity in a phylogenetic context. BMC Bioinformatics **7**: 371.

Lozupone, C., and R. Knight (2005). UniFrac: a new phylogenetic method for comparing microbial communities. Appl Environ Microbiol **71**(12): 8228–35.

Lozupone, C., M. E. Lladser, et al. (2011). UniFrac: an effective distance metric for microbial community comparison. ISME J **5**(2): 169–72.

Luckey, T. D. (1970). Introduction to the ecology of the intestinal flora. Am J Clin Nutr **23**(11): 1430–32.

Lynch, S. V., and K. D. Bruce (2013). The cystic fibrosis airway microbiome. Cold Spring Harb Perspect Med **3**(3): a009738.

Mazmanian, S. K., C. H. Liu, et al. (2005). An immunomodulatory molecule of symbiotic bacteria directs maturation of the host immune system. Cell **122**(1): 107–18.

Morgan, X. C., and C. Huttenhower (2012). Chapter 12: human microbiome analysis. PLoS Comput Biol **8**(12): e1002808.

Morgan, X. C., and C. Huttenhower (2014). Meta'omic analytic techniques for studying the intestinal microbiome. Gastroenterology **146**(6): 1437–48, e1.

Morgan, X. C., T. L. Tickle, et al. (2012). Dysfunction of the intestinal microbiome in inflammatory bowel disease and treatment. Genome Biol **13**(9): R79.

Muegge, B. D., J. Kuczynski, et al. (2011). Diet drives convergence in gut microbiome functions across mammalian phylogeny and within humans. Science **332**(6032): 970–74.

Munoz-Tamayo, R., B. Laroche, et al. (2010). Mathematical modelling of carbohydrate degradation by human colonic microbiota. J Theor Biol **266**(1): 189–201.

Ó Cuív, P., D. Aguirre de Carcer, et al. (2011). The effects from DNA extraction methods on the evaluation of microbial diversity associated with human colonic tissue. Microb Ecol **61**(2): 353–62.

Parks, D. H., and R. G. Beiko (2010). Identifying biologically relevant differences between metagenomic communities. Bioinformatics **26**(6): 715–21.

Pompei, A., L. Cordisco, et al. (2007). Folate production by bifidobacteria as a potential probiotic property. Appl Environ Microbiol **73**(1): 179–85.

Pruesse, E., C. Quast, et al. (2007). SILVA: a comprehensive online resource for quality checked and aligned ribosomal RNA sequence data compatible with ARB. Nucleic Acids Res. **35**(21): 7188–96.

Pull, S. L., J. M. Doherty, et al. (2005). Activated macrophages are an adaptive element of the colonic epithelial progenitor niche necessary for regenerative responses to injury. Proc Natl Acad Sci U S A **102**(1): 99–104.

Qin, J., R. Li, et al. (2010). A human gut microbial gene catalogue established by metagenomic sequencing. Nature **464**(7285): 59–65.

Rossi, M., A. Amaretti, et al. (2012). Folate production by probiotic bacteria. Nutrients **3**(1): 118–34.

Salminen, S., C. Bouley, et al. (1998). Functional food science and gastrointestinal physiology and function. Br J Nutr **80**(Suppl 1): S147–71.

Salonen, A., J. Nikkila, et al. (2010). Comparative analysis of fecal DNA extraction methods with phylogenetic microarray: effective recovery of bacterial and archaeal DNA using mechanical cell lysis. J Microbiol Methods **81**(2): 127–34.

Santacruz, A., M. C. Collado, et al. (2010). Gut microbiota composition is associated with body weight, weight gain and biochemical parameters in pregnant women. Br J Nutr **104**(1): 83–92.

Schloss, P. D. (2010). The effects of alignment quality, distance calculation method, sequence filtering, and region on the analysis of 16S rRNA gene-based studies. PLoS Comput Biol **6**(7): e1000844.

Schloss, P. D., S. L. Westcott, et al. (2009). Introducing mothur: open-source, platform-independent, community-supported software for describing and comparing microbial communities. Appl Environ Microbiol **75**(23): 7537–41.

Segata, N., D. Boernigen, et al. (2013). Computational meta'omics for microbial community studies. Mol Syst Biol **9**: 666.

Segata, N., S. K. Haake, et al. (2012). Composition of the adult digestive tract bacterial microbiome based on seven mouth surfaces, tonsils, throat and stool samples. Genome Biol **13**(6): R42.

Segata, N., J. Izard, et al. (2011). Metagenomic biomarker discovery and explanation. Genome Biol **12**(6): R60.

Stein, R. R., V. Bucci, et al. (2013). Ecological modeling from time-series inference: insight into dynamics and stability of intestinal microbiota. PLoS Comput Biol 9(12): e1003388.

Strozzi, G. P., and L. Mogna (2008). Quantification of folic acid in human feces after administration of Bifidobacterium probiotic strains. J Clin Gastroenterol 42(Suppl 3 Pt 2): S179–84.

Suez, J., T. Korem, et al. (2014). Artificial sweeteners induce glucose intolerance by altering the gut microbiota. Nature 514(7521): 181–86.

Suttie, J. W. (1995). The importance of menaquinones in human nutrition. Annu Rev Nutr 15: 399–417.

Tang, W. H., Z. Wang, et al. (2013). Intestinal microbial metabolism of phosphatidylcholine and cardiovascular risk. N Engl J Med 368(17): 1575–84.

Tringe, S. G., and P. Hugenholtz (2008). A renaissance for the pioneering 16S rRNA gene. Curr Opin Microbiol 11(5): 442–46.

Turnbaugh, P. J., F. Backhed, et al. (2008). Diet-induced obesity is linked to marked but reversible alterations in the mouse distal gut microbiome. Cell Host Microbe 3(4): 213–23.

Turnbaugh, P. J., and J. I. Gordon (2009). The core gut microbiome, energy balance and obesity. J Physiol 587(Pt 17): 4153–58.

Turnbaugh, P. J., M. Hamady, et al. (2009). A core gut microbiome in obese and lean twins. Nature 457(7228): 480–84.

Tyler, A. D., M. I. Smith, et al. (2014). Analyzing the human microbiome: a how to guide for physicians. Am J Gastroenterol 109(7): 983–93.

Viaud, S., F. Saccheri, et al. (2013). The intestinal microbiota modulates the anticancer immune effects of cyclophosphamide. Science 342(6161): 971–76.

Wang, Z., E. Klipfell, et al. (2011). Gut flora metabolism of phosphatidylcholine promotes cardiovascular disease. Nature 472(7341): 57–63.

Weinstock, G. M. (2012). Genomic approaches to studying the human microbiota. Nature 489(7415): 250–56.

Weng, M., and W. A. Walker (2013). The role of gut microbiota in programming the immune phenotype. J Dev Orig Health Dis 4(3): 203–14.

White, J. R., N. Nagarajan, et al. (2009). Statistical methods for detecting differentially abundant features in clinical metagenomic samples. PLoS Comput Biol 5(4): e1000352.

Wu, G. D., J. Chen, et al. (2011). Linking long-term dietary patterns with gut microbial enterotypes. Science 334(6052): 105–8.

Xu, J., M. A. Mahowald, et al. (2007). Evolution of symbiotic bacteria in the distal human intestine. PLoS Biol 5(7): e156.

Yuan, S., D. B. Cohen, et al. (2012). Evaluation of methods for the extraction and purification of DNA from the human microbiome. PLoS One 7(3): e33865.

Zhang, A. Q., S. C. Mitchell, et al. (1999). Dietary precursors of trimethylamine in man: a pilot study. Food Chem Toxicol 37(5): 515–20.

Zhang, H., J. K. DiBaise, et al. (2009). Human gut microbiota in obesity and after gastric bypass. Proc Natl Acad Sci U S A 106(7): 2365–70.

Zhou, Y., H. Gao, et al. (2013). Biogeography of the ecosystems of the healthy human body. Genome Biol 14(1): R1.

Illustration Credits

Abbreviations

AA, Alcoholics Anonymous
Aβ, amyloid β
AD, Alzheimer disease
AIDS, acquired immunodeficiency syndrome
AP—MS, affinity purification followed by mass spectrometry
ApoE, apolipoprotein E
APP, Alzheimer precursor protein
ARACNe, Algorithm for the Reconstruction of Accurate Cellular Networks
ASPM, asp (abnormal spindle) homolog, microcephaly-associated
ATP, adenosine triphosphate
BBS, Bardet–Biedl syndrome
BLAST, Basic Local Alignment Search Tool
BMI, body-mass index
CCLE, The Cancer Cell Line Encyclopedia
CDC, Centers for Disease Control and Prevention
CDK, cyclin-dependent kinase
CGT, cellular and gene therapy
ChIP, chromatin immunoprecipitation
ChIP-seq, chromatin immunoprecipitation-sequencing
CLR, context likelihood of relatedness
CMAP, connectivity map
CML, chronic myeloid leukemia
CNVs, copy-number variations
CONEXIC, copy number and expression in cancer
CRP, C-reactive protein
CSF, cerebrospinal fluid
DAG, directed acyclic graph
DMC, data monitoring committee
DNA, deoxyribonucleic acid
EBI, European Bioinformatics Institute
EBV, Epstein–Barr virus
EGF, epidermal growth factor
EGFR, epidermal growth factor receptor
ENCODE, Encyclopedia of DNA Elements
ERGM, exponential random graph model
ERK, extracellular signal-regulated kinase
FBA, flux basis analysis
FIRM, Framework for Inference of Regulation by miRNAs

5mC, 5 methylcytosine
FKBP, FK506 Binding Protein
fMRI, functional magnetic resonance imaging
FPG, fasting plasma glucose
FTDP-17, frontotemporal dementia and Parkinsonism linked to chromosome 17
FWER, familywise error rate
GC, gas chromatography
GGM, Gaussian graphical models
GIMs, genetically informed metabolites
GlcNAc, N-acetylglucosamine
GPCRs, G-protein–coupled receptors
GPR, gene–protein reaction
GRB2, growth factor receptor–bound protein 2
GSK3, glycogen synthase kinase 3
GSMN, genome-scale metabolic network
GWAS, genome-wide association study
HbA_{1c}, gylcated hemoglobin
HCV, hepatitis C virus
HER2, human epidermal growth factor receptor 2
HIV, human immunodeficiency virus
HIV–AIDS, human immunodeficiency virus–acquired immunodeficiency syndrome
HMDB, Human Metabolome DataBase
HMP, Human Microbiome Project
HPV, human papillomavirus
HSPG, heparan sulfate proteoglycan
iHMP, Integrative Human Microbiome Project
INIT, Integrative Network Inference for Tissues
INR, international normalized ratio
IV, intravenous
KEGG, Kyoto Encyclopedia of Genes and Genomes
LC, liquid chromatography
lncRNA, long-noncoding RNA
LV, Lotka–Volterra
MAPK, mitogen-activated protein kinase
MARK, microtubule affinity-regulating kinase
MEK, methylethyl ketone
MEMo, mutual exclusivity module
MetaHIT, Metagenomics of the Human Intestinal Tract (European Commission)

MGWAS, metabolite GWAS analyses

MMCD, Madison Metabolomics Consortium Database

MOA, mechanisms of action

mRNA, messenger RNA

MS, mass spectrometry

MSEA, metabolite set enrichment analysis

MT, microtubule

MTB, *Mycobacterium tuberculosis*

MTBR, microtubule binding repeat

mTOR, mammalian target of rapamycin

MYC, v-myc avian myelocytomatosis viral oncogene homolog

NBS, network-based stratification

NCBI, National Center for Biotechnology Information

NGS, next-generation sequencing

NMF, nonnegative matrix factorization

NMR, nuclear magnetic resonance

NP, nondeterministic polynomial time

NSABP, National Surgical Adjuvant Breast and Bowel Project

OGA, β-N-acetylglucosaminidase

OGT, O-linked GlcNAc-transferase

OMIM, Online Mendelian Inheritance in Man

ORF, open reading frame

PAGE, polyacrylamide gel electrophoresis

PanCan, pan-cancer

PANDA, passing attributes between networks for data assimilation

PARADIGM, pathway representation and analysis by direct reference on graphical models

PCA, principal component analysis

PCoA, principal coordinates analysis

PHF, paired helical filament

PITA, probability of interaction by target accessibility

PLS-DA, partial least squares discriminant analysis

POC, proof of concept

ppERK, phosphorylated ERK

PPI, protein–protein interaction network

PRR, proline-rich region

PTEN, phosphatidylinositol-3,4,5-triphosphate 3-phosphatase

PTK, protein tyrosine kinase

PTM, post-translational modification

QTL, quantitative trait locus

RBCs, red blood cells
RNA, ribonucleic acid
RNAP, RNA polymerase
RNA-seq, RNA sequencing
rRNA, ribosomal ribonucleic acid
RT-PCR, reverse-transcription polymerase chain reaction
SAGs, significantly altered genes
SARS, severe acute respiratory syndrome
SBML, Systems Biology Markup Language
SDS, sodium dodecyl sulfate
SH3, SRC homology 3
S-I-R Model, epidemiologic model with three categories—susceptible,
    infected, and recovered
SNP, single-nucleotide polymorphism
SOS, son of sevenless
SPRT, sequential probability ratio test
SRM, selected reaction monitoring
STD, sexually transmitted disease
SV40, simian virus 40 polyomavirus
TCA cycle, the citric acid cycle
TCGA, The Cancer Genome Atlas
TF, transcription factor
TFBS, transcription factor–binding site
TGF, transforming growth factor
TMAO, trimethylamine-N-oxide
TRN, transcriptional regulatory network
TSS, transcription start site
VEGF, vascular endothelial growth factor
VKORC1, vitamin K epoxide reductase subunit
WBANs, wireless body area networks
WGCNA, weighted gene co-expression network analysis
WT, wild-type
X2K, Expression2Kinases
Y2H, yeast two-hybrid

Glossary

Adaptive design—A prospectively planned maneuver in an ongoing clinical trial in which the data are inspected during an interim analysis, modifications to the trial structure are made, and the trial is allowed to continue to completion.

Adjacency matrix—An approach to represent all of a network's relationships in a matrix format, including any weighting or directionality of edges.

Affinity purification–mass spectrometry (AP–MS)—A set of technologies for detection of co-complex physical associations by purification of an affinity-tagged molecular 'bait' followed by mass spectrometry for identification of proteins associated with the bait

Alternative splicing—differential inclusion of pre-mRNA exons into the final mRNA product, acting to increase mRNA structural complexity.

Bait protein—A protein used to find interactors in a protein interaction screen.

Bayesian network—An approach that uses a directed acyclic graph structure to model random variables based on their conditional dependencies. In transcriptomics network construction, variables are genes and their conditional relationships are determined from gene expression data.

Betweenness centrality—A measure of the importance of a network node based on how often that node occurs within the set of shortest paths in that network.

Biclustering—A statistical learning approach involving two-dimensional clustering of data that identifies sets of biomolecules (e.g., genes) whose abundance is correlated in a subset of conditions.

Binary interactome network—The collection of binary interactions mapped for a particular set of proteins.

Binary protein interaction—A direct physical interaction between two proteins.

Biological interaction—A mapped biophysical interaction that can be demonstrated to occur functionally in the cells or tissue under consideration.

Biomarker—Measurable indicator of a disease or physiological condition.

Biomarker-based clinical trial design—A range of clinical trial designs used to evaluate the response in subgroups of a trial population to a biomarker that measures an aspect of the disease state under study.

Bipartite network—A network that includes two different types of nodes, and in which edges can occur only between two nodes of different types.

Centrality—Characteristic of a network member that conveys the prominence or importance of that member in the network.

Chromatography—A technique that is used to separate metabolites from complex mixtures.

Chronic disease—Longer-lasting human disease or disorder that is influenced by behavioral and environmental risk factors.

Clinical trial—An experiment performed in humans to define the safety and/or efficacy of therapies (e.g., drugs, biologics, devices).

Cluster—Connected node group.

Clustering coefficient—Within a network, the probability that two nodes connected to a third node are directly connected themselves.

Co-complex interactome network—The collection of co-complex associations mapped for a particular set of proteins.

Co-complex protein association—A set of physical interactions between a bait protein and all proteins that stably interact with the bait protein, or associate indirectly with the bait through interactions with direct interactors of the bait.

Community—Densely interconnected node group.

Contact tracing—Data-collection and analytic technique used by epidemiologists to map out disease transmission routes.

Cyclic graph—A network structure in which edges form a loop (or cycle); for example, A points to B points to C points to A. In contrast, an acyclic graph cannot have cycles.

Degree—The number of links to the node.

Degree Distribution—Frequencies of the number of node connections within a specified network.

Directed network—A network in which edges have an associated direction (from node A to node B). A directed network can contain pairs of edges pointing in opposing directions (both A pointing to B and B pointing to A).

Disease module—A local neighborhood within the universe of the interactome that comprises integrated molecular interactions that underlie specific diseases.

Dose response—A description of the relationship between the blood levels of an agent (typically a drug) achieved at a given dose and the physiological effect of the agent on the subject.

Driver mutation—Mutations that play an important role in disease progression and development (especially cancer).

Edge—Connection between network nodes that represents a specific type of relationship based on the network model; also referred to as a "link." For example, correlation between nodes in a correlation-based network or an interaction between proteins in a protein–protein interaction network.

Edgetic perturbation—A mutation in a protein that destroys one or more interactions with other proteins but does not fully disable the protein.

Edgotyping—Systematic profiling of the interactions for a large set of mutant proteins to identify specific interaction defects.

Eigengenes—Set of vectors from a gene-by-sample matrix that summarizes a quantitative feature (such as gene expression or methylation) of genes across samples.

Endo(patho)phenotype—Shared biologic modules that, while upstream of the disease phenotypes, may be shared by multiple diseases. Consistency with traditional genetic terminology would also include pathological phenotype modules that are upstream of clinical phenotypes. The level of selection pressure for an endophenotype or endopathophenotype may be distinct from the baseline physiological state, as it may not be described by the same network architecture.

Endophenotype—A more penetrant but causally related trait. An endophenotype is associated with the respective phenotype in a relevant population; is heritable and state independent; cosegregates with the phenotype; and is causally related to the phenotype.

Enhancer—Similar to a promoter except that these regions are located distally, or far away, from the genes they regulate (as measured along the DNA sequence). Enhancer regions may be physically near their associated genes because of the three-dimensional structure of the genome and looping of DNA.

Epigenetics—The modifications, other than to the base sequence of DNA, that can affect the transcriptional potential of a genomic region. Examples include: (1) methylation marks, which modify CG-sequence elements and recruit MBPs (methyl-CpG binding proteins); MBPs physically prevent other proteins from binding to the DNA; and (2) histones, which combine to form nucleosomes, around which the DNA wraps. Different combinations of histones result in a different physical conformation of the DNA, which may affect its ability to be bound by regulatory proteins (if the affected genomic region is a promoter/enhancer) or transcribed (if the affected region is part of a gene).

Epigenome—Broadly defined as chromatin states across the genome and determined by cytosine methylation and histone modifications. The epigenome is sensitive to the environment of exposures. Non–sequence-based alterations in the epigenome may affect gene regulation/expression.

Epistasis—Interaction between genes or genetic variants.

ERGM—Exponential random graph model, which is a statistical model of the likelihood of tie formation in an observed social network.

Factor graphs—Graphical models that encode the independence relationships of random variables into a belief network.

Flux-balance analysis—Approach to investigating the theoretical properties of metabolism by analyzing metabolic conversion reactions based on a stoichiometric matrix of coefficients describing those reactions.

Forward edgetics—Determination of the specific interactome network perturbations that result from known disease mutations in proteins.

Gain-of-interaction—An alteration that causes a protein to have a protein interaction not found in the unaltered protein.

Genome-scale metabolic networks—Networks that encode knowledge about the metabolic reactions and catalyzing enzymes that exist in biological systems (e.g., organisms, cells, or tissues).

Genome-wide association study—Analysis of the statistical relationships between a phenotype of interest and a large panel of genetic variants selected to capture most of the common genetic variation within a study population.

Genotype—The state of the genome at any given locus.

Germline mutation—Alterations in genes of germ cells (e.g., eggs and sperm) that are heritable to subsequent generations.

H1N1—Influenza virus that caused a world-wide pandemic in 2009. Also called swine flu.

Homophily—Similarity of two or more network members on some relevant nodal characteristic.

Hub—A node that is connected to many other nodes in a network.

Infectious disease—Human disease caused by transmission of an infectious agent such as a virus.

Interaction domain—An independently folding region of a protein that is capable of interacting with a specific region in another protein.

Interaction motif—A short and evolutionarily variable stretch of amino acids in a protein.

Intermediate (Patho)phenotype—The underlying drivers of all pathobiology, these endotypes include inflammation, thrombosis, hemorrhage, fibrosis, apoptosis, and cell proliferation (also see endo(patho)phenotype).

Isoform—One of several protein forms produced by alternative splicing.

Isolate—Member of a social network who is not connected to any other network member.

Kinase inhibitor—A type of molecularly targeted drug that inhibits a kinase controlling important signaling pathways for cancer progression and survival.

Linear regression—An approach that models the outcome of a given variable as a function of the properties of other independent variables. In transcriptomics network reconstruction, the expression of a gene can be considered a function of the expression level of its upstream transcription factor regulators.

Link randomization—Methods in which the links between nodes are randomized while keeping the identity of the nodes intact.

Loss-of-interaction—An alteration that causes loss of a specific interaction of a protein.

Mendelian randomization—A study design that utilizes the known relationships between a genetic variant and a quantitative measure of interest (e.g., environmental exposure pattern or a quantitative biomarker) to determine whether that quantitative phenotype is causally related to a disease outcome.

Message passing—A form of communication between processes that is achieved by sending information between different components. In transcriptomics networks, this approach can be applied to synthesize information from network models representing multiple, complementary data sources by iteratively updating each of the models with information from the others.

Messenger RNA (mRNA)—Produced through the transcription of DNA by RNA polymerase II. Translation of mRNA by the ribosome produces the protein encoded by the RNA.

Metabolic reaction network—In this network, nodes represent metabolites and links represent enzymes connecting metabolites. Genome-scale metabolic reaction networks are available for human as well as several model organisms (e.g., mouse and yeast).

Metabolome—The entire complement of low-molecular-weight molecules (molecular weight <2000 amu) in a biological sample or organism.

Metabolomics—Study of metabolite levels in a biological specimen.

Metabotype—The sum of the measured metabolites that exist in a biospecimen at a given point in time.

Metagenome—The entire collection of genomes and their genes from a mixed community of organisms.

Metagenomics—The study of the metagenome. In metagenomic studies of the microbiome or virome, sequencing is performed on the collection of genomes derived from bacteria and fungi (microbiome) and/or viruses (virome).

Methyltransferases—Enzymes that catalyze the transfer of a methyl group.

Microbiome—Originally defined as the collection of genomes of the microorganisms that share a body space. More recently, this term has been used interchangeably with the term *microbiota*.

Microbiomics—Study of the microbial composition and/or abundance in a biological sample.

Microbiota—Originally defined as the collection of microorganisms that share a body space. More recently, this is used interchangeably with the term *microbiome*.

Microenvironment—The normal cells surrounding a tumor (e.g., immune cells, fibroblasts, cells forming blood vessels).

Micro-RNA (also called **miRNA)**—RNA fragments that bind to mRNAs and target them for degradation, preventing protein translation.

Mod-form—Specific pattern of reversible modifications on all modifiable residues in a protein.

Mod-form distribution—Proportion of the molecular population with a given mod-form.

Modular structure—In a network with modular structure, links within the same modules are much denser than those among different modules. Several algorithms (e.g., Guimerà–Amara algorithm) are available to find modules in a network.

Modules—A collection of nodes that contribute to a shared cellular function or a shared disease and/or have more links between the nodes of the module than to nodes outside that module.

Molecularly targeted therapy/drug—Therapies target and inhibit a specific enzyme or a protein that are important for cancer survival and progression or that enhance host immune systems to eliminate tumor cells.

Monoclonal antibody—A type of molecularly targeted drug and an antibody to target a specific antigen in tumor cells. If an antigen in tumor cells is targeted by the antibody, the host immune system is recruited to attack the tumor cells.

Motif—Recurrent node connectivity patterns, such as triangles.

Multi-omic network integration—Combining large-scale characterizations of different biomolecules to aid generation and interpretation of networks.

Mutual information—A nonlinear measure of the correlation between two variables that accounts for complex relationships by comparing the joint probability distribution for pairs of variables to the products of their corresponding marginal distributions. In the context of transcriptomic network reconstruction, mutual information is often applied in a similar way as Pearson correlation.

Negative feedback amplifier—A system that includes both control by negative feedback loops and an amplification process; this design provides reduced impact of noise in the input signal while providing smoother output responses.

Network—An abstract formalism that describes the interactions among numerous components in a system. Networks in biological systems are defined by experimentally characterized or statistically inferred associations.

Network (of a cellular process)—A representation of the interactions between cellular elements (such as those in a pathway or involved in gene regulatory processes) in which cellular elements are represented by "nodes" and interactions by "edges." Inferring networks and using them as tools to understand cellular processes is one of the most active areas of methods development in biology.

Network-based stratification—A method originally developed to cluster patients based on mutations in similar network regions in gene interaction networks.

Network map—Graphical depiction of social network showing nodes and ties.

Network marker—Specific topological and statistical features in a molecular interaction network (e.g., protein–protein interaction and metabolic reaction networks) under a condition of interest (e.g., under a disease state or drug compound).

Network medicine—The application of network science and systems biology to disease mechanisms and pharmacotherapeutics.

Network motif—Network subgraph, typically composed of a small group of nodes and edges, that has a specific biological function.

Network reconstruction—Bottom-up generation of a network based on compiling information from typically hundreds of research articles and experiments.

Next-generation phenotypes—Measurable characteristics of an individual that are digital (quantitative), are dynamic (with a broad dynamic range), have a defined responsiveness (with specified perturbations), are multiscale (molecular, cellular, tissue, organismal), are multidimensional (unconstrained by existing disease silos), and are translatable (accessible in multiple different species and cell types).

Node—A network component that in network medicine often represents a biological entity; also referred to as a "vertex."

Node in social networks—Member of a social network.

Node randomization—Methods in which the identity of the nodes in a network is randomized.

Nonnegative matrix factorization—A linear algebra approach in which a matrix is factorized to contain only nonnegative elements to ensure that each input vector is represented as a purely additive combination of "parts.".

Off-target drug effects—Consequences of a pharmacological agent related to actions on biochemical entities or pathways that were not the intended sites of pharmacological impact.

-omics—Comprehensive characterization of different biomolecules within a particular biological system (e.g., genomics measures the DNA; transcriptomics measures the RNA; proteomics measures the proteins; metabolomics measures the metabolites).

Operational taxonomic unit (OTU)—A group of organisms with ribosomal RNA (rRNA) gene sequences that show a certain level of identity. For instance, 16S rRNA gene sequences with 97% sequence similarity are often grouped together and considered a surrogate for a species-level taxon.

Opinion leaders—Members of a social network who by their position in the network have greater influence on the spread of information through the network.

Origons—Pathways featuring a transcription factor and its direct and indirect regulatory targets.

Pandemic—An epidemic of global or otherwise large-scale proportions.

Passenger mutation—Mutations randomly occurring in tumors that are not important for cancer progression and development.

Pathophenotype—Systems-level consequences of disease genotype and all other factors.

Pathways—A set of biomolecules known to interact with one another to produce a cumulative biological function.

Pearson correlation—A measure of the linear relationship between two variables. In transcriptomic networks the variables in question are genes, and this relationship is determined by comparing two genes' expression levels across a set of experimental conditions.

Penetrance—Proportion of those with a genotype who exhibit a phenotype.

Petri net—A graphical model wherein objects (which have initial concentrations and decay rates) are connected by transitional relationships.

Pharmacodynamics—Study of the effects of a particular drug on the person who takes the drug.

Pharmacokinetics—Study of the changes in distribution and metabolism of a drug after an individual takes that drug.

Pharmacometabolomics—The study of metabolites and biological pathways that are activated with exposure to a pharmacologic treatment.

Phenotype—A measurable characteristic of an individual; the final outcome of genotype and all other factors.

Plasticity—The adaptability or the capacity for alteration in the presence of environmental perturbations and/or exposures.

Pleiotropy—Range of phenotypic outcomes of the same genotype.

Post-translational modification—Chemical modification of a protein by enzymatic action on the polypeptide after translation. Post-translational modification (PTM) can be reversible (e.g., phosphorylation) or irreversible (e.g., proteolytic cleavage) and is caused by the balance between enzymes that modify the protein or remove the PTM. Mass spectrometry is currently the method of choice to detect PTMs; PTMs can modify the interaction pattern of the protein and/or its molecular function. Evidence from many contexts suggests that different mod-forms can have different effects.

Prey protein—Interactor of a bait protein identified in a protein interaction screen.

Promoter—A region of DNA, containing target recognition sequences, to which transcription factors can bind and mediate the expression of a "nearby" gene. Promoters are located proximal, or directly next to, the start of a gene.

Protein—Amino acid polymers linked by amide ester bonds (linear polypeptides) that are the primary constituents of cells and perform many different cellular functions. Proteins are produced as a result of the translation of messenger RNA.

Protein–protein interaction network—High-throughput experimental techniques (e.g., yeast two-hybrid method) have been used to investigate interaction between two proteins at a genome-wide level in several model organisms (e.g., human, mouse, fly, worm, and yeast). In a protein–protein interaction network, nodes represent proteins, while links represents interaction between two proteins.

Proteoform—specific pattern of modifications, allowing for both reversible and irreversible modifications.

Proteome—The collection of all proteins in a cell.

Proteomics—Study of protein levels in a biological sample.

Pseudo-interaction—A reproducible biophysical interaction that may not occur physiologically (also referred to as a "noisy" or "fortuitous" interaction).

Quarantine—Strategy to isolate infected or susceptible individuals to limit spread of a disease outbreak.

Rational polypharmacy—The use of combinations of drugs that target one or more pathways in the disease module.

Reverse edgetics—Alterations in a protein that exhibit specific interaction defects are produced, and these altered proteins are reintroduced in vivo to investigate the function of the corresponding interaction..

Scale-free network—A network in which the degree distribution follows a power law.

Separation—A measure to quantify the extent to which two groups of nodes do or do not overlap in a network.

Shot-gun sequencing—The process of randomly fragmenting long segments of DNA (often by shearing) and sequencing the shorter fragments produced, each of which derives from a different and potentially overlapping section of the original DNA molecule.

Signaling networks—Sets of biomolecular components that contribute to signal transduction and connect extracellular receptor inputs to metabolic or transcriptional regulatory consequences.

16S rRNA gene—Encodes the 16S segment of bacterial ribosomal RNA (rRNA). The 16S rRNA gene contains both conserved and hypervariable regions, making it useful for amplification, sequencing, and taxonomic identification of microbial communities.

Social influence—Process of behavioral influence based on social relationships.

Social network—Social entities (such as people, organizations, etc.) connected to one another by a specific relationship or social tie.

Social selection—Process of forming new social relationships.

Somatic mutation—Alterations in genes of any cells except for germ cells that are not heritable by subsequent generations.

Statistical network inference—Top-down generation of network interactions based on statistical associations extracted from biomolecular measurements.

Stoichiometric matrix—A matrix that represents the metabolic network connectivity. The matrix contains the stoichiometric coefficients of the biochemical reactions being described. The rows represent the metabolites, and the columns represent the reactions.

System Biology Markup Language (SBML)—The de facto standard format based on extensible markup language (XML) to represent various biological phenomena (e.g., metabolic reactions, gene regulation, and signaling pathways). Various software, especially CellDesigner modeling software, support SBML. CellDesigner can conduct simulation based on a computational model of biological processes stored in SBML format by using an ordinary differential-equation solver engine that supports the SBML format.

Targeted metabolomics—The generation of a set of known, identifiable metabolites in a biological sample.

Therapeutic misconception—Occurs when research subjects believe that the purpose for participating in a clinical trial is to receive "treatment" for their disease—failing to appreciate the distinction between the imperative of clinical research for gaining new knowledge and the process of ordinary clinical treatment.

Tie—Relationship that connects two nodes in a social network.

Transcription factor—A protein that can regulate gene expression by binding to the DNA and facilitating (or impeding) the recruitment of RNA polymerase II and the subsequent production of mRNA.

Transcriptional regulatory networks—Networks that encode the interactions between transcription factors and the target genes whose mRNA expression levels they influence.

Transcriptome—The sum total of all the RNA molecules expressed in a cell, including non-coding RNA, micro-RNA (or mi-RNA), and messenger RNA (mRNA). The measured abundance levels of RNA molecules is commonly referred to as "gene expression" and is widely used as the primary input values for algorithms that seek to model transcriptional networks. Measurements of gene expression are dependent on many factors, including the measurement technology used.

Transcriptomics—Study of gene expression levels, typically mRNA, in a biological sample.

Untargeted metabolomics—The measurement of all endogenous metabolic signals in a biological sample.

Virus–host interaction—A physical interaction, whether binary or indirect, between a viral protein and proteins resident in the host cell.

Wireless body area networks (WBANs)—A network that transmits real-time physiological data from research subjects. Investigators can thus assess the dynamic response to an intervention and are freed from the extrapolations that must be made from periodic snapshots of a clinical response as might be recorded during a routine clinic visit. A WBAN system can be connected to a monitoring hub and transmit data over WiFi, Bluetooth, or mobile networks. It allows the subject to be mobile and is location-independent.

Yeast two-hybrid (Y2H)—A set of technologies for detection of binary interactions by genetic reconstitution in yeast of a split transcription factor.

Contributors

Elliott M. Antman, M.D.
Professor of Medicine
Associate Dean for Clinical and
  Translational Research
Harvard Medical School
Brigham and Women's Hospital
Boston, MA

Albert-László Barabási, Ph.D.
Distinguished Professor and Director,
  Center for Complex Networks Research
  and Department of Physics, Northeastern
  University
Center for Cancer Systems Biology and
  Department of Cancer Biology,
Dana Farber Cancer Institute
Brigham and Women's Hospital
Lecturer in Medicine, Harvard Medical
  School Boston, MA
Professor, Center for Network Science
Central European University, Budapest

Michael A. Calderwood, Ph.D.
Interactome Group Leader/
  Senior Scientist
Center for Cancer Systems Biology and
  Department of Biology
Department of Genetics
Harvard Medical School
Dana–Farber Cancer Institute
Boston, MA

Benoit Charloteaux, Ph.D.
Senior Scientist
GIGA-Genomics Core Facility
University of Liège
Liège, Belgium

Clary B. Clish, Ph.D.
Director, Metabolite Profiling
Broad Institute of MIT and Harvard
Cambridge, MA

Michael E. Cusick, Ph.D.
Smith Research Lab
Center for Cancer Systems Biology
Dana–Farber Cancer Institute
Boston, MA

Dawn L. DeMeo, M.D., M.P.H.
Associate Professor of Medicine
Harvard Medical School
Associate Physician, Brigham and Women's
  Hospital
Channing Division of Network Medicine
Boston, MA

John C. Earls, M.S.
Ph.D. Student
Department of Computer Science and
  Engineering
University of Washington
Seattle, WA

James A. Eddy, Ph.D.
Bioinformatician
Benaroya Research Institute
Seattle, WA

Samik Ghosh, Ph.D.
Senior Scientist
Systems Biology Institute
Tokyo Medical and Dental University
Tokyo, Japan

Kimberly Glass, Ph.D.
Instructor in Medicine
Harvard Medical School
Channing Division of Network Medicine
Brigham and Women's Hospital
Biostatistics and Computational Biology
Dana–Farber Cancer Institute
Department of Biostatistics
Harvard School of Public Health
Boston, MA

Jeremy Gunawardena, Ph.D.
Associate Professor, Systems Biology
Harvard Medical School
Boston, MA

Takeshi Hase, Ph.D.
Member, The Systems Biology Institute
Tokyo Medical and Dental University
Tokyo, Japan

David E. Hill, Ph.D.
Research Associate in Genetics
Dana–Farber Cancer Institute
Boston, MA

Isabelle Huvent, Ph.D.
Centre National de la Recherche
  Scientifique, UMR 8576
University of Lille 1
Villeneuve d'Ascq, France

Hiroaki Kitano, Ph.D.
The Systems Biology Institute
Tokyo Medical and Dental University
Tokyo, Japan

Isabelle Landrieu, Ph.D.
Research Director, Centre National de la
  Recherche Scientifique, UMR 8576
Université de Lille 2
Institute Pasteur de Lille
Lille Cedex, France

Jessica Lasky-Su, Sc.D.
Assistant Professor of Medicine
Associate Statistician
Channing Division of Network Medicine,
  Brigham and Women's Hospital and
  Harvard Medical School
Boston, MA

Arnaud Leroy, Ph.D.
Associate Professor
Université de Paris-Sud
Faculté de Pharmacie à Châtenay-Malabry
Châtenay-Malabry, France

Guy Lippens, Ph.D.
CNRS Research Director
LISBP
University of Toulouse
Toulouse, France

Augusto A. Litonjua, M.D., M.P.H.
Associate Professor of Medicine
Harvard Medical School
Channing Division of Network Medicine
Associate Physician, Brigham and Women's
  Hospital
Boston, MA

Joseph Loscalzo, M.D., Ph.D.
Hersey Professor of the Theory and
  Practice of Medicine
Harvard Medical School
Chairman, Department of Medicine and
  Physician-in-Chief
Brigham and Women's Hospital
Boston, MA

Douglas A. Luke, M.D.
Professor and Director
Center for Public Health Systems Science
Director, Doctoral Program in Public
  Health Sciences
Professor, Brown School
Washington University
St. Louis, MO

Shuyi Ma, Ph.D.
Postdoctoral Scientist
Center for Infectious Disease Research
University of Washington
Seattle, WA

Calum A. MacRae, M.D., Ph.D.
Associate Professor of Medicine
Harvard Medical School
Chief, Cardiovascular Division
Brigham and Women's Hospital
Boston, MA

Jörg Menche, Ph.D.
Principal Investigator
CeMM
Research Center for Molecular Medicine
  of the Austrian Academy of Sciences
Vienna, Austria

Sucheendra K. Palaniappan, B.Eng., Ph.D.
Postdoctoral Fellow
Inria Rennes–Bretagne Atlantique
  Research Center
Campus Universitaire de Beaulieu
Rennes Cedex, FR

Benjamin Parent, Ph.D.
Teacher
Institut Supérieur d'Electronique du
  Nord
Lille, France

Sudhakaran Prabakaran, Ph.D.
Postdoctoral Fellow
Department of Systems Biology
Harvard Medical School
Boston, MA

Nathan D. Price, Ph.D.
Professor and Associate Director
Institute for Systems Biology
University of Washington
Seattle, WA

John Quackenbush, Ph.D.
Professor of Computational Biology and
  Bioinformatics
Harvard T. H. Chan School of Public Health
Professor of Cancer Biology
Professor of Biostatistics and
  Computational Biology
Director, Center for Cancer Computational
  Biology
Dana–Farber Cancer Institute
Senior Scientist
Brigham and Women's Hospital
Boston, MA

Thomas Rolland, Ph.D.
Postdoctoral Fellow
Human Genetics and Cognitive Functions
  Lab
Institut Pasteur
Paris, France

Martin W. Schoen, M.D., M.P.H.
Fellow, Division of Hematology/Oncology,
  Department of Medicine
St. Louis University School of Medicine
St. Louis, MO

Edwin K. Silverman, M.D., Ph.D.
Physician, Brigham and Women's Hospital
Professor of Medicine, Harvard Medical
  School
Chief, Channing Division of Network
  Medicine
Brigham and Women's Hospital
Boston, MA

Caroline Smet-Nocca, Ph.D.
Assistant Professor
Université de Lille 1
Institute Pasteur de Lille
Lille Cedex, France

Joanne E. Sordillo, Sc.D.
Assistant Professor of Medicine
Associate Epidemiologist
Harvard Medical School
Channing Division of Network Medicine
Brigham and Women's Hospital
Boston, MA

Marc Vidal, Ph.D.
Professor of Genetics
Department of Genetics
Dana–Farber Cancer Institute
Boston, MA

George M. Weinstock, Ph.D.
Professor and Associate Director,
  Microbial Genomics
The Jackson Laboratory for Genomic
  Medicine
Farmington, CT

Scott T. Weiss, M.D., M.S.
Professor of Medicine
Harvard Medical School
Director, Partners HealthCare
  Personalized Medicine
Associate Director, Channing Division of
  Network Medicine
Boston, MA

Index

Note: Figures are indexed in italic.